"Heartfelt admiration and appreciation to Sharon Chaiklin and Hilda Wengrower as they envision and co-create a completely new edited collection together with leading members of the international Dance/Movement Therapy community. The reader is a privileged witness."

Joan Chodorow, PhD, BC-DMT, author of
Dance Therapy and Depth Psychology: The Moving Imagination

"The editors offer a precious and original contribution to the development of new perspectives for DMT in the contemporary world. It is an effective tool to update as a dance therapist and also to dialogue with colleagues from other professions in light of shared scientific acquisitions. New research and applications testify to the vitality of this discipline within different cultures. This book represents an important didactic support for dance movement therapists and a stimulating encounter for other experienced professionals."

Vincenzo Puxeddu, MD, PhD, DMT, EADMT President (European Association Dance Movement Therapy), co-director DMT Master program Paris University

DANCE AND CREATIVITY WITHIN DANCE MOVEMENT THERAPY

Dance and Creativity within Dance Movement Therapy discusses the core work and basic concepts in dance movement therapy (DMT), focusing on the centrality of dance, the creative process and their aesthetic-psychological implications in the practice of the profession for both patients and therapists.

Based on interdisciplinary and multidisciplinary inputs from fields such as philosophy, psychology, anthropology and dance, contributions examine the issues presented by cultural differences in DMT through the input of practitioners from several diverse countries. Chapters blend theory and case studies with personal, intimate reflections to support critical descriptions of DMT interventions and share methods to help structure practice and facilitate communication between professionals and researchers.

The book's multicultural, multidisciplinary examination of the essence of dance and its countless healing purposes will give readers new insights into the value and functions of dance both in and out of therapy.

Hilda Wengrower, PhD, DMT, is co-editor with Sharon Chaiklin of *The Art and Science of Dance Movement Therapy: Life is Dance* and has published papers and chapters in multiple languages on subjects related to dance movement therapy. She teaches internationally.

Sharon Chaiklin, BC, DMT, is a founding member and past president of the American Dance Therapy Association and past president of the Marian Chace Foundation. She has worked clinically for many years and taught internationally.

DANCE AND CREATIVITY WITHIN DANCE MOVEMENT THERAPY

International Perspectives

Edited by Hilda Wengrower and Sharon Chaiklin

Routledge
Taylor & Francis Group

NEW YORK AND LONDON

First published 2021
by Routledge
52 Vanderbilt Avenue, New York, NY 10017

and by Routledge
2 Park Square, Milton Park, Abingdon, Oxon, OX14 4RN

Routledge is an imprint of the Taylor & Francis Group, an informa business

© 2021 Taylor & Francis

The right of Hilda Wengrower and Sharon Chaiklin to be identified as the authors of the editorial material, and of the authors for their individual chapters, has been asserted in accordance with sections 77 and 78 of the Copyright, Designs and Patents Act 1988.

Library of Congress Cataloging-in-Publication Data
A catalog record for this book has been requested

ISBN: 978-1-138-33751-0 (hbk)
ISBN: 978-1-138-33752-7 (pbk)
ISBN: 978-0-429-44230-8 (ebk)

Typeset in Baskerville
by Apex CoVantage, LLC

In loving memory of Harry Chaiklin. Grateful for all the support and memories.

Sharon

To Tany, Tamara, Noam and Shir, may there be much dance in your lives.

Hilda

CONTENTS

EDITORS

Sharon Chaiklin, BC-DMT, is a founding member and past president of the American Dance Therapy Association. A student of Marian Chace, one of the first dance therapists in the United States, she worked for over 34 years in psychiatric hospitals and private practice. Sharon taught in the Graduate Dance/Movement Therapy Program at Goucher College, Baltimore, MD, and has authored several articles. She was co-editor of the book *Foundations of Dance/Movement Therapy: The Life and Work of Marian Chace*. Invitations to teach brought her to Israel, Argentina, Japan, Korea and the Philippines. She currently serves as trustee on the board of the Marian Chace Foundation. She received the ADTA Lifetime Achievement Award in 2012. She co-edited with Hilda Wengrower the book *The Art and Science of Dance/Movement Therapy: Life is Dance*. The book was published in English, German, Hebrew, Korean, Russian and Spanish.

Hilda Wengrower, PhD, DMT, teaches and lectures in Israel at the School for Arts and Society-Ono Academic College and internationally. She maintains a private practice that includes supervision. Hilda has published papers and chapters in several languages on subjects related to arts therapies in educational settings, Dance Movement Therapy (DMT) with children with behavioral disorders, migration, arts-based research and DMT, and DMT and psychiatry. She is the Head of the DMT section at the Israeli Association for Arts Therapies and is a delegate to several international associations. Hilda is book reviews editor of the international journal *Body, Movement and Dance in Psychotherapy* and co-edited the book *Traditions in Transition in the Arts Therapies*. She co-edited with Sharon Chaiklin the book *The Art and Science of Dance/Movement Therapy: Life is Dance*.

CONTRIBUTORS

Beatrice Allegranti, DMP, PhD, has 25 years of professional experience as a choreographer, dance movement psychotherapist (UKCP reg.), educator and award-winning feminist scholar. Beatrice holds the position of Reader/Associate Professor in Dance Movement Psychotherapy and Choreography at the University of Roehampton and is involved in UK and internationally funded work encompassing choreography and filmmaking as well as clinical practice, supervision, mentoring, consultancy and shaping policy across dance, biomedical health and education sectors. Examples of UK and international facilitation include dance movement psychotherapy conflict resolution and trauma support with young people from Palestine and Israel (Arts for Peace and The Irish Defense Forces); UK, NHS clinical practice in mental health; young onset dementia; learning disabilities; autism as well as training medical staff in kinesthetic communication. Through her work, Beatrice brings the arts, humanities and sciences into interdisciplinary conversation and her portfolio includes extensive peer reviewed publications, keynotes, films and dance theatre performances—all with a focus on activism (see www.beatriceallegranti.com).

Iris Bräuninger, DMT, PhD, is a senior researcher and lecturer at the University of Applied Science of Special Needs Education in Zurich, Switzerland, where she is also the co-director of the BA program in Psychomotor Therapy. She received her PhD from the University of Tübingen, Germany, and studied DMT at the Laban Centre/City University of London, England. She teaches internationally and at the DMT Master Program at the Autonomous University of Barcelona, Spain. Iris formerly was researcher and deputy head of the DMT department at the University Hospital of Psychiatry, Zurich, and a postdoctoral researcher at the Stress and Resilience Research Team at the University of Deusto in Bilbao, Spain. Iris is a DMT supervisor with the German BTD and Spanish Association ADMTE. She is a KMP notator and holds the European Certificate of Psychotherapy (ECP). Her research focuses on DMT's and psychomotor therapy interventions. Iris has published extensively (see www.researchgate.net/profile/Iris_Braeuninger/research).

Marja Cantell, PhD, psychology (University of Lancaster, UK), postgraduate diploma dance movement therapy (Roehampton University, UK) and postdoctorate human movement science (UWA, Australia). Her multidisciplinary research on movement development and observation, as well as research capacity building among health care professionals, has been published, for example, in *Body, Movement and Dance in Psychotherapy*, *Canadian Art Therapy Association Journal*, *Research in Developmental Disabilities* and *Scandinavian Journal of Medicine and Science in Sports*. In 2000, she was a co-founding member of the Finnish Dance Therapy Association. For many years, she performed with MoMo Dance Theatre in Calgary, Canada. Since 2010 she resides in the Netherlands, working as an assistant professor in inclusive and special needs education at the University of Groningen and a research coach and teacher in the master of arts therapies, Codarts University of the Arts in Rotterdam. In her private practice she applies the concept of "Movement for All" (see www.movementcantell.com).

Zeynep Çatay, PhD, is a clinical psychologist, Dance/Movement Therapist and Somatic Experiencing Practitioner from Istanbul who is now living in New York City. After completing the Expressive Therapies program at Lesley University, she received her PhD in clinical psychology from the Long Island University in New York. She was a faculty member at the Psychology Department of Istanbul Bilgi University between 2005 and 2019, where she also founded the Certificate Program in Creative Movement and Dance/Movement Therapy in collaboration with Marcia Plevin. She also served as the co-Chair of the Arts Psychotherapy Association in Turkey. In addition, she has been in private practice working with adults and children. She is currently a visiting scholar and lecturer at the New School for Social Research in New York City and a candidate at NYU Postdoctorate Program for Psychoanalysis. Her current research interests focus on the nonverbal bodily dynamics in psychotherapy and development.

Sohini Chakraborty, PhD. Sohini is an Ashoka fellow, sociologist, dance activist, dance movement therapist and the founder-director of Kolkata Sanved. For more than 22 years, Sohini experimented with breaking the barriers of traditional dance and introduced dance movement therapy as a tool for psychosocial rehabilitation in South Asia. This unique and innovative methodology was developed by Kolkata Sanved under her leadership. Honed over the past two decades, Kolkata Sanved's Sampoornata' model is a pioneering concept in South Asia. Sohini has received various national and international awards for outstanding achievement and inspiration. She has been felicitated by the Department of Women and Child Development and the Department of Social Welfare of the government of West Bengal in 2016. She received the prestigious True Legend Award in 2015 and the Diane von Furstenberg Award in 2011 for transforming the lives of other women.

Rona Cohen, PhD, teaches at Tel Aviv University and *Kibbutzim College's* School of Dance. Her research interests and publications focus on the problem of the body in continental philosophy and the question of the body in aesthetics, psychoanalysis and dance. She has published essays in *Philosophy Today* and *Kant Akten*, among other places, and in the volume *Psychoanalysis: Topological Perspectives*. She is currently engaged in writing a book on the body in dance from a philosophical aesthetic perspective and co-editing a forthcoming special issue of *Angelaki* on philosophy and death. In recent years she has worked closely with dance students and dancers on theorizing dance creative processes.

Elena Cristóbal Linares is a mother and psychologist who holds a master's in dance movement therapy from the Autonomous University of Barcelona, Spain, and a master's in psychology of assisted human reproduction from the University of Barcelona. She also studied in Seville, attending the PhD Program "Flamenco: A multidisciplinary approach to its study." Currently she lives in Tenerife, but she was born in Córdoba in 1977. It is Córdoba which bequeathed her flamenco core and the *duende* (goblin) soul, which as Lorca says, "lives in the last rooms of the blood." She has long tried to connect dance movement therapy and flamenco to offer them to others because they are a good combination of feeling, awareness and expression. For 12 years she has worked with people with severe mental disorders through this type of creative therapy. Currently, she has a private space where she works in clinical psychology, accompanying women and couples who have fertility problems and assisting with reproduction treatments. Within this multidisciplinary program, she and her patients sometimes open group processes through the DMT.

Sondra Fraleigh is Professor Emeritus of Dance at the State University of New York (SUNY Brockport), a Fulbright Scholar and an award-winning author of nine books. Some of them: *Back to the Dance Itself: Phenomenologies of the Body in Performance* (2019); *Moving*

Consciously: Somatic Transformations through Dance, Yoga, and Touch (2015), and *Dance and the Lived Body* (1987). Sondra was chair of the Department of Dance at SUNY Brockport for nine years, later head of graduate dance studies and selected by SUNY as a university-wide Faculty Exchange Scholar. She received the Outstanding Service to Dance Award from CORD in 2003. Her choreography has been seen in New York, Germany, Japan and India. She was a teaching fellow at Ochanomizu University in Tokyo and at the University of Baroda in India. She also has numerous chapters in books on culture, aesthetics, ecology and cognitive psychology. Sondra is the founding director of *Eastwest Somatics Institute* for the study of dance, yoga and movement (see www.eastwestsomatics.com).

David Alan Harris, MA, BC-DMT, NCC, LCAT, LPC, specializes in dance/movement therapy (DMT) with survivors of human rights abuse and war, and he has lectured on the subject on five continents. When supervising a mental health team in Sierra Leone in the wake of a ruthless civil war, David introduced counselors there to DMT and its methods. He launched what were apparently the first DMT groups in West Africa—including the first anywhere for former child combatants. David later accepted the Freedom to Create 2009 Youth Prize at London's Victoria and Albert Museum on behalf of the boy soldiers' DMT group. The American Dance Therapy Association has bestowed on David both its research award and its Leader of Tomorrow award. In 2017, he shared its President's award with Dr. Christina Devereaux for a special issue of the *American Journal of Dance Therapy*, which they co-edited from 2014 to 2017.

Rainbow T. H. Ho has been working as a professor, researcher, dance therapist, expressive arts therapist, dance teacher and dancer for many years. She is the associate dean of the Faculty of Social Sciences, professor of the Department of Social Work and Social Administration, Director of the Centre on Behavioral Health and the director of the Master of Expressive Arts Therapy program at the University of Hong Kong. She has published extensively in refereed journals, scholarly books and encyclopedias, and she has been the principal investigator of many research projects related to dance/movement therapy, expressive arts therapy, mind-body medicine, spirituality and physical activity for healthy and clinical populations. In 2015, Rainbow received the Outstanding Achievement Award and Research Award from the American Dance Therapy Association and the Outstanding Teaching Award from the University of Hong Kong. She also received the Research and Development Award from the Australia, New Zealand and Asian Creative Arts Therapies Association in 2016.

Susan Dee Imus, MA, LCPC, BC-DMT, GL-CMA, is an associate professor and former director of the Dance/Movement Therapy & Counseling MA and Arts in Health minor program at Columbia College Chicago (CCC). She has worked at numerous hospitals across the United States and has been a consultant to universities, hospitals and corporations worldwide. At CCC she created the MA program in Dance/Movement Therapy & Counseling, where she chaired the Department of Creative Arts Therapy for 19 years. She co-founded the Graduate Laban Certificate in Movement Analysis (GL-CMA) program in 2001 and founded the Shannon Hardy Making Connections Suicide Prevention Program in 2002. Susan served for nine years on the Committee of Approval for the American Dance Therapy Association (ADTA) and chaired the committee from 2006–2009. She earned the first annual ADTA Excellence in Education Award in 2006 and chaired the Education, Research, and Practice Committee of the ADTA between 2012 and 2016.

Emilie Jauffret-Hanifi, DMT, dancer and dance-therapist, graduated with a master's degree in dance-therapy from Paris Descartes University (Sorbonne). After starting in Paris with France Schott-Billmann with Parkinson's patients, Emilie continues today her work as a dance-therapist with different publics in the south of France.

Kyung Soon Ko, Ph.D., LCPC, BC-DMT, GL-CMA, NCC, is assistant professor at Soonchunhyang University in Korea. She began as a Korean traditional dancer, receiving her master's in Dance Education in Korea. She received her second master's in Dance/Movement Therapy and Counseling at Columbia College Chicago and her PhD in Expressive Therapies at Lesley University. She worked for Asian Human Services in Chicago, providing clinical services for Asian clients with chronic diseases; she also served as a field supervisor for DMT interns at Columbia College. Ko received the 2015 Award for Journalism by The Marian Chace Foundation and is a member of the Committee of Research & Practice with the ADTA.

Sabine C. Koch is Psychologist and Dance Movement Therapist, BC-DMT, Professor of DMT at SRH University Heidelberg and of Empirical Research in the Arts Therapies, Alanus University Alfter (AU), and Director of the Research Institute for Creative Arts Therapies (AU). She specializes in embodiment research, evidence-based research, Kestenberg Movement Profiling (KMP), Capoeira and active factors of creative arts therapies. She has contributed meta analyses and systematic reviews in DMT and CATs, primary studies on DMT for schizophrenia, autism, depression, trauma, Parkinson's, phenomenological approaches to therapy, theory and method development (e.g. in arts-based research).

Donna Newman-Bluestein BC-DMT, Certified Movement Analyst, mental health counselor, educator, trainer, author and performer with the intergenerational dance company Back Pocket Dancers. She has provided DMT to people aged 3 to 109, helping them cope with mental illness, physical disabilities, chronic pain, coronary artery disease and dementia. Donna co-authored *The Dance of Interaction: An Embodied Approach to Nonverbal Communication Training for Caregivers of People with Dementia* with Dr. Meg Chang. An international trainer, speaker and presenter, Donna's passions are twofold: (1) advocating for the field of DMT, and (2) transforming the culture of care for people with dementia through dance and embodied caregiving. To motivate people, particularly those with dementia, to interact, she created the Octaband®, a tool to foster a sense of connection through movement.

Svetlana Panova, DMT, professional dancer, choreographer, dance teacher and dance-therapist, graduated from La Sorbonne. Svetlana has been conducting Primitive Expression workshops for Parkinson's patients within the France Parkinson Association and at the Salpêtrière Hospital in Paris for six years.

Marcia Plevin, BC-DMT and psychologist, is an American former professional modern dancer, teacher and choreographer working in Italy since 1986. In 1998 she co-founded the Association of Creative Movement method Garcia-Plevin ® with Mariaelena Garcia in Rome, with trainings presently in Italy, Turkey and China. She is a member and supervisor of dance movement therapy for the American Dance Therapy Association and the Italian Dance Therapy Association. She is presently a teacher and supervisor of dance movement therapy for Art Therapy Italiana; Institute of Expressive Psychotherapy, Bologna; Bilgi

University psychology department, Istanbul and the Inspirees Institute, Beijing, China. Presently, she is on the Circles of Four, Discipline of Authentic Movement faculty. Her articles have been published in specialized journals: *Arts and Psychotherapy*, *The American Journal for Dance Therapy*, *Body/Mind and Psychotherapy* and in books published by Jessica Kingsley and Oxford University Press. The Italian version of *Creative Movement and Dance* was published in 2006 and has been translated into several languages.

Kristine Purcell, MA in Dance/Movement Therapy from Drexel University, Board-Certified Dance/Movement Therapist and Licensed Graduate Professional Counselor, has worked for the last seven years as a dance/movement therapist in a number of settings. These include outpatient, school and special education programs with children with neuro-developmental diagnoses; with older adults in a nursing home; with adult members of clergy in a residential setting and with a spectrum of ages and diagnoses in acute inpatient settings, partial hospital and residential settings. Kristine grew up with a passion for dance, studying with her mother and sister at their studio in Annapolis, MD. This passion carried through into her graduate studies and professional life, in which she is intent on keeping alive the creativity and art of dance/movement therapy and recognizing the heart of dance in each individual.

Ulf-Dietrich Reips, Ph.D., is a full professor at the University of Konstanz, Germany. He received his PhD in 1996 from the University of Tübingen and worked at universities in Switzerland, Spain, California (US), and the UK. His research focuses on Internet-based research methodologies, the psychology of the Internet, measurement and development. In 1994, he founded the Web Experimental Psychology Lab, the first laboratory for conducting real experiments on the World Wide Web. Ulf was a founder of the German Society for Online Research, was elected the first non-North American president of the Society for Computers in Psychology and is the founding editor of the free open access journal *International Journal of Internet Science*. He is involved with both clusters of excellence recently awarded to the University of Konstanz by the Excellence Strategy of the German Federal and State Governments. Ulf and his team (http://iscience.uni-konstanz.de/) develop and provide methods and free Web tools for researchers, teachers, students and the public. They received numerous awards for their Web applications (available from the iScience Server at http://iscience.eu/) and methodological work serving the research community.

Ruth Ronen is professor of Philosophy at Tel Aviv University. She graduated from the University of Toronto in 1984 and joined the faculty of Tel Aviv University in 1985 and the Philosophy Department in 1997. She was head of the Philosophy department between 2014 and 2018. Her areas of research are: philosophy of art, philosophy and psychoanalysis. Among her books: *Lacan with the Philosophers*, *Art Before the Law: Aesthetics and Ethics*, *Aesthetics of Anxiety*, *Art and its Discontents* (in Hebrew), *Possible Worlds in Literary Theory*. She is currently engaged in projects on the philosophy of dance and on aesthetic communities.

Yukari Sakiyama, PhD, BC-DMT, KMP Certified Analyst, earned her PhD at the Graduate School of Humanities and Science of Nara Women's University in 2005, focusing on touch in dance/movement therapy. She is currently a full associate professor at Mukogawa Women's University, Junior College Division of Early Childhood Education. She was also visiting scholar at Long Island University, Department of Health Physical Education and Movement Science from September 2014 to March 2015. She teaches Physical Education for children, focusing on early childhood development based on KMP. She is also vice president of the Japan Dance Therapy Association (JADTA) and chair of the Credential Committee. She received an award from Marian Chace Foundation for valuable contributions to Dance Movement Therapy in Japan and continuing generosity to the membership of the American Dance Therapy Association in 2002.

Rosemarie Samaritter, DMT, Ph.D., is a licensed senior dance movement therapist and supervisor. She has been working in outpatient settings in the Dutch Mental Health Services and in private practice for more than 30 years, with an emphasis on dyadic DMT intervention in personality disorders, trauma and psychopathologies with a disturbed sense of self (attachment trauma, autism). Rosemarie has been involved in the development of one the first professional DMT programs in the Netherlands in 1986 and was founding chair of the dance therapy chapter of the Dutch Association of Creative Arts Therapies. Throughout her career she has also been teaching and presenting DMT theory and methodology in various DMT programs in Europe and at international conferences. As a researcher at *Codarts Arts for Health Rotterdam* (NL) and *KenVaK* Research Centre for the Arts Therapies (NL) she is involved in intervention research and the development of innovative DMT research projects with a specific focus on dance-informed research strategies.

France Schott-Billmann, PhD in psychology, is a dance teacher, dance-therapist, and dance-therapy teacher at the Master of Dance Therapy at Paris Descartes University (Sorbonne), a researcher in dance anthropology and author of several books about social and therapeutic functions of dance, including, in English: *Primitive Expression and Dance-Therapy: When dancing heals* (Routledge, 2015).

Jane Wilson Cathcart, BA, Adelphi University; MSW, New York University; Board Certified Dance/Movement Therapist (BC-DMT); Licensed Clinical Social Worker (LCSW-R); Certified Movement Analyst (CMA); and Certified EMDR Practitioner. Ms. Cathcart's early clinical training was in dance therapy at Turtle Bay Music School and with therapist Marian Chace at Bellevue Medical Center. She has had 50 years of clinical experience in settings such as Manhattan Children's Psychiatric Center and Little Meadows Early Childhood Center with children, adolescents, physically challenged and developmentally delayed populations. She taught in the Wesleyan University Graduate Liberal Studies Program for 17 years. Her work is shown in the ADTA film *Dance Therapy: The Power of Movement*, where she is identified as "Jane Downes." Jane has been a trustee of the Marian Chace Foundation of the ADTA since 1996. In 2018 Jane received the ADTA Lifetime Achievement Award. She maintains a private practice in New York City and Cold Spring-on-the Hudson, NY.

FOREWORD

"We dance to know who we are." I recorded this statement from Mary Wigman in my notebook when I studied with her in 1965–1966 in Berlin, Germany. Dance and cultural scholars know her as the early modern dancer and teacher who spurred understanding of the importance of dance in human development. Wigman's exploratory methods were carried further by many international students who studied with her after the reestablishment of the Wigman School of Dance following World War II.

Opportunities to dance in any inquisitive way were rare then and only gradually opened up as the entire world engaged in renewal. Beginning in 1985, I felt drawn to the postwar Japanese dance of *butoh*, also called "darkness dance". There I found the same yawning hope for depth of experience that Wigman had shared in her teaching, and I was not surprised to learn that butoh founders Hijikata Tatsumi and Ohno Kazuo had studied in the lineage of Wigman. Ohno's butoh taught me not to fear the shadows so that I might be able to see more light. His classes respected group experiment and created space for failure. Dance experience and process were important at his studio in Yokohama, Japan. Today Ohno's son Yoshito cultivates the same intrinsic awareness of dance experiences. As with the Ohnos, Wigman's classes in Berlin were nonjudgmental and generous in spirit. Such awareness begins with *dance as process*, not in emphasizing product. From the time of early modern dance through butoh and beyond, dancers have created aesthetic (affective) pathways for personal discovery and group cohesiveness in creative dance processes.

Now the creative therapeutic methods of dance have a solid identity. Through its international proponents, Dance Movement Therapy proliferates around the globe, developing in diverse mental health settings. In their foundational work, *The Art and Science of Dance/Movement Therapy: Life is Dance* (2016), Sharon Chaiklin and Hilda Wengrower shared their broad engagement with the international field of Dance/Movement therapy. *Dance and Creativity within Dance Movement Therapy: International Perspectives* expands the scope of Chaiklin and Wengrower's original inquiry. This work delineates the global reach of DMT, and it is just as pioneering as Chaiklin and Wengrower's first foray into cultural consciousness through dance and movement therapy.

The book in your hands shows that therapeutic dimensions of dance have existed in various contexts of dance globally and that they continue to evolve with cultural diversity. Dance/Movement Therapy in this century has grown in the wake of an immense amount of exploration and courage to create, where *the aesthetic as the affective* provides a difference to the often-objectifying gaze of concert dance. The values of DMT are not concerned with perfection in stage performance, yet they still involve creativity and rudimentary elements of performance. Dancers who promote the values of movement for everyone know what is at stake in sharing dance widely and directly. Many populations benefit from DMT in light of physical and mental health, as this book addresses. Dance/movement therapeutic processes can affirm the importance of affectivity in recovering a life worth living. The risk and trust involved in dance improvisation permeates many of the processes of DMT. To put the potentials of dance improvisation simply in my own words:

My movement comes as a surprise to me
When I don't stop its emotional flow, but let it be.

In letting be, I get to know myself in movement,

In owning my own irreplaceable existence.

Students and practitioners as well as researchers in the field of DMT will benefit from the viewpoints in this book. The editors and contributors bring a comprehensive view to creative standpoints and practices of dance and movement in therapeutic settings. Chapters address the study of dance as art and its implications for therapy. Contributors integrate knowledge stemming from dance studies, neuroscience, phenomenology, psychotherapy and philosophy of art. They research DMT through dance aesthetics and specific techniques, using aesthetics as a therapeutic tool.

Because aesthetics is just now being addressed in the burgeoning field of DMT, and has been lacking in dance scholarship in general, I would like to develop a sketch of an *aesthetics of care*; this book attests such a thing. Since the time of Plato, aesthetics has been the study and appreciation of beauty, and to some extent it still is, but the parameters have expanded along with new ways of defining and understanding aesthetic phenomena. It seems that beauty has a history as lengthy as that of aesthetics.[1] In contemporary life, aesthetic perception invokes more than beauty in art. As a case in point, *the whole of this book brings an aesthetics of care to light*. The combined work of many authors develops *affective/aesthetic* concerns of care in dance and movement. They document care as embodied in DMT processes—care for those who suffer loss, victims of human trafficking, young onset dementia, the elderly, Parkinson's disease and much more. The work of DMT cares to assist clients through dance experiences of well-being through new awareness and life improvements.

Aesthetikos from the Greek, points to *affectivity*, as this involves sense perception in both its active and receptive phases. Put in less theoretical terms, aesthetics is a word that speaks to affective life and how we relate to feelings: the things that make us feel good and the things that make us feel bad. The first is conducive to well-being, and the second might lead to depression and other maladies. "Things" that help create feeling and emotion can come from anywhere—events, relationships, illnesses, fears, abuse, and so on.

Accordingly, I walk my puppy every day and watch her cavort. Now in retirement from academe, I still dance. I write. I try to surround myself with things that make me feel good. My house is a menagerie of antiques, gifts, stuff from my travels, Zen paintings, people I love and good memories. My clothes are colorful and remind me of my travels. My piano that I seldom play nevertheless reminds me of many hours in flow with music. I call my home "house of light", because it has a wide view of the desert where I live in touch with light. When I'm in the dark, the light is within reach. I'm lucky that way and hope to share my luck in whatever way I can. Sharing connects me to others and makes me feel good. Even so, there is much that slips beyond my control, no matter what I do, and at best, antiques only last so long. When I'm forced to admit life's contingencies, I strive to focus on what seems right and good.

Feeling good is the most basic of aesthetic values. Acts of taking care and giving care can feel very good, but care is theoretical until it manifests in some action, feeling or dance. Care is part of empathy and palliates suffering. In empathizing with others, we listen, and listening with the heart is an aesthetic experience. As such, listening is an aesthetic value of care. Donna Newman-Bluestein turns aesthetics of care toward vision in her chapter, "Seeing with the heart: The aesthetics of dance/movement therapy with the elderly". Readers will discover an aesthetics of care in her chapter and on every page of this book.

When we are healthy, we are disposed toward good experiences, at least in theory. Ethically speaking, perhaps we even want to do good. At times, my education in idealism breaks down, however, because I know that some people want to feel bad and to behave badly. They have told me so. And I ask myself, is this how life is supposed to be? In the asking, even idealists know that life sometimes finds us in the dark, falling down and feeling bad. Aesthetic values are felt in wide expressive ranges. As intrinsic values, they are experiential by definition. And if they are valued, they are good, even when they are ugly. How wonderful—we get to feel what we feel and not turn away. This I learned at the Wigman School, famous for exploring the grotesque in dance. Bad feelings were not disallowed. All of this came back to me in butoh. In workshops, my mentor Ohno-sensei said, "Don't turn away from the messiness of life."

I know this is circular thinking, but in aesthetic discourse, the wheel stops on experience, not beauty or idealism. Aesthetics (as though this were a person) is not afraid of the dark. Carl Jung, whose work provided one of the threads of DMT, taught that what we deny in life manifests as fate.[2] He promoted healing through dream work and active listening. There are better ways to see into the shadows than those of glaring confrontation. Many better ways are shown in the case studies of this book. Dance is the better way, the embodied way toward experiencing the truth of existential suffering, joy and healing.

I came to see aesthetics this experiential way through extensive study of this matter during a sabbatical leave in 1980. I wanted a philosophical approach because I couldn't find anything substantive about aesthetics in dance scholarship at that time. What distinguishes dance movement from other kinds? What are the root values of dance upon which all other values depend (including sociopolitical values)? A phenomenologist would say that a thing (like dance) appears in consciousness first pre-reflectively as *what it is*. Aesthetic values are the affectively lived qualitative dimensions we experience in dance and recognize as such, and they are all around and within us. In dance, aesthetic values are *the good we experience in movement*. When we dance darkness, we revalue it and accept the shadows in ourselves and others. Black is a beautiful color. Through my studies I learned that all values are rooted in aesthetics, because the aesthetic is affective and experiential.[3] Further, affective movement experiences in dance are without end. They belong to movement and movers in the moment, and it is this belonging that matters more than the words that describe it.

~

As I read the emerging chapters of the present work, I track my impressions in a scattered way and then organize them in light of a story that comes to me. It emerges in an image of hope, one that has wings and heart, and finally a whole body. Presently, I imagine someone ageless, who nevertheless has dementia and carries a scarf to waft in the wind. She could also be *he*, and as part of a group, this person takes chances, learning how to share space and how to build group-speak dynamically while maintaining individuality. She owns her own body, even before thought, tapping into authenticity through Heideggerian "unconcealment", so to speak. For the sake of cultural and connective memes, let me give this gender-fluid imaginary person a therapist and adaptive dancer called, "Lore".

"Where did dance go", Lore asks? Where did the dance of dance/movement therapy go after penetrating in the hinterlands of psychology and clinical objectives? This is what this book asks, traversing fascinating territory in pursuit of the answers to the questions. I am not surprised that the book discovers differences in cultural constructions of body, space and time and that it uses Laban's dance-specific theories in this pursuit. What I might not have anticipated is the book's pragmatic examples of cultural differences in DMT. Asia has its own dance styles, of course, and habitus. I learn from Lore that Koreans respect containment of emotion, not overt expression, while Westerners are more comfortable with expressing emotion openly. I observed the same thing when I lived in Japan.

In time, I understand how Lore's dances relate temporally and spatially to experiential dimensions of life, past time and future unknowns. If that isn't enough, she creates dances with metaphors from nature (trees, perhaps) as guides toward renewal, but not because she is romantic about nature. Using practical wisdom, she discovers through experiment that many people can relate to nature images, especially those who are ill or aging. Lore learns from the people she works with; she moves at their pace and in their frame of reference. She doesn't force or forge ahead of them.

> Lore stays with clients in what happens.
>
> Being OK together with them, not forcing solutions,
>
> She uses movement to create unanticipated space for progress,
>
> Focusing also on positive memories in dancing.
>
> Moving together with others
>
> In touch with darkness,
>
> Is the aesthetic path of Lore.

Congratulations to Lore and to Sharon and Hilda on this accomplishment and to all contributing authors who share their experiences, research and talents so willingly.

Sondra Fraleigh

NOTES

1. "The Great Theory of Beauty and its Decline". Wladyslaw Tatarkiewicz. *The Journal of Aesthetics and Art Criticism* 31 (Winter 1972): 156–80.
2. Carl Jung cited by Joseph Campbell in his workshops on mythology and psychology at the Theater of the Open Eye in New York City, 1981. Jungian psychology provides an important basis for free association and art in DMT.
3. I explain this perspective with extensive source material in "Witnessing the Frog Pond," my chapter on phenomenology and aesthetics in *Researching Dance*, Eds. Sondra Fraleigh and Penelope Hanstein, Pittsburgh: University of Pittsburgh Press, 1999, 188–224.

ACKNOWLEDGMENTS

All the contributors were very giving of their ample knowledge and wholeheartedly collaborated with us in making this book the best it could be.

We would like to express our gratitude to Dr. Joan Chodorow, Dr. Silvio Gutkowski, Dr. Heather Hill, Mrs. Elina Matoso (University of Buenos Aires), Dr. Eva Marxen (School of the Art Institute of Chicago), Roberto Serafide Fratini (Institut del Teatre, Barcelona) and Ms. Jane Wilson Cathcart (Marian Chace Foundation of the ADTA), for kindly reading some chapters or giving especially helpful information. Each one of them was generous, open and thorough.

The librarians at the School of Society and the Arts at Ono Academic College—Henya Levy, Elana Eitan, Noga Dvir, Ktam Wahesh—have been tremendously cooperative and quickly answered our calls for help; we extend our warm thanks to them.

Mrs. Dalia Ben Shoshan, the general director of the School of Society and the Arts has been supportive of the work on this book, and we offer her our indebtedness. Our expression of thanks is also extended to the Scientific Committee of the School.

Ms. Amanda Devine and Ms. Grace McDonnell at Routledge were always quick and clear in answering our questions and our requests for assistance. It was a pleasure to work with them.

Students and supervisees throughout the years have been partners in a fruitful dialogue, and their questions and observations helped clarify and deepen the book's ideas. Patients of all the ages called our attention to the capital contribution dance and creative movement brings to their lives.

INTRODUCTION

There has been a fair amount written about Dance Movement Therapy (DMT)—often about its connections with various branches of psychology as well as psychotherapy, neuro-science, education, and other disciplines. DMT practitioners have written about their ideas and techniques while working with people of all ages with various physical and emotional needs. With other disciplines making use of movement in various ways, it becomes import-ant to differentiate more clearly what is unique about Dance Movement Therapy and its applications, since there are other therapies that also make use of the body but with a dif-ferent focus.[1] The questions to be answered are: What is the practice of Dance Movement Therapy? What makes it different from other therapeutic techniques, and what is its impor-tance in working with different therapeutic need or age groups? DMT practice is growing in range and international scope. Is there a commonality among practitioners that identifies them as belonging to the same profession, even with cultural differences? What is the core of the practice and would those practicing agree upon basic concepts from which we all work? Allowing for different theoretical bases and techniques, is there an agreement as to what is necessary in order to practice the profession of Dance Movement Therapy?

DMT is continually expanding and developing internationally. In reviewing its many aspects and locales, we became aware that therapists become interested in new ideas and related disciplines that support the dance therapy work done in the profession. However, we are also aware that these ideas frequently subsume the basic core of our work so that the strength of what we do becomes lost, less defined, or underestimated.

It is important to cast aside the viewpoint of dance as frivolous and unimportant and to identify its many attributes so that its vital connection to growth and healing is recognized. The art of dance as a root of the DMT profession, the creative process, and aesthetics as well as the necessity of mind-body-spirit integration have to be fully recog-nized. It is the art form contained within the therapeutic relationship that both the ther-apist and the individual/group make use of in DMT and which enables the therapeutic process. The art of dance is profound in its many aspects, and these are discussed by all the authors throughout the chapters of this book. The authors also explore variations in DMT's use as viewed through cultural differences and the specific needs of the patients and settings.

This book examines these issues through the input of practitioners from several coun-tries. Included are three sections which comprise theory, research, and practice based on case studies to illustrate basic concepts that support new ideas. It is our hope that these many var-ied accounts lead to a broad understanding of how the creative processes in dance and dance in its many forms suggest interventions that enable therapeutic change. We believe dance to be a powerful and sometimes, a joyful modality that needs to be better comprehended. This book is addressed to dance movement therapists (dmt), students, and colleagues in the health professions as well as dance scholars, performers, and choreographers who may find interest and inspiration within these diverse chapters.

Being an international book, there are various ways to designate the profession: dance/movement therapy, dance therapy, dance movement psychotherapy, and so on. These dif-ferences may relate to legal or licensing issues or to how the profession developed in each country. In order to simplify reading, the term Dance Movement Therapy is denoted frequently with the initials DMT. The clinician, the dance movement therapist, is indicated by the lowercase initials dmt.

OVERVIEW OF THE CHAPTERS

The chapters in this book will provide different experiences to the reader. Some of them will inspire action as a professional; others will challenge well-established ideas and practices; several may open paths of personal reflection. The reader may not only find material to think about but may also encounter material that elicits emotional responses.

We are very happy that Sondra Fraleigh accepted our invitation to write the Foreword. Her life trajectory integrating dance and the study of the phenomenology of the dancing person, make her very suitable person for introducing this book.

Consistent to the purpose of the book, the first chapter, by Hilda Wengrower, focuses on dance and aesthetics through phenomenological and psychoanalytical theories, including the contributions to DMT stemming from the perspective of positivity in psychoanalysis. Its purpose is to look at and think about dance as well as its intrinsic aesthetic and creative potentials, connecting the former with psychological life and highlighting specific factors that promote (mental) health and well-being.

Rainbow T. H. Ho takes the reader into a voyage through the planet and along history to learn how cultures have been using dance for healing. Ho distinguishes three movement attributes that are effective in DMT: aesthetics, contemplation, and poetics. She notes that they converge with some of the healing factors in arts therapies identified by Koch, that is also mentioned by Wengrower's chapter. Ho supports her text with references from the fields of cognition, neuroscience, clinical research, and vignettes from her own work.

Rona Cohen was invited to write an exploration of the concept of the authentic in the form of Authentic Movement and the homonymous term in Heidegger's work. Especially since the rise of the paradigm of social constructionism (Guba & Lincoln, 1994), the psychological meaning of authenticity has been debated. This chapter offers an introduction to the core concepts of Heidegger and links them to Authentic Movement and DMT. The chapter by Ruth Ronen focuses on the visual experience of the onlooker and is based mostly on French perspectives in the aesthetics of dance. This chapter is thought-provoking because it challenges the strongly grounded holistic idea of the visual experience of a dancing body through concepts such as "detachment". Part I of the book, then, not only presents the work of contributors from different parts of the world but also brings different philosophic considerations most relevant to DMT.

Part II of the book collects research papers. Iris Bräuninger and Ulf-Dietrich Reips investigate how new therapists appraise the importance of dance in their work and profession, comparing their answers to those offered by more experienced colleagues. The researchers also contrast the situation from the first decades of the development of DMT to its current state. Then, Zeynep Çatay and Marcia Plevin, who created Transformational Body Tracings (TBT), discuss how this method enhances embodiment in training and in practice of DMT. TBT takes two to three long sessions or more and entails the integration of drawing a full body outline, coloring it, moving, reflecting, and writing. TBT becomes a kind of visual diary, a facsimile of the self upon which the participants are able to reflect and understand many issues about themselves and their bodily experience. The authors analyze the process through multidisciplinary knowledge.

Continuing with her research on the aesthetic factors active in DMT, Sabine C. Koch presents the construct of *being moved*, the study of which is being developed as an emotion in aesthetics and psychology. In DMT there is a feedback process between moving and being moved that deserves to be looked at carefully in order to deepen knowledge of DMT's specificities and workings. Some of the aesthetic aspects presented in the first chapter from phenomenological and psychoanalytic theories can easily be compared with some of the aesthetic factors identified by Koch through the lens of social and cognitive psychology, thus strengthening their validity.

Next, Rosemarie Samaritter and Marja Cantell select published studies to identify the varieties of information brought by the therapists when describing methods and specific interventions in DMT. Based on the reviewed data, they offer a structural and conceptual outline that allows for systematizing the material in order to thoroughly describe, understand, apply, and teach interventions and their theoretical/meta-theoretical foundations.

Since DMT's are connected to theories and concepts, Susan Dee Imus's chapter offers a taxonomy of the structural components of clinical work. She goes into detail about how to look at one's practice and to describe it in order to establish a meaningful communication with colleagues and students. Her discussion also enables practitioners to look at their methods of working and the methods' relationship to their goals. The author also introduces a theoretical framework for teaching denominated A-FECT, which illustrates the use of her model.

After looking at interventions and the process of DMT sessions in the previous two chapters, Kristine Purcell guides us to stare at the creative process of the patient during the therapeutic process. Although it is considered a core aspect of DMT, we do not yet have a model of its elements, stages, and how they manifest themselves. Purcell's model is based on her scrutiny of theories on creativity that contemplate both unconscious and conscious material, delineating how stages and components of the creative process lead to therapeutic change. A case study about a group in an inpatient psychiatric unit demonstrates the application of her model.

Beatrice Allegranti's chapter opens Part III of the book. She extends the clinical perspective of DMT to its use for social and cultural change. Based on her knowledge of dance and choreography, she describes her work with families in which a member has early onset of dementia. Her unusual methods engage dancers who collaborate with her and the families. The next chapter delves into work with persons in the advanced stages of dementia. The reader will find Donna Newman-Bluestein's courageous sharing of her own process undergone after many years of work with this population and her judicious and sensitive working through it. Her chapter is a testimony to her integration of art and science in DMT. She uses the term aesthetics as a cluster of principles in the work of an artist, and from there she takes us through her journey with this special population. Therapists working with other kind of clients will also profit from this text, because the issue of personal aesthetic preferences is dealt with, as they exist ubiquitously even without our noticing them. The contribution of Emilie Jauffret-Hanifi, Svetlana Panova, and France Schott-Billmann on dance-rhythm therapy with patients with Parkinson's disease describes the use of rhythms, drumming, movement/dance, and voice to enable these patients to deal with their motor and non-motor, as well as with the psychological/emotional.

The next three contributors speak about the need for cultural specificity and sensitivity in DMT by examining how they have transformed DMT practices through specific cultural values in their home countries of India, South Korea, and Japan. India is known for its important contributions in spiritual practices and classical dance, but as with every country, it also has social problems. Sohini Chakraborty has spent many years working at combining her experience in dance in order to respond to the needs of victims of sexual trafficking and abuse. Her chapter describes a unique rehabilitation center she founded with a group of survivors that enables change and support for women and children who have gone through traumatic experiences. Through the use of dance and self-reflection, her model enables participants to be accepting of themselves and reintegrate into society.

The two following chapters from South Korea and Japan open our eyes to their ways of understanding, living and making use of body, dance, and communicating emotions. Both chapters delineate the meaning of body and mind, psychotherapy, verbalization, culture-specific emotions, and traditions. Knowing a different culture allows one to ponder about similarities and divergences with one's way of life. Through the presentation of a case study, Kyung Soon Ko portrays the use of Salpuri, a traditional Korean dance, in the treatment of a woman suffering from *haan*, a specific Korean feeling. It was through her joining to her patients' culturally embedded way of feeling and behaving that the therapy developed and effectively helped the woman. Yukari Sakiyama speaks of the influence of Japanese body culture as well as its rituals and imagery related to nature and how they merge in DMT practices. Traditionally, the body is not sinful but respected, she explains. Also discussed is the effect of Butoh and other dances upon DMT's practice. The concept of Hogushi relating to the passive stance of the body in order to let it be what it is, is thought-provoking, and we can see some link to this attitude in the practice of Authentic Movement. Sakiyama gives us a culture-based explanation to the avoidance of verbalization: Japan as a homogeneous nation permits individuals to share common meanings of many symbolic events. They have the same understanding of events that do not demand verbalization; they are conveyed through nonverbal processes.

Transitioning from East Asia to Spain, we learn of the integration of flamenco's dance/culture in DMT work with persons with chronic and severe mental disorder. Elena Cristóbal Linares brings to the sessions her comprehensive, embodied knowledge of this culture and describes moments imbued in flamenco's poetry. In this case, the inclusion of flamenco for the patients is also a way to strengthen their belonging to society. The therapeutic use of the structural/aesthetic components of flamenco rhythm, weight, and space can inspire dance movement therapists in other parts of the globe.

David Alan Harris developed dance/movement therapy to assist former child soldiers in war-torn African Sierra Leone. His understanding of how dance and movement were employed within the culture and his awareness of the trauma in these youths' lives enabled the development of creative and therapeutic movement. He further narrates how this was later used to enable the community and the youths to gather and facilitate transformation among themselves through symbolized and ritualized action.

Although many dmts start as relatively young dancers in the profession, persons of course age, and their bodies change. Jane Wilson Cathcart describes nicely and openly the process she underwent and how she dealt with some of it. She gives valuable information about some of the early dmts and their work as elders. Her vignettes talk about her fully embodied presence as a "dancing" dance movement therapist that can be inspiring also for young therapists.

We are hopeful that the material within the book will create a dialogue among colleagues to further build our knowledge. The pronouns –they/themselves- are used instead of she/he, according to the most recent changes in linguistic use instituted by the American Psychological Association.

Hilda Wengrower and Sharon Chaiklin

NOTE

1. See the journal *Body, Movement and Dance in Psychotherapy*, 2016, Vol. 11, 2–3.

REFERENCES

Guba, E. G., & Lincoln, Y. S. (1994). Competing paradigms in qualitative research. In N. Denzin & Y. Lincoln (Eds.), *Handbook of qualitative research* (pp. 105–117). Thousand Oaks, CA: Sage.

Part I

ABOUT DANCE

CHAPTER 1

DANCE COMES TO THE FRONT STAGE IN DANCE MOVEMENT THERAPY

Hilda Wengrower

INTRODUCTION

This chapter brings to the fore specific aspects of dance and aims to raise ideas about dance's intrinsic potential for therapy, i.e. to promote development as well as maintain/ regain well-being in a therapeutic process. The study of dance as a personal experience or as an artistic media and the inclusion of positive psychodynamic psychotherapy may lead to innovations in the conception and practices of dance movement therapy (DMT), thereby restating the role of embodied/danced experience and demarcating its uniqueness as psychotherapy.[1]

Dance movement therapy is interdisciplinary, as it defines itself as the therapeutic use of dance movement that integrates psychology, and observational skills, converging into the theory and practice of the profession.

Seligman (2011, p. 868) asserted that psychoanalysis would achieve broader sight when including wisdom from "the surrounding *arts* [emphasis added by author] and sciences." He brought up Freud's call for making use of knowledge from more than one direction. If predicated on these concepts, together with the study of psychology in its different branches we can fortify our field's root in art. This chapter invites us to turn to dance again and what comes with it, to feel it in new ways and consider it with new resources.

DANCE AS IMAGE OR METAPHOR

Images and metaphors common in cultures or uttered by prominent figures who have an impact in their society reveal meanings and values attributed to some issue—in this case dance. Dance has been used as a metaphor for different meanings. Nietzsche utilized it for light-free thought and life-attitude (Nietzsche, 1998/2008); the idiom "it takes two to tango" denotes the idea that conflicts are based on the responsibility of two parts in relationship. Dance has also been used as an image for tasks or phenomena that demand clever and fine coordination of numerous factors as in research, i.e., "the choreography of qualitative research design" (Janesick, 2000), and I am sure readers remember many more metaphors and images of dance.

As Lakoff and Johnson (2008) demonstrated, metaphors emerge from our body and movement experiences. The image of dance in Western culture has been in a process of transformation through history, beginning in the last years of the nineteenth century. Dancers and dance scholars have coined the term *bodily knowledge* indicating the knowledge germinated in the practice of dance, as is the case of the dancers who created Dance Movement Therapy (DMT). For example, Chace's dancing and bodily knowledge led her to practice kinesthetic empathy when communicating with psychotic patients, thus anticipating what experimental psychology and neuroscience discovered later as embodied simulation (Gallese, 2005; Wengrower, 2010).

Nietzsche (1872/1910) used dance as an image to reclaim the body from oblivion and repression in rationalistic, authoritarian culture and as a metaphor for free/light thinking. He also related to dance itself and saw in the dancer somebody who knows how to listen to the body and transform strength and power (Santiago Guervós, 2008). In spite of its evanescence (movement disappears at the very moment it is executed), dance manifests the interplay of its constituent elements only limited by anatomy and gravity. To dance is to transform oneself into another body without changing skin; it is to discover another one in oneself, to become movement and to *feel alive*. As Santiago Guervós explained, for Nietzsche dance is also a symbol of living creatively – contemplating the horror of the depths and the harshness of life, overcoming both of them through dance.

The essence of dance is the balance between the basic forces of the body and the spiritual powers in constant fluidity, in continuous threat and recovery: life itself. Nietzsche's Zarathustra wants to teach people to transcend themselves, using their legs to dance. He exhorted that those who want to learn to fly have to learn to stand, walk, run, spring, climb, and dance. Dance, then, opens new paths, new discernment and a new possibility of life. It is stability in instability (Santiago Guervós, 2008, p. 6).

DANCE MOVEMENT THERAPY: OFFSPRING OF DANCE

While Nietzsche used dance as metaphor, dancers saw its contribution for the individual within the dance itself. For Mary Wigman (1886–1976), one of the salient figures in modern dance history who impacted much of DMT, dance was a "means toward self-knowledge—not a disclosure of personality but a construction of it, not self-expression as self-indulgence but a creation of self in expressive action" (Fraleigh, 1987, p. xxii). Wigman centered her work on the question, "Who am I?" However, her dance wasn't self-centered but an embodiment of the expressive range of movement (Fraleigh, 1987, p. 28), which often included the exploration of the obscure sides of self, as can be seen in her Witch Dance from 1926 (Mooiman, 2014).

During her childhood, Trudi Schoop, one of DMT's forerunners, suffered from fears that she tried to control with obsessive-compulsive rituals until finally she could no longer control them: "My infatuation with life's elements—rhythm, melody, space, shapes, forms— kept me somehow in balance and made me dance. . . . When I danced, I was happy, I had no fears" (qtd. in Berrol, 2012, p. 187). As Berrol analyzed, through her improvisational, exploratory movement, Schoop the girl began to appease the demons threatening her and ignited the possibility of emotional transformation through dance. From then on, Schoop's dreads transformed into structured dances that became part of the ground for her work as an artist and later as a dance movement therapist (dmt).

Similarly, Mary Whitehouse graduated in dance, then studied with Wigman in Germany and was later part of Martha Graham's company. During World War II, she worked in an aircraft factory. In this position, she observed and experienced the repetitive movements of the women as they worked. She got the idea to form a troupe and later went on to produce performances, thus ratifying her belief that every person can dance from an unfettered and self-connected attitude. Gradually, she developed her professional work on the basis of her study of Jung's theories and the idea that creativity in movement is healing (Sullwoold & Ramsay, 2007). And of course there is Marian Chace, a dancer who used dance knowledge to relate to people and develop a theory and practice of dance movement therapy that is part of the foundations of DMT (Sandel, Chaiklin, & Lohn, 1993).

As noted in these examples (and as is true of others not mentioned here) (Levy, 1988), DMT's Western pioneers and their disciples were dancers immersed in this art; their discoveries of the therapeutic use of dance were related to their own experience onstage and/or offstage. Feeling and reflecting on their own experiences with dancing and their students' dancing, each one of them concluded they had a powerful means to help people to enhance their self-awareness and personal development, assist children's maturational process, or help persons with psychological difficulties. Although I am not a pioneer, this resembles my process in some ways: I became interested in DMT because I was aware of the impact of dance, mainly improvisational, on myself and my students.

DANCE FOR ONESELF OR FOR THE GAZE OF ANOTHER PERSON?

Some of the arguments brought by some colleagues who have been deterred from using the term *dance* for the profession and choose to call it *movement therapy* stem from the belief that there is a connotation of performance with the term *dance*, as if it were something done for others and appraised by them or something that's focused on pleasing an onlooker. Sharon Chaiklin and I thought that this view comes from a narrow understanding of dance, and so we proposed the following definition:

> Dance is used in the broadest sense of body movement, which may involve a small gesture or the total use of self. It lasts over time, perhaps merely a brief moment, and may use rhythms or not. It may spread out over space or use only that which one's body inhabits. However, in all cases, it is a motor action that emanates from an individual in response to internal sensations or perceived external stimuli.
>
> (Chaiklin & Wengrower, 2016, p. xxx)

Contemporary concert dance has for a long time blurred the barriers between addressing an audience in a theater, non-professional dance, and daily life movement. The sociocultural movement of education through arts (Laban, 1963; Read, 1943) and the explorations of choreographers and dancers stressing movement freedom have led to a sense that dance is to be danced and felt. This new conceptualization thus lowers the place of narrative in dance, as it was used in classical ballet, and offers new possibilities for everyone to dance. Now the differences between professional and amateur dancing lie in the mastery of the movement and its sophistication, intention, motivation, context, and structuration.

Reading Fraleigh (1987), who focuses on the self-awareness of the professional dancer, it is easy to associate with the experience of the person dancing for themselves. The dancer is/must be connected with themselves; if they is concentrated on the scrutiny of the spectator, the emotional impact on the audience is lost. The performer gets to know themselves through their work in a dance on a universal level; their being is part of the collective of dancers and they also gains self-awareness on the individual level as a unique person. In some psychotherapeutic practices in DMT, the universal is considered in therapy without neglecting the focus on the individual.

Dance: Forms of Feelings, Vitality, and Presence

Having established that the dancing experience serves a person's self-awareness which is one of the fundamental tenets in probably all psychotherapeutic schools, we shall introduce elements of this experience as they are identified by some dancers and philosophers in a phenomenological perspective: forms of feeling, vitality, and presence. These characteristics stem from two indissoluble traits: dance's ephemerality and the fact that it is executed through the body's movement. These elements are cardinal for the use of dance in therapy and as therapy.

Cunningham wrote that dance is simultaneously movement and stillness in space and time. This constant fluidity, this permanent impermanence (or the transitory character of dance in which each movement vanishes the very moment it has been performed) furnishes the attraction that it exerts on dancers, choreographers, teachers, and spectators. Dance "is its own necessity, not so much as a representation of the moving world, rather as a part of it, with inherent springs" (Cunningham, 2015, p. ix). Dance movement therapists connected to their dancing selves feel this necessity. Permanent impermanence, stability in instability— can we find better images for life? However, is dance as evanescent as described and usually conceptualized? Visually dance is fleeting, but certainly its kinesthetic and emotional impact in the mover and in the witness stay for longer.

Dancing as well as watching dance connect to vitality, as mentioned by performer and scholar Johannes Birringer (2005) and psychoanalyst Daniel Stern (2010). Birringer wrote that we go to see dance because we love movement and relish dancing "as it is a *vital part of our physical and sexual culture*, and perhaps *the oldest sense we have of feeling alive in our bodies*" (Birringer, 2005, p. 10). On a similar thread of thought, Stern (2010) stated that dance moves us by the experience of *vitality*, which then reverberates in us. Trudi Schoop (in Dieste, 2008) said: "When you dance you are alive." We shall see that vitality when dancing is a felt experience, as reported by DMT students and professionals.

Philosopher Susanne Langer wrote about dance from the standpoint of a viewer; several of her texts have been very influential on the study of the arts, especially music and dance. In this section, her analysis that enriches a dmt's understanding of dance is brought in. She integrated the aspects of vitality and forms of feelings; they are an intricate connection, not easily pulled apart. For Langer, dance is a *virtual realm of power*, a magic magnetism between dancers and/or between them and the onlooker, a subjective experience of will and volition, of *vital power* (Langer, 1953). Studying Langer's work, Weber asserted that dance is "a means of intersubjectivity, a genuine path of interbeing" (Weber, 2002, p. 195). Probably many of this book's readers have felt this mentioned magnetism, the realm of power while dancing in a group or with another person. In other text, Langer alluded to dance as an *apparition* of active powers, an effect that is something more than what dancers do. What the viewer sees is a display of intermingling forces "by which the dance seems to be lifted, driven, drawn, closed or attenuated . . . whirling like the end of a dervish dance, or slow, centered, and single in its motion" (Langer, 1976, p. 78). Being lifted, attenuated, and so on, are the forms of vitality that Stern coined after Langer's (1953) "forms of feelings" as shall be discussed in the next section. The powers perceived are not physical forces embodied by the muscles. These powers seem to correspond to the flow of human experience or "life as it feels to the living" (Langer, 1976, p. 79), not always being articulated as narrative or anecdote (Stern, 2010, p. 75). In a DMT session, the therapist might see power in the gaze of a patient, or in a group interaction; on the other hand, they might see lack of powers in a weakened/bound form or a missed grounding.

A very important contribution of Langer for DMT is her referring to *forms of feelings*; to her, everything that can be felt—arousal and rest, pleasurable physical sensations or pain, complex emotions and intellectual strains—is the subjective aspect of experience (Reese, 1977). Dance expresses experiences that are difficult to scrutinize because they may be ambiguous or complex, varying and transforming. Descriptive words do not always help to get the intensity and specificity of the subjective experience. There are endless ways to feel joyful, sad, and so on. Emotional life is complex and fluid, multilayered and polyphonic; dance is very suitable to approach this complexity. Dance, Langer asserted, is a form that conveys feeling: the rhythms and relations, crises and disruptions, the complexity and richness of what is sometimes called man's "inner life," the stream of experience, life as it feels to human beings. In a dance, she said, there is a display of

> the way feelings, emotions, and all other subjective experiences come and go—their rise and growth, their intricate synthesis that gives our inner life unity and personal identity. What we call a person's "inner life" is the inside story of his own history; the way living in the world feels to him.
>
> (Langer, 1976, p. 79)

Other testimonies present a more radical stance in the discussion about the experience of the dancing person and are even closer to some tenets of DMT. For instance, Fraleigh (1987) wrote,

> I am the twisting, the stretching. My body is me. Thinking, feeling, moving. Body is myself in my lived concreteness. It is who I am and the way in which I am. The lived body refers to my personal way of existing and the meanings attached to this manner of existing in a world in which I experience presence.
>
> (p. 32)

Fraleigh's ideas are somehow echoed by Caldwell (2018), who asserted: "The body is not something we have, rather *an experience we are* [emphasis added]" (p. xix). This experience is not always verbalized, "because most of its components are nameless, and no matter how keen . . . [it] may be, it is hard to form an idea of anything that has no name" (Langer, 1976, p. 79). Langer argued these feelings are nameless because there is no *handle* for them in the mind (Ibid., p. 80).

In DMT we can associate the nameless components of the experience in different ways. One is that the nameless has never been symbolized because it pertains to a pre-symbolic normal developmental stage or to an early developmental trauma that continues to impact the person's life. In DMT there is another kind of situation as well: after an exploratory/introspective improvisation, the mover does not find words to communicate their experience or chooses to stay silent, keeping the embodied state of mind. There is a sense that to put into words what has been an inner experience might take away its power. In verbal communication we use signs, specifically words, which aspire to get to the highest level of generalization and therefore establish a distance from the original experience (Noy, 1999). Psychoanalyst Noy wrote that arts fill the need of expression of these experiences that words cannot provide. Both Noy (1999) and Stern (2010) stated that although achieving verbal communication implies an advancement in development, it entails the loss of the richness of the nonverbal, the analogic mode of communication (Wengrower, 2016), referred to by Noy as the primary mode of communication. Simply put, not everything can/has to be verbalized, as Isadora Duncan said: "If I could tell you what it meant, there would be no point in dancing it" (qtd. in Duncan & Rosemont, 1981). Some of the nameless experiences can be transmitted and represented through the systems of movement analysis or the feelings of vitality (Laban, 1963; Loman & Sossin, 2016; Stern, 2010; Tortora, 2016)

Important contributions to the study of dance were made by Maxine Sheets Johnstone and Sondra Fraleigh, who integrate in their lives a dance career with scholarship in philosophy. In her phenomenological description of dance, Sheets Johnstone (2015) asserted that it is a kinetic form that is seen; it appears to the viewer but is nonetheless foremost a lived, unreflective, and embodied experience (p. 22–23). It is a total phenomenon in which the mover/dancer is "one with the dance, pre-reflectively aware of their body as a form in the making" (p. 31).[2] It is only when the dancer is completely one with the dance that they exists in the dance, and then they experiences *vitality* and force. Sheets Johnstone exhorted onlookers to be in the same experiential position.

Sondra Fraleigh (1998) wrote:

> When I dance, I am subtly attuned to my body and my motion in a totally different way than I ordinarily am in my everyday actions. That is, I seldom take notice of my ordinary comings and goings. . . . But, when I dance, I am acutely aware of my movement. I study it, try out new moves, study and perfect them, until I eventually turn my attention to their subtleties of feeling and meaning. Finally, I feel free in them. In other words, I embody the motion. . . . *And in this, I experience what I would like to call "pure presence," a radiant power of feeling completely present to myself and connected to the world* [emphasis added].

> (p. 140–141)

These descriptions present one of the therapeutic objectives dmts aspire to help their patients achieve, namely, being embodied, being present in the moment with one's vitality.

Forms of Vitality

Psychoanalyst and researcher Stern (2010) was influenced by Langer's concept of forms of feelings and coined the term "forms of vitality" based on it. Langer conceived the notion "forms of feeling" to relate to feelings evoked by music and dance or expressed through these arts, which are not related to the distinct emotions (Ekman, 1999) and are not a specific action: fading, exulting, easiness, and so on. During his observations of infants and their caretakers, Stern noticed these forms and along different of his publications created diverse designations until he arrived at "forms of vitality." He introduced vitality as the sensation of being alive[3] and the modes people have of feeling it. It takes on different forms in the same individual and across persons; it is felt by oneself consciously and non-consciously and is perceived by others. Vitality can be understood as the way to feel/express emotions: somebody laughs inward, producing a soft sound, while another or the same person in a different situation produces a strong cascade of laughter (Stern, 2010, pp. 27–28). So forms of vitality are the colors of life, especially but not only in intersubjective relations, or as Stern put it, without them life would lack much of its interest; it would be digital and dispossessed of its analogical characteristics.[4] Many persons experience vitality while moving, through kinesthesia and proprioceptivity, i.e., the inner experience of movement of one's self and others, or as Birringer cited earlier, while watching dance. Stern noted these are main indicators of feeling alive and animate. Movement brings with it the perception/sensation of force within it, which is strongly connected to experiencing vitality. When mentioning movement, dance comes to mind. As previously stated, one of the main changes produced in dance during the second half of the 20th century was the shift from performed stories to the exploration of movement's dynamics, including daily actions and objects, non-linear forms, and non-narrative forms. Laban's movement observation and notation system, as well as improvisation, contributed greatly to this search (White, 2016).

The dynamic forms of vitality are related to the quality, the "how" of the lived experience. They are different from the discrete emotions, cognition, and sensations, and the last ones are modality-specific (related to the specific senses). This concept is also connected to identification and empathy; forms of vitality are mainly nonverbal processes by which individuals share/exchange experience by means of body–mind interactivity. In therapy they constitute part of somatic resonance or countertransference. Forms of vitality are also a cardinal element in implicit relational knowing; they have constituent elements as seen in the time-based arts (dance, music, theater, cinema): movement, tempo, intention, force, and space, thus making dance a "royal road" to take to approach this experience.[5] Therapist and patient bring them to the therapeutic encounter (Seligman & Harrison, 2012).

Dynamic forms of vitality are part of episodic memories; they are their zest. In psychotherapy they afford an access to non-conscious experiences, be they past, dissociated, or implicit relational knowledge never verbalized nor psychologically represented, as the nameless stated by Langer. Stern held that they allow for verbalization when evoking the past. However, in my own practice his concept of forms of vitality and Langer's notion of forms of feelings have gone in a different direction: instead of aiming to verbalize an unknowable feeling/experience, patients and the therapist learn to accept the inability (temporary or not) to name it, for example, during/after a movement experience. Besides the need of some patients and their therapists to find words for their feelings, one has to accept that there are also nameless experiences for the time being and/or forever. They can be worked through nonverbally; one can empathize, showing understanding by reflecting or attuning to the movement. The therapist can suggest describing the experience through a body part gesture, movement, or vocalization, allowing patients to understand that not everything needs to be verbalized or uttered.

AESTHETICS AND DANCE MOVEMENT THERAPY

Since dance is art, the ties between aesthetics and mental health should be delineated. The word aesthetics has different meanings, and one of them refers to the branch of philosophy that deals with the arts, their characteristics, and their workings (or mechanisms). Aesthetics also relates to discussions about beauty, the qualitative evaluation/judgment of the perception of a specific piece of art or perhaps an occurrence in nature. It is a subjective experience marked by the culture in which the individual is embedded as well as in early developmental exchanges (Bollas, 1978). Aesthetics is not only related to (classical) beauty, especially in contemporary art. Nevertheless, most persons are influenced by aesthetics in daily life, and we bring it to the clinic, so it is important to be aware of it.[6] In this section, I shall introduce other meanings of aesthetics that are even more pertinent to DMT. Koch (2017) stated the ground for a model of embodied aesthetics in the arts therapies; the ideas presented here are close to her work and stand near to the conceptual tools psychodynamic dmts use.

Aesthetics, Perception and Knowledge

The word "aesthetics" derives from the Ancient Greek word *aisthetikos*, signifying sensitive, sentient, relating to sensorial perception, and knowing through the senses. Hence, aesthetics discusses sensorial-emotional processes. In 1735 the philosopher Baumgarten used this term to convey that arts are a way of knowing, an idea that has been furthered in the arts-based research model and its variations. This concept finds a home in the arts therapies, i.e., concerning self-knowledge and self-awareness through artistic activity. Dance provides a context for self-knowledge. Attention shifts from the functional body, and routine tasks shift towards presence. The experience of the dancer moves from exploration, creativity, and aesthetics to changes in body–self awareness that happen in and through the dance (Fraleigh, 1987, pp. 28–29). Fraleigh departed from an existential phenomenological angle by stating that she came to know herself (and her *possible self*) through the actions she takes in dance: "Dance works express not so much the self as the seemingly endless ways in which our bodily lived existence can be aesthetically (or affectively) moved" (p. 33). This statement resonates with the Spanish philosopher Trías who, according to the phenomenological tradition, conveyed that psychology should admit another aspect to the ways of being, apart from what one wishes to be or what the subject thinks has to be and the one the person is. Trías added "the possible self"[7], or the possibilities one has to be (Trías in Wengrower, 2016, pp. 24–26).

Psychoanalyst Summers (2005) proposed to enrich the therapeutic process by adding a step after insight was achieved: to accompany the patient to find new manners of being and relating that to the integration of a new sense of self. He argued moving from understanding the present into helping the patients create a new future and giving them an active role in this quest. In DMT, we can escort our patients to discover/try the possibility of other ways of being through exploring movement and its effects on them in a path of self-creation.

Two examples from my own practice come to my mind to further illustrate the benefits of dance and creativity in therapy, experiencing different ways of being as pointed earlier. The first is of Elaine, an eleven-year-old girl who was thin, pale, and frequently rejected by her peers. Her usual movement was contained, her neck stiffly held, and her eyes simultaneously transmitted fear and sensitivity. In the DMT group sessions, she was joyful, alive, and had a leading role. Her teacher in the special school Elaine attended was completely surprised when I told her about this. She thought I might be confusing her with another girl. Dancing awakened the vitality that was turned off in other situations, and this child could experience another way of being in the world. Another example is embodied by Tomer, a 15-year-old boy who had learning difficulties based on emotional problems and some learning disabilities. He signed up for an inclusive movement and drama group I led in his junior high mainstream school. His creativity and humor in movement and acting was so great that he attracted the interest of the "best girl students" of his age group, "the queens of the group." Obviously, he experienced another way of being in school that, for the first time (according to the counselor), allowed him a positive experience of himself. Months later he was accepted in an acting training for adolescents organized by the section of youth services at the municipality. These are examples of discovering different ways of being, possible selves as mentioned earlier.

Aesthetics and Creative Living

Aesthetics is part of our daily life, and we pay attention to it because we want to enjoy ourselves and our surroundings—sometimes even depressed persons do. This is manifested in our clothing choices, how we arrange our homes, how we serve our meals, and in many other situations of our daily life both intra- and interpersonal. The way we organize the place where we work, the manner in which we talk with our patients (intonation, wording, pitch of voice, gestures) are aesthetic forms consciously chosen or not. Alternately, as Bollas (1978) wrote, in "life, the aesthetic . . . constitutes the subject's manner of holding and transforming internal and external realities" (p. 394). This is one of the possibilities DMT offers.

Winnicott's (2005) concepts of creative apperception or creative living clearly relate to aesthetics. They allude to a non-submissive attitude towards life, a proactive full living, creating the world as a baby does: "being able to live the life one has, and to be oneself"

(Caldwell & Joyce, 2011, p. 261). Although Winnicott doesn't use the word aesthetic experience, it is clear he refers to it and to its emotional effect when he shares this clinical vignette:

> One can look at a tree (not necessarily at a picture) and look creatively . . . How often I have been told: "There is a laburnum outside my window and the sun is out and I know intellectually that it must be a grand sight, for those who can see it. But for me this morning (Monday) there is no meaning in it. I cannot feel it. It makes me acutely aware of not being myself real.
> (Winnicott, 1986, p. 43)

Thus, an aesthetic approach to life and creative living are indicators of mental health.

Years before reading this excerpt of Winnicott, I worked with a woman in her thirties who was going through long physically and emotionally demanding medical processes; therefore, one of the foci in her therapy was to psychologically accompany her and help her to stand through this challenge. Here is a transcription of how one of our sessions ended:

H: Be good to yourself, look for something pleasant.

R: I do not have money to go to cinema.

H: You live in a rural area, surrounded by trees, open your door, walk around, look, feel them.

Her response sadly shows how people don't always feel they can access art and beauty immediately and are thus limited in their creative living.[8]

Aesthetics and Emotions

Emotional experiences may have aesthetic aspects, and aesthetic experiences have emotional implications. Fraleigh sees them as one, as can be read in her foreword to this book. There are aesthetic experiences in therapy sessions or in daily life while discovering something about ourselves, a new meaning, the emotion of an insight, or in an intimate conversation, realizing the connection of a movement with a feeling, moments of harmony in a group, and so on. Possibly the aesthetic emotion we feel in many of these moments is what is called "being moved."[9] Somebody once told me that when walking in the streets after his first psychotherapeutic session, surprisingly he felt that the light was stronger and colors brighter than usual. What a wonderful example of seeing life hopefully clearer and in a new light!

As in the earlier example, we can see the overlapping of aesthetic experience and emotion in different situations. When we do something we feel is positively experienced and appreciated by others, it affects self-image and our sense of agency, and sometimes this comes with a sense of beauty. For instance, I remember David, an eight-year-old boy with a rigid, rough aggressive/defensive presence and hoarse voice. Once, while dancing to a waltz, he exclaimed smilingly, "They should come from the TV to watch at us!" The waltz wasn't part of his cultural repertoire; however, the balancing-flowing movement shared with his group, colored by light scarves aroused in him an aesthetic experience of being beautiful, probably capable as well, and deserving an admiring gaze (Kohut, 1977). During this time, his expression was soft and his movement smooth.

Aesthetic Experience/Moment

An aesthetic moment is "an occasion when time becomes a space for the subject. We are stopped, held, in reverie, to be released, eventually back into time proper" (Bollas, 1978, p. 385) Bollas said this about literature and poetry; however, I think we can extend his theory to dance.[10] A profound rapport is felt between a person and an object of art in an aesthetic moment. It affords an illusion of deep connection; it arouses a memory that is not cognitive nor visual but existential, and it is lived as an experience of being. Psychoanalyst Bollas indicated the origin of this aesthetic moment in early infancy when the baby lives the experience of being within intimate dialogue with the caretaker. The experiences of distress, hunger, and so on are dissipated/transformed into peacefulness/satisfaction, and the way these processes elapse and are managed by the caretaker through their own aesthetics are transformational for the baby. The acts of early care are carried out through time qualities, intensities, flow, and so on, which are primarily aspects of the performing arts and dance (Wengrower, 2016). Subsequently, "[T]he aesthetic experience is not something learned by the adult, but is an existential recollection of an experience where being handled by the maternal aesthetic made thinking irrelevant to survival" (Bollas, 1978, p. 388).

In a DMT session, this experience is probably lived during moments of a dance/movement encounter with the therapist, with a member of the group, or the minutes after the encounter. As said earlier, it is probably unnecessary to talk about this moment, although sometimes sharing it through a nonverbal medium can give it validity when acknowledged by the partner/s in the experience.

WHAT IS DANCE FOR ME: DMT STUDENTS' DESCRIPTIONS OF THEIR EXPERIENCE WHILE DANCING

At the beginning of the introductory course to DMT that I teach in a master's program, students are invited to explore, through an improvisation, what dancing means for each one of them. The aim is to reflect on the experiential significance of dance for themselves and integrate it with theoretical and research-based knowledge. The second step is to write a self-report that is shared verbally and discussed in the group. I also teach a course for experienced professionals (10–20 years in DMT), and the purpose is to bring them back to their motives for choosing to study this profession and to refresh the value of dance for them and for their clients.

In this section, I shall present the thematic analysis of students' answers to the question about their experience while dancing. The order of presentation is based from higher to lower frequency of the themes mentioned. Each line brings expressions from a different student, and most of the respondents wrote answers that fit into more than one category. The final theme, serenity, was only mentioned by one individual but has been included because it is often seen and expressed during therapy.

The answers from the professionals' group carry the knowledge accumulated along their years of study and work; the influence of the practice of Authentic Movement[11] and Winnicott's concept of true self are transparent. Three professionals and five students in the regular track of learning allowed the use of their texts. All excerpts are included with the written permission of the authors. Similarities with the testimonies of professional dancers and early dmts already discussed in this chapter can be found in these discussions.

Authenticity

Authenticity as experiencing a self true to itself, a "wholeness of being" (Koch, 2017, p. 89; Cohen, her chapter in this book).

> It is an opportunity to feel and revive the linkages between me and *me being* in this moment, between parts of myself, between me and significant persons in my life, between me and what surrounds. An authentic encounter with the present and history.

To move in an authentic way. Without wanting to please anybody or to be aesthetic.

Connection to the authentic, to myself.

The freedom to be who I want to be the way I want to be, without thinking or asking myself: is this right? Is this correct? When I know there is no correct-incorrect, it releases me from pleasing, I trust my body and whatever it brings is received with love.

I feel sincere and genuine when I dance, without masks.

Way of life. My natural place.

Vitality and Positive Affects

As mentioned earlier, vitality's core meaning relates to feeling positively alive (Birringer, 2005; Stern, 2010) and present in the moment (Fraleigh, 1998).

> I connect to my *bones*, my *strengths*, *myself*. Interesting these words are connected in Hebrew [they have the same root, three basic letters[12]]. Liveliness. Groove in my body. Rising mood. Body work uplifts my mood.

> Dance for me is life, life's joy, the essence of life.

> Joy.

> Serenity.

> Adrenalin entering into the body, bursting energy.

> Support, daring, jump, strength, playing, intensiveness, young girl.

> An invitation to the movement of life.

> It reassures me. Strengthens me. Pleasure, joy, spontaneity, creativity.

> My existence in the world is confirmed, it gets meaning, vitality.

Presence/Embodiment

Presence as being entirely in the moment (Fraleigh, 1998) has been considered healing "in and of itself" (Sheperd, Brown, & Greaves, 1972 in Geller & Greenberg, 2002) which obviously includes being in the body, one of the meanings of the construct of embodiment.

> Femininity, passion, both.

> My existence in the world is confirmed, it gets meaning, vitality.

> Dance is the space where my body isn't a slave to the mind's will and to social norms, it can move freely, rounded, confused, reversed, connected and disconnected to its own wish, and be a significant presence, existing and supporting my life, my life's meaning in present matchless moments.

> To flow regulated with less exertion, this teaches me to trust and accept.

> Connection\disconnection, touch, sensation, balance\unbalanced, weight shifting, leaning, floor, supported.

> Feelings and sensations move in me incessantly, and the body moves with them.

Healing

Dancing provides experiences of healing, which is clearly manifested in the following answers:

> Dancing allows me to go on and surpass obstacles and challenges on the way.

> Movement heals me.

> To flow regulated with less exertion, this teaches me to trust and accept

Freedom

People dancing experience freedom through bodily self-awareness, self-assurance, and self-expression (Frichtel, 2019)

> The freedom to be who I want to be.

> Move freely

> Freedom to listen to body-mind and express . . .

> Makes me feel free

Self-Awareness

> Freedom to listen to body-mind and express . . .

> I learned to listen to my body that said to me to separate from my boyfriend.

> I feel.

> . . . dynamics, weariness, pain, disappointment because unfulfilled expectations of a dance that did not get to be what I wanted.

Expression of Feelings

> A way to express feelings. From childhood until now I find it difficult to express myself or to articulate a critique verbally.

> Freedom to listen to body-mind and express . . .

BRIEF DISCUSSION

Professionals recalled authenticity with higher frequency than students. Their responses and conceptualizations of authenticity clearly connect to Winnicott's concept of true self and strengthen Koch's (2017) identification of art making as contributing to authenticity or having an integrative function. Vitality appears recurrently in the sample presented. It is felt while dancing and is communicated both in bodily and emotional terms (adrenalin, bones) and more frequently in psychological terms (daring, the essence of life, strengthens, and so on). Vitality also appears in sentences written by Sondra Fraleigh (1987, 1998) and Langer

(1953), especially in Langer's concept of virtual power. She mentions the magnetic power between the dancers; Weber, who studied her work, stated that dance is a means for intersubjectivity, interbeing. Curiously enough, there is no mention of the experience of dancing in a group or with another person in the texts received from the students. Maybe the question asked and the fact that the movement exploration was a solo improvisation focused respondents on their experience of moving alone.

Other statements on vitality in dance as a vital part of culture, either watching or actively dancing, come from Birringer (2005), an artist and scholar, and Daniel Stern (2010) who wrote that the arts dedicated more attention to this aspect of experience than psychology. "They have had to do so, as they want to express the aliveness and vitality of human movement and sound" (Ibid., p. 89). Sheets Johnstone (2015) wrote about dance as a total phenomenon in which the dancer only arrives at the experience of vitality when they is completely one with the dance. Fraleigh (1998) asserted that there is a feeling of "radiant power," of being wholly present and connected to the world when the dancer is intensely aware of their movement. As if echoing this sentiment, one student said that her presence in the world is confirmed when dancing. This expression can be seen as one of the precious moments experiencing pure presence, as Fraleigh (1998) wrote, or feeling alive and real as another respondent explicitly stated. Dance, with its simultaneous connection to the ground and its emotional appeal, allows for self-perception and enhances it. Presence, vitality, and aliveness are closely linked in the experience of the dancing person.

Healing was experienced while dancing, it encouraged confrontation of challenges, and acceptance of facts and emotions. Summarizing: the verbal expressions of the students resonate with several of the ideas about the dancing experience brought before. Further research will look into patients' dancing experience.

POSITIVITY IN PSYCHOANALYSIS AND DMT

Positive psychology chose to research health mechanisms, positive experiences and traits in personality, and integrated them in clinical work. Psychoanalyst Mariam Alizade (2002/2010) proposed to persist with the traditional psychoanalytical work while at the same time consolidating healthy aspects of the person.

Alizade asserted that together with tears, treatment should be open to laughter and joy. Pulling on her reading of Spinoza, Nietzsche, Bergson, Castoriadis, and other philosophers who wrote about vitality, creation, and becoming, she amalgamated their thoughts against predetemination or unique paths of development as an affirmative conception of being human. Alizade related to constructive aspects of the person, both conscious and unconscious, the capacity not to stick to conflict, and stated that building health in treatment is as important as confronting mental illness. She found that positivity spreads through associations, cannot be touched/translated verbally, and it is not always representable and thinkable: it is apparent in actions. We can conclude that positivity demands the therapist to be open to perceive it. According to her, the ideology of focusing on suffering during therapy has iatrogenic risks and acts as an epistemological barrier that blinds professional sight. Western culture and psychodynamic psychotherapy have often focused on seriousness, sorrow, and verbalization. Cheerfulness and trivial things have been considered meaningless/superficial, expecting that positive affects will arise by themselves as an effect of healing; therefore, their study was neglected. After reviewing research in neuroscience and in developmental and social psychology, psychoanalyst Music (2009) asserted that psychotherapeutic work on the hopeful and positive aspects of the person has to be promoted.

DMT is well equipped to incorporate positivity in its scope: it accesses the non-verbal, encompassing the positive aspects of the person, enabling playful and creative exploration and performing different ways of being and seeing in the present and imagining the future (Summers, 2005), accompanying the patient in a process of healthy vital embodiment.

CLOSING REFLECTIONS

The immanent and irreplaceable aspects of dance are above all, sensed. They include vitality, authenticity (the sense of being true to oneself), self-integration, presence/embodiment, affinity between persons moving in attunement, aesthetics and its psychological values. All these aspects are fundamental in life; dance is a way of accessing and enhancing them in mental health in a psychotherapeutic setting such as Dance Movement Therapy. When they are an empathized experience, they can be reflected upon (although this is not always necessary, as said earlier, since sometimes empathy might be enough), verbally shared, or expressed in other ways. Dance movement therapists can create specific modalities of practice that do not necessarily echo verbal psychotherapy and merge aspects, structures, and forms of dance. Experiences offered may have different degrees of structuration according to the needs of the patients. Remember Bollas's assertion that the aesthetic is the subject's way of "holding and transforming internal and external realities" (Bollas, 1978, p. 394).

Freud's saying that the ego is first a bodily experience is still valid—no matter how the concept of ego has been metamorphosed. We begin being in our bodies and continue to be our body when we develop and add important components to our being. We embody and perform, unconsciously, our history, emotions, sufferings, and happiness, and we can actively be aware, imagine, explore, and change them. Through dance/movement the patient can explore and enact possibilities of being in the world and with others, as philosophers mentioned here asserted. Psychoanalysts like Alizade and Summers include widening the possibilities of being in their weltanschauung

Vitality in its various forms (Stern, 2010) can help to confront predicaments and be part of our resilient presence; the recognition that feelings have forms and are not always speakable but can still be expressed and worked through is crucial. Aesthetics and dance have a core place in DMT's practice because they are part of well-being/mental health. Looking at positivity in psychotherapy has been legitimated, asserting the efficacy of a therapeutic approach that sees exploring joy as important as delving into sadness.

This is not a complete study of all the values intrinsic to dance, nor has empirical research been introduced here. One of the purposes of this chapter is to lay the groundwork for reflection and encourage new lines of investigation and practice unique to our roots in dance. This does not mean leaving aside the knowledge acquired and built upon during the last decades incorporating psychological understanding. As Kelso (1997) wrote: "the aim of science is not things themselves . . . but the relations among things; outside these relations there is no reality knowable." Therefore, this chapter suggests delving onto the dance experience, thereby contributing valuable and unique gains in the field of Dance Movement Therapy.

NOTES

1. Sabine C. Koch has been developing research on the active and specific factors in arts therapies. See Koch (2017).
2. The stability in the instability and the permanent impermanence mentioned earlier, which refer to the transient characteristic of dance: movement is performed and disappears to give space to another one.
3. Thus coinciding with Nietzsche, Birringer, and Schoop, mentioned earlier.
4. Watzlawick, Beavin, and Jackson (1967) distinguished between two modes of communication: the digital mode and the analogical mode. The first mode is mainly verbal language in which the relationship between significant and signified is a matter of convention. Digital has rich and complex syntax, but alone is less efficient in expressing emotions or conveying relationships, and in this aspect is semantically limited. In contrast, the analogical mode is more closely related to the signified; it is based on similitude and equivalence and has more freedom from conventions but is far from being univocal. This is the case of gestures, movements, body posture, the use of space and interpersonal distance (proxemics), and the nonverbal aspects of speech (speed, modulation, and so on). Various authors agree that analogical patterns are the privileged mode of emotional expression (Wengrower, 2016, pp. 26–28).
5. These component elements of forms of vitality make them dynamic and were first studied almost a century ago by Rudolf Laban (White, 2016), who laid the groundwork for several systems of movement observation used in DMT.
6. See Donna Newman-Bluestein in this book and Wengrower (2017) for more information on this argument.
7. For more, see the chapter "On the Possibility of Authentic Movement: A Philosophical Investigation" by Rona Cohen in this book.
8. I am thankful for Jane Wilson Cathcart's reading of this chapter and her comments; this idea is inspired by her.
9. For more on being moved as an aesthetic emotion, see the chapter "Being Moved as a Therapeutic Factor of Dance Movement Therapy by Sabine C. Koch in this book.
10. As said elsewhere, most psychoanalysts writing about aesthetic experiences do not relate to dance (Wengrower, 2016).
11. Authentic Movement is self-exploratory movement practice based on inner impulses.
12. עצם, עצמי

REFERENCES

Alizade, M. (2002). *Lo positivo en psicoanálisis. Implicaciones teórico-técnicas* (Trans. 2010). Buenos Aires: Lumen (Psychoanalysis and positivity, Karnac Books).
Berrol, C. (2012). Discourse: Trudi Schoop and Vaslav Nijinsky, and dance as healer. *Body, Movement and Dance in Psychotherapy, 7*(3), 185–199. doi:10.1080/17432979.2011.633101
Birringer, J. (2005). Dance and not dance. *Performing Arts Journal, 27*(2), 10–27.
Bollas, C. (1978). The aesthetic moment and the search of transformation. *Annual of Psychoanalysis, 6,* 385–394.
Caldwell, C. (2018). *Bodyfulness.* Boulder, CO: Shambhala Publications.
Caldwell, L., & Joyce, A. (2011). *Reading Winnicott.* Oxford, UK: Routledge.
Chaiklin, S., & Wengrower, H. (2016). Introduction. In S. Chaiklin & H. Wengrower (Eds.), *The art and science of Dance Movement Therapy: Life is dance* (2nd ed.). New York: Routledge.
Cunningham, M. (1965/2015). Foreword. In M. Sheets Johnstone (Ed.), *The phenomenology of dance.* Philadelphia: Temple University Press.
Dieste García da Rosa, E. (2008). Experiencias límites en danza. In H. Wengrower (Ed.), *Terapia a través del movimiento y la danza.* Chile: Univ. Bolivariana de Chile.
Duncan, I., & Rosemont, F. (1981). *Isadora speaks.* San Francisco: City Lights Books.
Ekman, P. (1999/2000). Basic emotions. In T. Dalgleish & M. Power (Eds.), *Handbook of cognition and emotion* (pp. 45–60). London: Wiley and Sons.
Fraleigh, S. (1987). *Dance and the lived body: A descriptive aesthetics.* Pennsylvania: University of Pittsburgh Press.
Fraleigh, S. (1998). A vulnerable glance: Seeing dance through phenomenology. In A. Carter (Ed.), *The Routledge dance studies reader.* London and New York: Routledge.
Frichtel, M. J. C. (2019). Discovering freedom in dance education. In *Dance and the quality of life* (pp. 347–364). Cham: Springer.
Gallese, V. (2005). Embodied simulation: From neurons to phenomenal experience. *Phenomenology and the Cognitive Sciences, 4*(1), 23–48.
Geller, S. M., & Greenberg, L. S. (2002). Therapeutic presence: Therapists' experience of presence in the psychotherapy encounter. *Person-Centered and Experiential Psychotherapies, 1*(1–2), 71–86.
Janesick, V. (2000). The choreography of qualitative research design: Minuets, improvisations and crystallization. In N. K. Denzin & Y. S. Lincoln (Eds.), *Handbook of qualitative research* (pp. 379–400). London: Sage.

Kelso, J. A. S. (1997). *Dynamic patterns: The self-organization of brain and behavior*. Cambridge, MA: MIT Press.

Koch, S. (2017). Arts and health: Active factors and a theory framework of embodied aesthetics. *Arts in Psychotherapy, 54*, 85–91.

Kohut, H. (1977). *The restoration of the self*. New York: International Universities Press.

Laban, R. (1963). *Modern educational dance*. Revised by L. Ullmann. London: MacDonald and Evans (First published 1948).

Lakoff, G., & Johnson, M. (2008). *Metaphors we live by*. Chicago: University of Chicago Press.

Langer, S. (1953). *Feeling and form: A theory of art*. New York: C. Scribner and Sons.

Langer, S. (1976). The dynamic image: Some philosophical reflections on dance. *Dance, 33–34*, 76–82.

Levy, F. (1988). *Dance/movement therapy: A healing art*. Maryland, USA: AAHPERD Publications.

Loman, S., & Sossin, M. (2016). The Kestenberg Movement Profile in dance/movement therapy: An introduction. In S. Chaiklin & H. Wengrower (Eds.), *The art and science of Dance Movement Therapy: Life is dance* (pp. 255–284). New York: Routledge.

Mooiman, M. (2014). *The witch* [video file]. June 23. Retrieved from www.youtube.com/watch?v=AtLSSuFlJ5c.

Music, G. (2009). What has psychoanalysis got to do with happiness? Reclaiming the positive in psychoanalytic psychotherapy. *British Journal of Psychotherapy, 25*(4), 435–455.

Nietzsche, F. (1872/1910). *The birth of Tragedy*. The Project Gutenberg. Retrieved December 30, 2019, from www.gutenberg.org/files/51356/51356-h/51356-h.htm

Nietzsche, F. (1998/2008). *Thus spake Zarathustra*. Retrieved December 30, 2019, from www.gutenberg.org/files/1998/1998-h/1998-h.htm

Noy, P. (1999). *Psychoanalysis of art and creativity*. Tel Aviv: Modan (Hebrew).

Read, H. (1943). *Education through art*. London: Faber and Faber. Retrieved from https://archive.org/details/in.ernet.dli.2015.460970/page/n3/mode/2up

Reese, S. (1977). Forms of feeling: The aesthetic theory of Susanne K. Langer. *Music Educators Journal, 63*(8), 45–49.

Sandel, S., Chaiklin, S., & Lohn, A. (Eds.), (1993). *Foundations of dance/movement therapy: The life and work of Marian Chace*. Columbia, Maryland: The Marian Chace Memorial Fund.

Santiago Guervós, L. E. (2008). Nietzsche y la danza. *Danza ballet*. Retrieved June, 2009, from www.danzaballet.com/nietzsche-y-la-danza/

Seligman, S. (2011). Book review: Forms of vitality: Exploring dynamic experience in psychology, the arts, psychotherapy, and development. *Journal of the American Psychoanalytical Association, 59*(4), 859–868.

Seligman, S., & Harrison, A. (2012). Infancy research, infant mental health, and adult psychotherapy: Mutual influences. *Infant Mental Health Journal, 33*(4), 339–349. https://doi.org/10.1002/imhj.21330.

Sheets Johnstone, M. (2015). *The phenomenology of dance*. Philadelphia: Temple University Press.

Stern, D. (2010). *Forms of vitality: Exploring dynamic experience in psychology, the arts, psychotherapy and development*. Oxford: Oxford University Press.

Sullwold, E., & Ramsay, M. (2007). A dancing spirit: Remembering Mary Starks Whitehouse. In P. Pallaro (Ed.), *Authentic movement: Moving the body, moving the self, being moved* (Vol. 2, pp. 45–49). London: Jessica Kingsley Publishers.

Summers, F. (2005). *Self creation: Psychoanalytic therapy and the art of the possible*. New York: Routledge.

Tortora, S. (2016). Dance movement psychotherapy in early childhood treatment and in pediatric oncology. In S. Chaiklin & H. Wengrower (Eds.), *The art and science of Dance Movement Therapy: Life is dance* (2nd ed., pp. 159–182). New York: Routledge.

Watzlawick, P., Beavin, H., & Jackson, D. (1967). *Pragmatics of human communication: A study of interactional patterns, pathologies and paradoxes*. New York: W.W. Norton & co.

Weber, A. (2002). Feeling the signs: The origins of meaning in the biological philosophy of Susanne K. Langer and Hans Jonas. *Σημειωτκή-Sign Systems Studies, 30*(1), 183–200.

Wengrower, H. (2010). I am here to move and dance with you. In V. Karkou (Ed.), *Arts therapies in schools: Research and practice* (pp. 179–197). London: Jessica Kingsley Publishers.

Wengrower, H. (2016). The creative-artistic process in Dance Movement Therapy. In S. Chaiklin & H. Wengrower (Eds.), *The art and science of Dance Movement Therapy: Life is dance* (2nd ed., pp. 13–32). New York: Routledge.

Wengrower, H. (2017). The interweaving of the personal and professional dances with immigrants and refugees. In R. Hougham, S. Pitruzzella, & S. Scoble (Eds.), *Cultural landscapes in the arts therapies* (pp. 63–80). Plymouth: University of Plymouth and An ECArTE Publication.

White, Q. E. (2016). Laban's movement theories: A dance/movement therapist's perspective. In S. Chaiklin & H. Wengrower (Eds.), *The art and science of Dance Movement Therapy: Life is dance* (pp. 235–254). New York: Routledge.

Winnicott, D. W. (1986). Living creatively. In C. Winnicott, R. Shepard, & M. Davies (Eds.), *Home is where we start from: Essays by a psychoanalyst* (pp. 39–54). New York: Norton.

Winnicott, D. W. (1971/2005). Creativity and its origins. In *Playing and reality* (pp. 87–114). New York and London: Routledge.

CHAPTER 2

BACK TO BASICS

The Aesthetic, Poetic, and Contemplative Movements'
Attributes That Heal in Dance Movement Therapy

Rainbow T. H. Ho

DANCE AND MOVEMENT IN DANCE MOVEMENT THERAPY

Dance Movement Therapy uses dance movements in a therapeutic context to achieve an integration of mind, body, and spirit that can enhance the emotional, social, cognitive, and physical integration of a person (ADTA, 2019) or facilitate the acquisition of new inspirations or new perspectives that can broaden an individual's habitual thinking pattern or behaviors (Wengrower, 2016). During the process, dance movement is the most basic medium that helps foster a therapeutic relationship as well as promote potential changes. If, however, the dance/movement is used in a projective way or as a stand-alone movement—for example, if the therapist asks the participant to make a gesture or a movement for whatever reason and all other processes are conducted in the traditional verbal therapeutic approach with or without relating to the movement presented—can this still be considered DMT? In fact, using creative arts in counseling, social work, and the psychotherapeutic context has become more and more popular (Gladding, 2011). While we have to admit that psychotherapy skills and counseling techniques do help, my questions are how should we use dance/movement to impact the healing process more, and what qualities or attributes of dance/movement should DMT possess to ensure effective healing?

DANCE MOVEMENT ACROSS CULTURES AND HISTORY IN HEALING

Several authors have conducted reviews and summaries on how dancing has been used across time as a means for healing in different cultures. Among them, Stewart (2000) reviewed the history of using dancing as ritual and spiritual experiences around the world. Although the review started with a focus on how women have historically used their body movements to access sacred experiences, it also examined the whole world history of dancing as a healing method regardless of gender. Rueppel (2002) summarized what she referred to as the "inherent healing aspects of dancing" throughout the world, paying particular attention to the spiritual experiences that the dancers or the observers would gain. She described and explained how dancing has been used in different geographical regions and cultures for communicating with God, recreating myths, expressing the Divine, and in religious practices and worship that help to heal people. In particular, the Spiral Dance, Whirling Dervish, and Ran-Eu-Rhythm, and so on, and dance practices from Egypt, India, South Asia, and North America were presented as examples to show how dances were used to achieve the purposes of connecting with the spirit and getting transformative energy. She also described dances as a release of emotions that facilitates the improvement of mental conditions or specific diseases like cancer (Rueppel, 2002).

A dance performance can bring the audience to excitement, joy, or a new experience, and recreational dancing can be enjoyable for both the dancer and the observer. However, these experiences may not be termed as "healing." Therefore, what are the qualities or attributes in dance movements that heal, and how have these attributes been used in DMT? Revisiting the major practices and characteristics of dancing in relation to their function and dancing's involvement in the healing process in different cultures may help us to understand the common attributes of dancing that are cardinal to its therapeutic effects.

Dances in Africa

In most African cultures, an individual's health and illness are closely linked to his/her spirit. The occurrences of physical and psychological illnesses are due to the breakdown of the equilibrium in the natural human connections in the spiritual world or the lack of connection with God and the Supreme Being (Monteiro & Wall, 2011). In traditional African cultures, spiritual and ritual practices which focus on realigning or reconnecting the individual with the social and spiritual worlds are used for healing (Sow, 1979). Dance movement is usually included in those spiritual and ritual practices. Vodoun (Vodon), a nexus of dance ceremonies related to the spirits, has been commonly practiced in different areas of Africa (LaMothe, 2001). As described by LaMothe, "In Vodoun, the dancing is a catalyst for healing with the community" (LaMothe, 2001).

Dances in Europe

The earliest dances in prehistoric Europe were used with spiritual or societal meaning (Ernst, 2011). "Dithyramb," a song and a dance by a group of people to honor Dionysus, the god of wine and fertility in Ancient Greece (D'Angour, 2013), and the Spanish dance Danza de los Zancos (a stilt dance) (Armstrong, 1978) are two examples of these early dances. By the effort of a 17th-century German ballet master, Bernhard Wosien, the Sacred/Circle Dance, a dance form originally from traditional folk dance patterns, was developed into a more spiritual-like dance practice (Scott, 2017). The Sacred/Circle Dance was very popular all over the United Kingdom and Western Europe and is still performed (Watts, n.d.). Folk dances and country dances were very popular during the 18th and 19th century, mainly for recreation and social purposes (Pate, 2017). The appearance of the Romantic Ballet after the 1700s, and later, the modern form of dancing, led to the development of interpretive dancing, where the dancers tried to convey their emotions through dance movements (Ernst, 2011).

Dances in North America

Dancing in North America is mainly from three origins: the Native American dances, dancing traditions carried from Europe by immigrants, and African American dances. While most Native American dances relate to religious rituals or celebrate hunts, harvests, and so on (Weiser, 2018), dances originating from Europe mainly served social and entertainment purposes. From 1774 to the 1850s, the "American Shaker" was developed as a dance form in the Christian context (LaMothe, 2001). Due to their historical roots from slave dancers, the African American dances, on the other hand, are more emotional and soulful (Meade, 2006).

From these three traditions came hybrid dance traditions and movements. For instance, tap dance was developed from African dance and Irish clog dancing (Meade, 2006). Modern dances, however, particularly those developed in the early 20th century, represent a rebellion from European classical dance in terms of techniques and started to focus more on emotional expressions (Kahlich, 2011).

Dances in South America

The early indigenous dances in this area were mainly performed in ritual festivals and were also incorporated into spiritual practices related to honoring the natural forces, animal spirits, and celebration of events (Cashion, 2017). Alternately, the dance traditions carried from some upper-class, European immigrants were more for social or entertainment purposes. The strong infusion of the African culture between the 16th and 19th centuries brought new developments in Latin American dances. Since then, dancing has become "a mechanism for escape from emotional stress" and a mean to "restore the emotional and physical well-being of the individual and community" (Cashion, 2017). For example, the Argentine Tango, which combined the characteristics of African *candombe* dances and the Spanish-Cuban *habanera* rhythm as well as the European dances such as *waltz, polka*, and *mazurka*, was popular in the working class districts in the 19th century. It was danced with close physical contact between partners and gradually became an expression of passion and desire (Marshall, 2017).

Dances in Asia

Dances in different geographic areas, such as East Asia, South Asia, and Central Asia, vary in styles and traditions; just like they do in other places of the world, in all areas of Asia dances play an important role in ritual and spiritual practices and frequently are part of celebrations of harvests or prayers to ancestors. The Japanese folk dance, the *Bon Odori*; the lion dance and dragon dance in China; the shamanic fan dance *Buchaechum* in Korea; the *Unicorn* dance in Vietnam; and the *Pemdet* dance in Bali (Indonesia) and in Bhangra and Garba in India are only a few examples of the frequently performed dances during traditional festivals or spiritual/religious practices in the region (Crawford, n.d.). Dances in Asia also carry a strong relationship with different religious practices, particularly for the Buddhist, Hindu, and Islamic religions as practiced in this region.

Dances in Australia and New Zealand

Dances of indigenous Australians and New Zealanders share purposes similar to those in other places of the world; they are for use in worship, rituals, religious or spiritual practices, ceremonies and harvests. The *Haka*, one of the famous traditional dances of the indigenous Maori people in New Zealand, is a celebratory dance but is also performed to represent the preparation for battle, worship, and is even danced at funerals (Kings, 2017). In Australia, traditional indigenous dances have been performed to represent "the reality of the Dreamtime" where the dancers imitate particular animals and play stories related to their society and the environment (Brock, 2015). Other dances have also been developed in Australia and New Zealand with strong influences from European

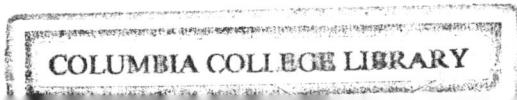

folk dances, and later, modern dances; and there are also locally developed dances like the Melbourne Shuffle and New Vogue. These dances are more for performance, recreation, and social purposes (Eiss, 2013).

Movement Attributes that Heal Across Cultures and History

Across the continents and time, dances have served some common and important purposes, including being part of rituals, worship, and spiritual practices; documentation of events; celebrations of success and harvests; enjoyment and social bonding; and emotional expression. Dancing is also the moment that dancers, and sometimes also observers, experience the contentment of communicating with higher forces, a sense of transcendence, the excitement of moving, and the venting of emotions and feelings. When people dance, they are endowed with these experiences and healing may happen. The transformation and healing processes of dancing have particularly been emphasized in the Jewish culture, as it has been said that "the one who cannot dance cannot heal" (Maron, 2010). Indeed, in Hebrew, the word for dance (*ma'cho'l*) actually relates to the word for illness or affliction (*machah'lah*). According to Maron (2010), dancing brings people into a state of happiness that will dissolve the negative energy caused by illness. Also, the reverse is true, for when someone is happy, they will dance-"his heart lifted his feet" (*Midrash B'reisheet Rabbah*). Even more, when one feels sad, the sadness will lead the person to dance. These all substantiate the innate power of healing in dance.

With a closer examination of the attributes of dance movements across cultures that lead to healing, some consistencies can be observed. Firstly, the aesthetic experiences of dancing and moving allow people a taste of enjoyment, satisfaction, and beauty. This quality can be found in all the dances that serve the entertaining, recreational, social, and even therapeutic purposes of dance. Secondly, the expressive power of movement enables the expression of feelings, emotions, and thoughts beyond language, or the poetic quality of dance. This can be observed in dances that are performed by people who are suffering or those who have emotions to convey, though this should be equally true for the expression of positive emotions. Thirdly, the spiritual or contemplative experience of movement leads to a sense of transcendence, an altered state of consciousness, or a metaphysical experience. This is more commonly found in dances performed for rituals, worship, religious, and spiritual practices.

In fact, the three movement attributes identified from the dances across different cultures and times contributing to healing align with some of the active factors pinpointed by Koch in arts therapies (Koch, 2017). Koch aimed to identify the factors that make arts therapies work and tried to understand what functions arts serve during the process. Her framework described a holistic picture about arts therapies built on a model of embodied aesthetics (Koch et al., 2016) and cognitive sciences. Several concepts similar to the ones already discussed can be found among Koch's active factors. Specifically, Koch's aesthetic factors can be seen in the sense of beauty and authenticity that are universal attributes of healing dance. Additionally, the nonverbal communication/metaphor that Koch described can be likened to affective symbolism for self-expression and transpersonal symbolism in connection with some bigger (spiritual) forces. Other active factors identified by Koch include hedonism, enactive transitional support, and generativity. The movement attributes described here offer support to Koch's theoretical framework. The three attributes are also the building blocks in dance movement that make it therapeutic and essential as a healing practice.

THE THREE MOVEMENT ATTRIBUTES IN DANCE MOVEMENT THERAPY

The Aesthetic Aspect of Movement That Satisfies One's Senses and Perception

To dance is to be out of yourself. Larger, more beautiful, more powerful. This is power, it is glory on earth and it is yours for the taking.

— Agnes De Mille

Research evidence in the past two decades has been rapidly accumulated to show the profound effects of DMT on the health and well-being of individuals in different populations and cultures. As an evolving health care profession, DMT has to demonstrate to other disciplines, as well as patients, its role in psychological, physical, and social outcomes. A lot of focus has been put on the effects of the DMT on changing individuals' psychological and physical symptoms, range of motion, thinking patterns, and social relationships in addition to their self-awareness and personal growth. Nonetheless, the discussion and focus on the artistic or aesthetic aspect of dance movement during the therapeutic process have gained less attention. The artistic and aesthetic aspects in dance movement during the therapeutic process usually do not refer to perfect dancing skills or body lines or the beauty of movement in performing or attaining a professional standard. The word "aesthetic," derived from Greek, has the meaning of "perceive," "feel," and "sense." In DMT, the aesthetic experience refers more to the appreciation of the perception and feeling of bodily movement. To put it another way, these aesthetics center on the enjoyment and awareness of moving and sensing through the body and the movement during the process as well as the sense of being authentic, of being able to connect to the self with the movements. This is also a process of sublimation (Merriam-Webster, 2019), understood as the transition from physical movement to the feeling of satisfaction in mind and spirit. It becomes a transformative process, regardless of form and skills, that produces a healing effect.

Hagendoorn (2011) discussed the aesthetic experiences of dancing and how dancing related to the cognitive functions of the brain, including perception, attention, prediction, and emotion (Hagendoorn, 2011). For dancing, he suggested that "aesthetic experience consists in an inclination, a disposition and a readiness to engage with an object's or event's formal, aesthetic, symbolic or expressive properties and to disregard any other function, purpose, meaning or qualities it might have" (p. 366). This assertion echoes Calvo-Merino's and her co-workers' neuroscience investigation of the aesthetic perception of dancing (Calvo-Merino, Jola, Glaser, & Haggard, 2008). They found that the bilateral occipital cortex and the right premotor cortex are involved in individuals' aesthetic response to dancing. Dancing might stimulate visual and sensorimotor responses, resulting in a feeling of beauty, pleasure, liking, or satisfaction. In DMT work with mothers and infants, Loughlin (2017) also observed how aesthetic experiences contributed to the pleasurable interactions, and thus the well-being, of the mothers and infants. In this sense, Hagendoorn (2011) suggested, not only does dancing have aesthetic properties but it also induces an observer's aesthetic experiences; that is, creates resonance in the observers which could be therapeutic.

Another important finding in Calvo-Merino et al.'s (2008) study was the increased activation in the aesthetically relevant areas in the brain when viewing the whole body movement or movement that involved moving across the space in a way that necessitated the movement of the core of the body and most of the body parts. The involvement of the core of the body, or the integration of the posture and gestural movement, is usually referred to as the "connected movement" (Hackney, 2002). In DMT, facilitating the development of more connected movement is one of its important therapeutic purposes; as more connected movement relates to a more connected mind and body in an individual. Hackney further related connectedness with the ability to access the emotions and feelings and to express them dynamically through body movements (p. 203). More connected movement also relates to the authentic expression in movements. Therefore, Calvo-Merino et al.'s study provided neuroscientific support to the value of the work of DMT on mind–body connection through promoting movement connectedness; their research also endorsed the importance of gaining aesthetic experiences through dance/movements in DMT.

The aesthetic experience in DMT succors people when they are suffering or in adversity, as it gives a new dimension within which they can perceive and establish connectedness within themselves or even with others and the universe. Over the years, I have witnessed this many times when working with cancer patients. On one occasion in a DMT session with a group of women with different types of cancer, after the improvisational movement with a piece of nature music, a woman described her experience as flying by herself in the sky. Originally, I thought that she might be feeling lonely; however, she described that experience as excellent and beautiful, as she has never moved with such freedom in her life. She felt that she could do away with focusing on others and with taking care of anyone but herself at that moment. She felt she was totally free but at the same time felt more connected with herself, nature, and the universe. I had never seen such energetic movement in a middle-aged woman who had never danced before and was in the final stages of cancer. She could move so freely and quickly but she also knew when to stop and recuperate. She kept closing her eyes, but she was smiling all the time with her face so relaxed. Without doubt, witnessing her was a beautiful moment, as I could feel her sense of freedom in her movement and felt more connected with her. She also stated that although she realized that she could not live long, she treasured the moment of being able to stay alone by herself and enjoyed it. She also related this with her experience of having cancer. She said that it was her cancer that made her stronger, and now she had the courage to face the remaining time left in her life alone by thinking positively—alone but not lonely, that was the insight she got from the dance/movement process in DMT.

In another DMT session, a childhood sexual abuse survivor described her experience: "I found that life and the body have their own rhythm. I need to slow down to experience, to sense and feel, and to listen to my own inner tempo" (Ho, 2015). For many sexual abuse survivors, losing contact with themselves and the bodily sensations is common, as such disassociation may help them cope with the overwhelming experiences and memories in the body (Young, 1992). However, long-term dissociation leads to difficulties in recognizing and expressing emotions even when they want to recapture them. After joining the DMT program, this lady regained the courage to reconnect with herself and her body. During the process, she was fully absorbed into the experience of dancing with her own rhythm. Her experience echoed the definition of aesthetics as she started to sense and perceive herself during the DMT process.

The Poetic Movement That Enables Expression

Dancing is very like poetry. It's like poetic lyricism, sometimes, it's like the rawness of dramatic poetry, it's like the terror—or it can be like a terrible revelation of meaning. Because when you light on a word it strikes you to your heart.

—Martha Graham

Dancing, like other art forms, can express meanings and ideas in a symbolic and metaphoric way. In DMT, as described by Chaiklin and Schmais (1993), symbolic body action has been used since the time when Chace, the DMT pioneer, worked with patients in psychiatric hospitals. Symbolic movement can serve as a medium through which "the patient can recall, re-enact and re-experience"(Chaiklin & Schmais, 1993, p. 97). It is also a medium where the therapist can meet and understand the client. Samaritter (2009) described another use of dancing as a metaphor; that is, metaphors or symbols can be the source for dance improvisation which allows for working from outside towards the inner movement and feelings of the dancer. In addition, she also explained that some movement metaphors and symbols are archetypical, meaning that they can be understood regardless of cultural backgrounds (e.g., a woman cradling a child).

The poetic quality of movement in DMT not only refers to emotional expression and understanding (Wengrower, 2016) but it is also closely linked to the aesthetic experience, as "poetic" literally means imaginative or "very beautiful or expressing emotion" (Merriam-Webster, n.d.). Margariti et al. (2012) described such a process in a DMT study with psychiatric patients where the participants were encouraged to dance and "seek for a quest for personal beauty in their movements, independent from social or other dance conventions" (Margariti et al., 2012, p. 97). As a result, the participants experienced a sense of fulfilment and happiness. Their study indicated that after a brief DMT program—which emphasized the Primitive Expression (PE) model's dance movements, rhythms, voice, and play—changes in psychological state, behavior, and brain physiology were observed. The authors regarded this as "a complex physical-cognitive-affective process of recollecting and releasing repressed emotions and tensions" (Margariti et al., 2012, p. 97), a state where the mind and the body are connected.

The poetic expression in dancing and moving in DMT can engender a new perception and understanding (Wengrower, 2016) as well as invoke the integration of an individual's cognition and emotion. A participant in a DMT group for cancer patients described her insights and feelings after an exploring of space in a symbolic and embodied way as "a real joy like going back to childhood". Through this experience, she "rediscovered her body self as well as her psychological self " (Ho, 2019). In a study with patients diagnosed with anorexia nervosa, Padrão and Coimbra described how symbolism helped the participants to pursue a more embodied and rich experience of both the internal and the external aspects of the self (Padrão & Coimbra, 2011). They emphasized that "dance/movement therapy should aim to increase patients' mastery of the symbolic system of dance so as to enable them to learn and make use of one more of the many "language" systems used to construct our world and make meaning" (p. 136).

The Contemplative Process of Moving That Allows for Transcendent Experience

> Dance is meditation in movement, a walking into silence where every movement becomes prayer.
>
> —Bernhard Wosien

> Dance is the movement of the universe concentrated in an individual.
>
> —Isadora Duncan

Contemplative practice in the Buddhist tradition is called *shamatha/vipashyana* (mindfulness/awareness) practice (Rockwell, 1989). In contemplative practice, the mind is trained to perceive the situations of each moment in a relaxed state and with a soft visual focus (*vipashy-ana*/awareness) (Trungpa, 1973). Since there is a synchronicity of the person's mind, body, and speech in the mindful state, the person is completely present in every moment. The soft focus also allows for developing clear and in-depth insights (Rockwell, 1989). Spiritual practice, a process of communicating with the higher force, usually involves contemplative practice, as the individuals should be fully present and devoted to the process.

Contemplative practice is usually a quiet and calm process. However, this only refers to the state of the mind. The word "contemplation" originally means "religious musing" and only later came to refer to an "act of looking attentively at anything" (Harper, 2001). Thus the concept as defined includes no clear direction on what the body or movement should be. A quiet mind can also be achieved in motion. Modern contemplative practices also include practices in movement such as walking, yoga (Bryant, 2015), and dancing (Buehler, 2015). Whether or not moving is the presentation of the contemplative process in different bodily actions; it is not the focus of contemplation itself. In dancing, the body is moving and not quiet at all, yet the dancer is fully present in the moment; thus, the process can be referred to as contemplative. In Dance Movement Therapy, contemplative experience in movement is cardinally important. It is also one of the goals of the therapeutic process, as the movement totally becomes the embodied expression of the mind—either in a quiet or vigorously moving body—through which the conscious and unconscious thoughts and feelings can unite, resulting in a sense of wholeness.

Authentic movement is a form of contemplative practice that dance therapists may use. Stromsted (2009) described authentic movement as the dance with the divine in which spiritual experiences may emerge when the repressed emotions and primitive instincts merge, allowing for a sense of resonance in both the mover and the witness. In her article, she demonstrated the transcendent power of the movement process by describing how a woman became aware of her prenatal trauma when witnessing another woman dancing while pregnant. Through the DMT process, she finally developed a sense of safety and healing by establishing a connection with the Virgin Mother. Smallwood (1978) and Farah (2016) also explained the practice of authentic movement as the movement in active imagination that allows for the bridging between the conscious and the unconscious that leads to a transcendent function as a sense of inner peace and energy flow from the unconscious.

Another form, or contemplative practice, that DMT uses is cathartic movements. Although catharsis involves vigorous movements in releasing strong and intense emotions, it can be regarded as contemplative practice by being an alternative presentation of contemplation in dynamic bodily action. Individuals in catharsis should be fully present and focused, and this may lead to an altered state of consciousness. Many spiritual dances or ritual dances use cathartic movements and processes to facilitate the entrance into such a state. Egypt's oldest trance dance, Zar, is one example (El Guindy & Schmais, 1994). DMT, or other expressive therapies, also use catharsis to facilitate emotional expression. As explained by El Guindy and Schmais (1994), the catharsis process is necessary in this context, as it will lead to an altered state of consciousness where conscious control of the mind and repressed emotions will loosen, self-criticism will be suspended, and new insights and observations may take place.

CONCLUSION

DMT utilizes the innate capacity of dance movement for healing. Across the time span and the history of dancing in different cultures, the contemplative process of moving in ritual dances has demonstrated the transcendent power of movement that leads to inner peace and new insights; the symbolic expression in movement helps emotional relief and expression; and the aesthetic experiences generate resonance and a sense of satisfaction. These three important attributes are, in fact, universal across arts modalities when arts serve a therapeutic purpose. Interestingly, these three important elements can coexist during the therapy process and are presented in the most basic form: the body movement in DMT, which enables and amplifies the healing effect. Although "dance alone is not enough"(Chace, 1993), without the dance and without attending to the fundamental or basic dance movement attributes that heal, DMT will lose its essence of being an arts-based creative therapy. Thus, the aesthetic, poetic, and contemplative movements are the most basic, but also the most cardinal, elements in DMT.

REFERENCES

American Dance Therapy Association. (2019). *What is dance/movement therapy?* Retrieved May 28, 2019, from https://adta.org/faqs/

Armstrong, L. (1978). Ritual dances. *Folk Music Journal*, *3*(4), 297–315.

Brock, F. (2015). *Dance tidbits: Dances of Australia.* Retrieved from https://fordneyfoundation.org/dance-tidbits-dances-of-australia/

Bryant, E. F. (2015). Hindu classical yoga. In L. Komjathy (Ed.), *Contemplative literature: A comparative sourcebook on meditation and contemplative prayer* (pp. 457–502). Albany, NY: State University of New York Press.

Buehler, A. F. (2015). Sufi contemplation. In L. Komjathy (Ed.), *Contemplative literature: A comparative sourcebook on mditation and contemplative prayer* (pp. 307–358). Albany, NY: State University of New York Press.

Calvo-Merino, B., Jola, C., Glaser, D. E., & Haggard, P. (2008). Towards a sensorimotor aesthetics of performing art. *Consciousness and Cognition*, *17*(3), 911–922. doi:10.1016/j.concog.2007.11.003

Cashion, S. V. (2017). Latin American dance. In *Encyclopedia britannica*. Retrieved from www.britannica.com/art/Latin-American-dance

Chace, M. (1993). Dance alone is not enough. In S. L. Sandel, S. Chaiklin, & A. Lohn (Eds.), *Foundations of dance/movement therapy* (pp. 246–251). Maryland: The Marina Chace Mermorial Fund.

Chaiklin, S., & Schmais, C. (1993). The Chace approach to dance therapy. In S. L. Sandel, S. Chaiklin, & A. Lohn (Eds.), *Foundations of dance/movement therapy: The life and work of Marian Chace* (pp. 75–97). Columbia, Maryland: The Marian Chace Memorial Fund.

Crawford, B. (n.d.). *Asian folk dance.* Retrieved from https://dance.lovetoknow.com/Asian_Folk_Dance

D'Angour, A. (2013). Music and movement in the Dithyramb. In B. Kowalzig & P. Wilson (Eds.), *Dithyramb in context* (pp. 198–210). Oxford, UK: Oxford University Press.

Eiss, H. (2013). *The mythology of dance.* Newcastle, UK: Cambridge Scholars Publising.

El Guindy, H., & Schmais, C. (1994). The Zar: An ancient dance of healing. *American Journal of Dance Therapy*, *16*(2), 107–120.

Ernst, T. (2011). *European dance history.* Retrieved from https://prezi.com/gow8fo-722cq/european-dance-history/

Farah, M. H. S. (2016). Jung's active imagination in Whitehouse's dance: Notions of body and movement. *Psicologia USP*, *27*(3), 542–552. doi:10.1590/0103-656420150121

Gladding, T. S. (2011). *The creative arts in counseling* (4th ed.). Alexandraia, VA: American Counseling Association.

Hackney, P. (2002). *Making connections: Total body integration through Bartenieff Fundamentals.* New York and London: Routledge.

Hagendoorn, I. G. (2011). *Dance, aesthetics, and the brain.* Tilburg: Tilburg University.

Harper, D. (2001). *Online etymology dictionary.* Retrieved from https://www.etymonline.com/

Ho, R. T. H. (2015). A place and space to survive: A dance/movement therapy program for childhood sexual abuse survivors. *Arts in Psychotherapy*, *46*, 9–16.

Ho, R. T. H. (2019). Embodiment of space in relation to the self and others in psychotherapy: Boundlessness, emptiness, fullness, and betweenness. In H. Payne, S. Koch, J. Tantia, & T. Fuchs (Eds.), *The Routledge international handbook of embodied perspectives in psychotherapy: Approaches from dance movement and body psychotherapies.* New York, NY: Routledge.

Kahlich, L. C. (2011). *Encyclopedia of American studies: Dance.* Retrieved from https://eas-ref.press.jhu.edu/dance.html

Kings, A. A. T. (2017). *5 traditions of New Zealand's Maori culture explained.* Retrieved from https://travel.startsat60.com/articles/5-traditions-of-new-zealands-maori-culture-explained

Koch, S. C., Mergheim, K., Raeke, J., Machado, C. B., Riegner, E., Nolden, J., . . . & Hillecke, T. K. (2016). The embodied self in Parkinson's Disease: Feasibility of a single Tango intervention for assessing changes in psychological health outcomes and aesthetic experience. *Frontiers in neuroscience*, *10*, 287.

Koch, S. C. (2017). Arts and health: Active factors and a theory framework of embodied aesthetics. *Arts in Psychotherapy*, *54*, 85–91.

Koch, S. C., Mergheim, K., Raeke, J., Machado, C. B., Riegner, E., Nolden, J., . . . Hillecke, T. K. (2016). The embodied self in Parkinson's disease: Feasibility of a single Tango intervention for assessing changes in psychological health outcomes and aesthetic experience. *Frontiers in Neuroscience, 10*.

LaMothe, K. L. (2001). Religion in motion: Sacred dance: A glimpse around the world. *Dance Magazine, 75*(12), 64.

Loughlin, E. (2017). Dance movement therapy: An aesthetic experience to foster wellbeing for vulnerable mothers and infants. In V. Karkou, S. Oliver, & S. Lycouris (Eds.), *The Oxford handbook of dance and wellbeing*. New York, NY: Oxford University Press.

Margariti, A., Ktonas, P., Hondraki, P., Daskalopoulou, E., Kyriakopoulos, G., Economou, N.-T., . . . Vaslamatzis, G. (2012). An application of the primitive expression form of dance therapy in a psychiatric population. *The Arts in Psychotherapy, 39*(2), 95–101. doi:10.1016/j.aip.2012.01.001

Maron, M. (2010). The healing power of sacred dance. *Tikkun, 25*(2), 61–64.

Marshall, E. (2017). *A guide to South America's most iconic dances.* Retrieved from https://theculturetrip.com/south-america/articles/a-guide-to-south-americas-most-iconic-dances/

Meade, M. (2006). *A history of social dance in America.* Retrieved from www.americanantiquarian.org/Exhibitions/Dance/about.htm

Merriam-Webster. (n.d.). Poetic. In *Merriam-Webster.com dictionary.* Retrieved April 5, 2019 from https://www.merriam-webster.com/dictionary/poetic

Monteiro, N. M., & Wall, D. J. (2011). African dance as healing modality throughout the Diaspora: The use of ritual and movement to work through trauma. *The Journal of Pan African Studies, 4*(6), 234–252.

Padrão, M., & Coimbra, J. (2011). The anorectic dance: Towards a new understanding of inner-experience through psychotherapeutic movement. *American Journal of Dance Therapy, 33*(2), 131–147. doi:10.1007/s10465-011-9113-7

Pate, E. (2017). *The history of European dance.* Retrieved from https://ourpastimes.com/the-history-of-european-dance-12324911.html

Rockwell, I. (1989). Dance: The creative process from a contemplative point of view. In L. Y. Overby & J. H. Humphrey (Eds.), *Dance: Current selected research* (Vol. 1, pp. 187–198). New York: AMS Press.

Rueppel, S. (2002). *The healing power of dance.* Retrieved from https://n.b5z.net/i/u/8000224/f/The_Healing_Power_of_Dance_by_Susan_Rueppel.pdf

Samaritter, R. (2009). The use of metaphors in dance movement therapy. *Body, Movement and Dance in Psychotherapy, 4*(1), 33–43. doi:10.1080/17432970802682274

Scott, R. J. (2017). *Sacred circle/world dance.* Retrieved from http://neskaya.com/about-circle-dance/

Smallwood, J. (1978). Dance therapy and the transcendent function. *American Journal of Dance Therapy, 2*(1), 16–23.

Sow, A. I. (1979). Introduction to African culture. In O. Balogun (Ed.), *Form and expression in African arts* (pp. 33–83). Paris: UNESCO.

Stewart, I. J. (2000). *Sacred woman, sacred dance: Awakening spirituality through movement and ritual.* Rochester, Vermont: Inner Traditions.

Stromsted, T. (2009). Authentic movement: A dance with the divine. *Body, Movement and Dance in Psychotherapy, 4*(3), 201–213. doi:10.1080/17432970902913942

Trungpa, C. (1973). *Cutting through spiritual materialism.* Berkeley: Shambhala Publications.

Watts, J. (n.d.). *About sacred circle dance.* Retrieved from www.junewatts.com/wwwcd.php

Weiser, K. (2018). *Legends of America.* Retrieved from www.legendsofamerica.com/na-dances/

Wengrower, H. (2016). The creative-artistic process in dance/movement therapy. In S. Chaiklin & H. Wengrower (Eds.), *The art and science of dance/movement therapy: Life is dance* (2nd ed., pp. 13–32). New York: Routledge and Taylor & Francis Group.

Young, L. (1992). Sexual abuse and the problem of embodiment. *Child Abuse & Neglect, 16*(1), 89–100.

CHAPTER 3

ON THE POSSIBILITY OF AUTHENTIC MOVEMENT

A Philosophical Investigation

Rona Cohen

INTRODUCTION

Imagine that you are a scientist or an explorer from outer space. You descend to Earth in the hope of finding new civilizations and understanding their culture. You quickly notice, among other things, that irrespective of whether you look at humans, trees, or animals, everything is in motion: people *stroll* down the street, cats *climb* on trees, trees *move* by the force of the wind, and, if you look closely enough through the lens of a microscope, you will see the movement of atoms.[1] But what is the nature of movement? Do all entities *move* in the same way? If we exclude *kinesis*, which is understood to involve a change of place, does movement have any existential significance? Is there a movement that is specific for the type of Being which we are? Furthermore, is there a movement that that is specific to each one of us?

Before approaching the question of the meaning of existential movement, let us look into our repertoire of movements. It is of course different for each of us, ranging from banal, instrumental or functional movements (e.g., reaching our hand to grasp an object), to the movement of dancers on the extreme end of the scale, who move in a way in which only a few of us are capable. In between lies the bulk of our repertoire: movements we imitated, identified with (consciously or unconsciously), learnt, and movements that are given to us by way of our *habitus*, in the sense intended by sociologist Pierre Bourdieu: "embodied dispositions that are shared by people with similar background" (Lizardo, 2004, p. 375). This background includes such identifiers as social class, religion, nationality, ethnicity, gender, education, and profession and it reflects the lived reality in which individuals are socialized. Thus, the *habitus* represents the way group culture and personal history shape the body, and as a result, shape the way we think and act. But is there a movement that *belongs* to each one of us *existentially*—that belongs to me as "*I am*", that is, prior to my movements as "I am a professor of philosophy"? If existence is prior to any of its characterizations, could there be a movement that is *mine* in an existential sense, before my movements are historically and socially situated in ways that are *given* to me? That is, could movement be an *existentiale*—a *mode of being*? Moreover, could we understand the meaning of Being by appealing to movement? If so, what would that movement consist in?

When Mary Starks Whitehouse came upon such movement she called it "authentic". This is because it was a movement that expressed a "truth of a kind unlearned", that is, movement that was genuine and *belonged* to a person and was *found* in the body, by contrast with a movement that was acquired, or, as Whitehouse put it, worn "like a dress or a coat" (Whitehouse, 1963/1999, p. 53). This chapter will address Whitehouse's insight visà-vis Martin Heidegger's notion of authenticity developed in his magnum opus *Being and Time* (1927). Before addressing the question of authenticity, and whether—philosophically speaking—movement could be authentic at all, a very brief introduction to *Being and Time* is required.

HUMAN BEING AS *DASEIN*

Being and Time centers upon the question of the meaning of Being: what is it *to be*? According to Heidegger, human beings, unlike other kinds of beings, such as trees, cats, and tables, differ in their *modes* of existence. Put differently, human beings *exist* differently from other kinds of entities. *Being and Time* is a study of the kind of being *we ourselves are*—a kind of being Heidegger designates with the term *Dasein*, which in German literally means both "existence" and "being-there" (*Da-sein*). In designating the type of being we ourselves are as "Dasein", Heidegger names the human being after its essence, namely, *existence*, thus "expressing not its 'what' (as if it were a table, house or tree) but its Being" (Heidegger, 1927/1962, §9, p. 67). Heidegger's method for exploring the question of being begins with tracing *Dasein's* existentials, i.e., *Dasein's* modes of being. This raises questions as to what belongs to *Dasein's* ontological structure (such as, for example, the fact that it is a being-towards-death, and a being-in-the-world), by contrast with what belongs to its *personhood*, which includes among other things its background, history, preferences, and psychological dispositions. Heidegger designates this latter dimension as "the ontic", whose domain is properly explored by anthropology, psychology, biology, and more (§10, p. 71).[2] Unlike other entities, *Dasein* is an entity that is concerned with its own Being, it is the entity that asks, interrogates, and is able to understand the meaning of its Being. This mode of inquiry is itself a mode of being "for those particular entities which we, the inquirers, are ourselves" (p. 27).

BOX 1   IN SUMMARY

According to Heidegger, the world of entities is divided into three types of beings, one of them is Dasein, the type of being human beings are. Other types of beings include instrumental objects (ready-to-hand) and objects of nature (present-at-hand). While ready-to-hand (objects) have properties, Dasein has *modes of being* (existentials) such as being-towards-death and being-with. Even asking the question of Being is an existentiale, since Dasein is the only type of being for whom the question of Being is an issue. *Existentials* are ontological, which is to say, given to Dasein by the sheer fact that it *is*, while *Existentiells* are ontic and are not given to us by the fact that we are, e.g., by our existence but rather by virtue of our biology, environment, culture and so on. While the former are the subject matter of philosophical study, the latter are a subject matter of the sciences, psychology, anthropology, and so on.

Authenticity: A Heideggerian Perspective

We all want to be authentic. And we all want to be true to ourselves, making our own choices freely. Or do we? Surprising though it may seem, Heidegger's answer to these questions is that the opposite is the case: *Dasein's* fundamental tendency is to turn away from itself, *to fall* (*Verfallen*). As Heidegger explains:

> Falling does not express any negative evaluation, but is used to signify that Dasein is proximally and for the most part *alongside* the "world" of its concern. This "absorption in" has mostly the character of Being-lost in the publicness of "the they" (*Das Man*). Dasein has, in

the first instance, fallen away (*abgefallen*) from itself as an authentic potentiality for Being its Self and has fallen into the "world"'.

(Heidegger, 1927/1962, §38, p. 220)

According to Heidegger, individuality "is not given for human, though all humans have a 'potentiality-for-Being' individuals" (Carman, 2005, p. 15). In our everyday existence, the human being as *Dasein* is not itself: it is proximally and for the most part the "They", or a "they-self", "doing what everyone would do in the common circumstances of life into which we are thrown" (p. 15). In this mode of being, our capacity for being individuals—that is, entities who are free to choose their own possibilities, to own up to what they are, *to their existence*—remains concealed. In being "absorbed in" the world, as Magda King remarks:

> Dasein understands himself not from the possibilities of its being, (which belong to each Dasein singly and uniquely) but from the worldish possibilities among other selves. In his everydayness, Dasein measures his own self by what the others are and have, by what they have achieved and failed to achieve in the world. This provides Dasein with a false sense of security and releases it from the burden of thinking or choosing for itself.
>
> (King, 2001, p. 81)

Before addressing the concept of *das Man*, we immediately see that for Heidegger the question of "being-with" is intimately connected to the question of "being-Self". According to Macann, the recognition of being-Self is both significant and paradoxical. It is significant in that it implies a concern with what it means for *Dasein* to be itself. Meanwhile, it is paradoxical since the aim of Heidegger's chapter is to demonstrate that, proximally and for the most part, *Dasein* is precisely *not itself* (Macann, 1992, p. 217).

BOX 2   IN SUMMARY

Although we'd like to think of ourselves as beings who strive for authenticity, Heidegger in fact argues that our fundamental tendency is to turn away from ourselves, he calls this mode of inauthenticity "Falling" or absorption. In its absorption in the world, *Dasein* is able to avoid standing authentically towards its own existence and in this way avoid the recognition and the responsibility it has towards itself. In being inauthentic, we understand ourselves not from our own possibilities but from the possibilities that are already given to us, structured, by society. This does not mean that when we make choices related to social issues we cannot be authentic; it simply means that when we let others choose for us or we accept at face value the norms and ideals of society (as Das Man), we risk losing our individuality, thus renouncing our unique and irreplaceable existence. However, "Falling" or being inauthentic is not a negative evaluation, or a tendency which only "weak" people have; it is a mode of being (existential) belonging to the type of being which we are, *Dasein*. Authenticity and inauthenticity coexist.

"Das Man" and Inauthenticity

According to Carel (2006), Heidegger uses *das Man* to refer to "an internal agency made up of social norms and conventions that eclipses the authentic self". She continues, claiming that "[it] is important to emphasize that Heidegger defines *das Man* as an *existentiale*, part of *Dasein*'s ontological structure" (p. 66). The German term *das Man* refers to an unspecified individual and is used in the same way as the English "one". To this extent, it is used to express views or actions without attributing them to any particular individual. Examples of such impersonal attributions are, "One would think that the president ought to resign", or "they say it is going to rain". As such, as Carel elaborates:

> [The] hegemony of *das Man* results in conformism and effacement of Dasein's self. The power of this control over a particular Dasein stems from its internalisation and acceptance by Dasein, and therefore from the inability to sense it as an external influence. As an internalised agency, *das Man* has complete power over any individual Dasein, and moreover compels Dasein to resist any opportunity to be released from its hold. *Das Man* is marked by mediocrity, fear of difference and flattening of possibilities.
>
> (Carel, 2006, p. 66)

Moreover, as Heidegger writes:

> The "they" even hides the manner in which it has tacitly relived us of the burden of choosing our possibilities. It remains indefinite who has "really" done the choosing. So Dasein makes no choices, gets carried along by nobody, and thus ensnares itself in inauthenticity.
>
> (§54, p. 312)

But *Dasein* has a choice. As Heidegger continues: "[T]his process can be reversed if Dasein brings himself from the 'they' . . . so that it becomes authentic Being-one's self" (p. 312). How is authenticity achieved? It begins with an understanding. According to King (2001, p. 29), Heidegger's argument that "the *'essence' of Dasein lies in its existence*" is the hardest to understand in *Being and Time*:

> The term *exist* can only mean the unique way in which man is: he *is* so that he understands himself in his being. To be in this way, that is, to exist, is according to Heidegger the essence of man.
>
> (King, 2001, p. 30)

Moreover, this understanding does not belong to *Dasein* in general but belongs to each *Dasein* singularly and uniquely. It is only in his own facticity—his existence—that a man can understand: "I myself am this man; this being is *mine*." According to Heidegger, "Dasein always understands itself in terms of its existence—in terms of a possibility of itself" (§4, 13). In other words, *Dasein* understands himself not through what he currently is, but through what he can be, through its potentiality-for-Being.[3] In this respect, *Dasein* does not have properties like an object but it neither does it have possibilities. Instead, *Dasein is* its possibilities. These possibilities do not exist apart from *Dasein* as something yet to be realized. To the contrary, he must be able to understand himself not only in that "I am", but in the possibility that "I can be". Thus, the fundamental characteristics of man's being are not properties and qualities, but *possibilities* of being. Moreover, since *Dasein* is in each case essentially its own possibility, it *can*, in its very Being, "choose" itself and win itself; it can also lose itself and never win itself; or only "seem" to do so (§9, p. 68). *Dasein* may choose to ignore the fact that he has possibilities: it may choose to ignore the fact that it is a "being-towards-death", for example, and hide in the safety of the tranquilization of the "They".[4] But these are only ways of *relating* to its possibilities by way of ignoring or disavowal. In clarification, Heidegger gives the example of hopelessness. On this point, as King elucidates it, even when *Dasein* "is sunk into hopelessness and expects nothing from life, he is still not cut off from his possibilities—he can change. His ability to become what he is not yet belongs essentially to his being (King, 2001, p. 145).

Thus, as Heidegger explains, hopelessness "does not tear Dasein away from its possibilities, but is only one of its own modes of Being *towards* these possibilities" (§46, p. 280).

BOX 3   IN SUMMARY

One of *Dasein*'s modes of being is Das Man (the They). In *Dasein*'s everyday reality as "the They", *Dasein* flees from its individuality, it flees from the fact that it has possibilities which are its own:" We take pleasure and enjoy ourselves as THEY take pleasure; we read, see, and judge about literature and art as THEY see and judge; likewise we shrink back from the "great mass" as THEY shrink back; we find "shocking" what THEY find shocking" (§54, p. 312). . According to Heidegger, in justifying our decisions by appealing to what THEY do, to what One does, we deprive ourselves of responsibility, of answerability, since "It remains indefinite who has really done the choosing. . . . *Dasein* makes no [independent] choices, gets carried along by the nobody, and thus ensnares itself in inauthenticity. This process can be reversed only if *Dasein* specifically brings itself back to itself from its lostness in the "they". (312)

The Meaning of Authenticity

What About Authenticity?

In §42 Heidegger writes:

> Dasein is essentially something that can be authentic [*eigentliches*], that is, something of its own [*zueigen*].

The concept of authenticity (*Eigentlichkeit*) lies at the center of Heidegger's thought. But it is significant, as McManus (2014) notes, that "in choosing to use '*Eigentlichkeit*', Heidegger passes over '*Authentizität*'", the latter which is the German term for what philosophers have traditionally meant by the English term. This 'passing over' is not accidental. Indeed, when choosing to use "*Eigentlichkeit*" Heidegger intentionally selects a term containing the word *eigen*, namely, "own". That is, "*Eigentlichkeit*" incorporates a term encompassing both what is real, actual, or genuine (as the word '*eigentlich*' means in ordinary, non-Heideggerian German), with the adjective '*eigen*', meaning 'own', i.e., "having a room or a mind of one's own" (p. 5).[5] Authenticity refers to what Heidegger characterizes as "mineness" (*Jemeinigkeit*), that which is our own, namely, our Being.[6]

Authenticity is the disclosure of one's irreplaceability. While I may be substituted or represented by other *Dasein* in my everyday life, for example, my partner can represent me in signing certain documents and my colleagues can substitute for me in a class I cannot attend, no one can substitute for me in what is *mine*, in other words, in my existence. Thus, as Heidegger explains, "[R]epresentability is not only quite possible but is even constitutive for our being with one another. Here, one *Dasein* (*das eine* Dasein) can and must, within certain limits, "*be*" another *Dasein* (*das andere "sein"*)" (§46, p. 285). Nevertheless, "this possibility of representing breaks down completely if the issue is one of representing that possibility-of-Being which makes up *Dasein*'s coming to an end" (§46, p. 285). The possibility of substitution completely breaks down if the issue is one of representing me in my ownmost [*eigenste*] possibility, in my being, or, in this case, in my dying. In other words, while the other can represent or substitute me in my "ontic possibilities", such as teaching a class, the other cannot represent or substitute me in the possibilities that are given me by the sheer fact that *I am*, such as the possibility of my death. No one can take death away from me because no one has given me death, the possibility of death is mine by virtue of my existence. So the possibility of substitution breaks down if at issue is a question of representing me existentially. This is simply impossible. In *The Gift of Death*, Derrida reflects on this issue:

> Once it has been established that I cannot die *for* another (in his place) although I can die *for* him (by sacrificing myself for him), my own death becomes this irreplaceability that I *must* assume. But this irreplaceability is the irreplaceability of my existence, my being. It is in this place that I am called to responsibility towards my being.
>
> (Derrida, 1995, p. 43)

Death, Heidegger argues, lays claim to an individual *Dasein* (§53, p. 308). If we think of death in terms of a possibility, we see that claiming this possibility as *mine* is at the same time realizing my irreplaceability. The key to understanding authenticity is understanding, not cognitively but existentially, that what is given to *Dasein* owing to the fact that he *is*, is something that no one can stand in for him. It is in these rare moments that we come to realize that our existence is utterly ours, irreplaceable and unexchangeable.

BOX 4   IN SUMMARY

Whereas Das Man aims at tranquilization, *Dasein* must disentangle itself from this very tranquilization, which encourages a "constant fleeing in the face of death" and a constant fleeing from itself, in order for it to face death authentically and by way of that, to face its own existence authentically. What does Being-toward-death mean? It doesn't mean thinking about death; this leads nowhere. Rather it means claiming my being as mine. Death individualizes *Dasein*, it is *Dasein*'s existential possibility which reveals to it that its *existence excludes any possible substitution*. When it comes to my existence, I am irreparable. It is here that we pass from the generality of the THEY to the particularity of the individual.

THE ONTOLOGY OF THE BODY

What, then, about the body? Could there be an existential-ontological meaning to the body? Does my body pertain to my existence, to my being, to my "*I am*", owing to which it should therefore be included in an ontological-existential philosophical analysis? Or does body merely characterize beings that already *are*, and not their Being? Furthermore, is the body "mine" in the same sense that Being is "mine? Do I "have" my own death and my own body in a fundamentally different way than I have my own money, for instance? That I cannot in principle jettison them, give them up, circumvent them, nor exchange them for new ones marks them as occupying a different ontological status in relation to me (Carman, 2015). Heidegger's existential analysis in *Being and Time* does not include a discussion of the ontology of the body, and in order to answer these questions, one has to go beyond Heidegger, looking instead to post-Heideggerian philosophers such as Jean-Luc Nancy and Maurice Merleau-Ponty, among others. For these thinkers, the body is not a material coat of arms, nor a Cartesian *res extensa* (extended substance, namely, the body), existing *partes extra partes* with the thinking substance (namely, the mind).[7] Nor, thereby, is the body a container of sense or meaning. Rather, "bodies are existence, the very act of ex-sistence, *being*" (Nancy, 2008, p. 19). In other words, the body boasts existential significance to the extent that our very existence—our being—cannot be understood without also analyzing the meaning of embodied existence.

The ontology of the body rests on the assumption that embodiment for the type of being that we ourselves are is different from the embodiment of other types of beings. Or to put it in non-Heideggerian terms: embodiment for human beings is different from that of animals, as well as from the materialism of inanimate objects and the "stuff" from which trees and flowers are composed. As beings defined by their relationship to their Being—as beings who in fact ask the *question* of Being—arguing that the body holds an ontological significance, that the body is not a quality added to existence but rather that the "*is*" is itself bodily, is already to say why *Dasein*'s relationship with its body is different from other type of entities' embodiment. The ontology of the body is thus primarily an exploration of the meaning of *existence as bodily*, since the body is, as Nancy claims in *Corpus*, "ontology itself", and "the Being of existence" (Nancy, 2008, p. 15).

But what is distinct about our ontological mode of embodiment? Human beings' embodiment is ontologically distinct insofar as the question of the Being of the body presents itself for *Dasein* as the question of the *body of the mind's* being. In other words, the ontology of the body is essentially the ontology of what, in Cartesian terms, we would call "the union". It makes no sense, writes Jean-Luc Nancy, "to talk about body and thought apart from each other, as if each could somehow subsist on their own" (p. 37). From this perspective, the mind–body relation is not something that is *added* to existence. To the contrary, it *is* existence. In *Belief and the Body*, Pierre Bourdieu, moreover, argues that "the body believes in what it plays at: it weeps if it mimes grief. It does not represent what it performs, it does not memorize the past, it enacts the past, bringing it back to life" (Bourdieu, 1990, p. 73).

AUTHENTIC MOVEMENT: "THE BODY BEFORE THE BODY"

Recently, I participated in a Gaga class: a movement language developed by the choreographer Ohad Naharin. For the majority of participants attending the session, it was their first experience of Gaga, and since it was late in the evening, most of us were tired after a long day at work, something that the instructor noticed immediately. The instructions that we were given initially sounded simple. At first we were asked to imagine ourselves floating freely and effortlessly over a sea of bubbles, becoming aware of the movement in our bodies as we delved into an almost meditative state. "If you look at an animal", Naharin explained in an interview, "how they move, shifting their weight, there is a letting go . . . to be explosive and quick, you must let go, you must collapse" (quoted in Subin, 2015). But what is it that we have to let go of? The thing I found most challenging in the session (and looking around me I could see that I was not the only one) was leaving behind, as it were, the body I "wore" all day, the postures I "used" at work, the movements I adopted when I met students in the university, taught a class, and so on. This body of *habitus*, of the Heideggerain *Das Man*, consisting in movements that were professionally appropriate, movements borrowed from the academic and social "repertoire" in the same way that I learned how to dress, the appropriate tone of voice and language to speak in class, and the appropriate way to address students. Recalling Heidegger's thesis that "Da-sein's fundamental tendency is to turn away

from himself to a self-forgetful absorption in his occupation in company with other people" (King, 2001, p. 41), most of that day I was absorbed in the world, and my movements
accordingly manifested that absorption. I was *Dasein* in its everydayness: a "they-Body". And
then there was Gaga, which demanded that I respond to the verbal cues of the instructor in
movements of my own, inventing or locating movements in my body instead of borrowing
those from a given repertoire, that is, from what I already knew.

The experience was intensive, and whether I succeeded or not is beside the point. What
the session so vividly demonstrated to me was the coexistence of two bodies: the body of
everyday *Dasein*, and its repertoire of movements, varied and many as they were. Then there
was something else: the search for a different movement: something of my own. This search
was neither active nor intentional: it *happened* as soon I began struggling to leave behind my
everyday movements and to experiment with something that was unknown to me. This 'letting go', as Naharin notes, is not about a loss of control. It is instead, I would argue, about
connecting with our intuitive knowledge that there is more to movement than what we are
familiar with. For me, it was about acting on the intuition that there is something that is *mine*
and yet is utterly unknown to me. Far from being a case of authenticity, this "experiment"
presented me with a question, a question that is at issue for each *Dasein*.

In analyzing Nietzsche's attitude to dance, philosopher Alain Badiou repeats the former's claim that the body in dance is the "body before the body" (Badiou, 2005, p. 57). This
before echoes the Heideggerian priority of the ontological, and, in this case, the priority of
the Being of the body that precedes any meaning or sense that is subsequently attributed or
given to the body. What, then, about movement? Paraphrasing this argument, we could say
that authentic movement is the "movement before the movement", that is, a *movement that is
not a quality that is added to an already given existence but rather the fact that being itself is in movement*.
In other words, movement is the way in which *Dasein is* rather than something that man as
entity *does*. However, this movement is not given: it is always something *Dasein* has to disclose
actively, as an invention that is, paradoxically, a discovery of one's ownmost being, or *mineness*.

In *Dance as a Metaphor for Thought*, Badiou distinguishes between two types of movement
according to their source: First, there is a movement that is caused by external forces acting
upon the body—whether necessary, like the force of gravity, or contingent, like the force of
the wind. Second, there is a movement that is instigated by an internal motive, whose source
is the mover herself. Badiou sees dance as a prime mover: "every gesture and every line of
dance must present itself not as a consequence, but as the very source of mobility" (Badiou,
2005, p. 58). "Dance is like a circle in space", he continues, "but a circle that is its own principle, a circle that is not drawn from the outside, but rather draws itself". This movement
is not the execution of a plan or design, nor a realization of finality, such as when I reach
my hand to take a glass because I want to drink. It is instead a movement that is a pure and
unintentional happening: a creation. This ontological analysis corresponds to Mary Whitehouse's insights gleaned from her experience:

> An early discovery in class or private work is that will power and effort impede movement.
> Gritting the teeth and trying inhibits the feel of the movement quality. . . . Whether it is a
> given exercise or free improvisation, one has to learn to *let it happen*, as contrasted to *doing it*.
> Since we are in general convinced that the body is our personal possession, an object, it feels
> strange to allow it, as subject, the independence of discovery.
>
> (Whitehouse, 1963/1999, p. 53)

Authentic movement is not a response to forces acting upon the body and therefore is
not a passive movement. Nevertheless, this movement is far from being the outcome of

intentionality, that is, as a product of the conscious will to move in a certain way. Rather, it is a movement induced by an unconscious will, by what psychoanalyst Jacques Lacan called "*it* speaks" (*Ça* parle), rather than "*I* speak", thereby differentiating between the conscious and unconscious ego, or Ça (in French, "it", a translation of Freud's "id"). As such, authentic movement transcends the dualism between mind and body and is essentially a psychic movement, an expression of unconscious desire. Authentic movement is movement that is irreducible to the materiality of the body and the forces that act upon it. Neither is it reducible to the ideality and abstraction of the mind. It is rather situated elsewhere and otherwise than in the traditional opposition between mind and the body, that is, in the "extension of the psyche" to refrain Freud's aphorism that transgresses the Cartesian separation between body and mind.[8] Furthermore, authentic movement transcends the opposition between passivity and activity. This is because the subject is active, in the sense of being the agent of the movement, but she is nevertheless not the conscious "I" who authors the movement. Psychoanalytically speaking, this movement is akin to a slip of the tongue (what Freud called "parapraxia"), or to the surprise and strangeness of the disclosure of an unconscious desire in speech, or, in this case, in movement.[9] A patient of Mary Whitehouse describes her experience thus:

> Once, for the first time I experienced "being moved" rather than moving. . . . Mary had said that we should rise in the simplest, most direct way we could without overtones. . . . I rose in one complete spiral movement . . . physically if I had been asked to do it, I could not have. "It" moved me, I did nothing.
>
> (Whitehouse, p. 53)

Badiou analyzes movement in dance in terms of a primary movement. As he puts it: "[I]t is like the first body . . . it is a new beginning, because the dancing gesture must always be some thing like invention of its own beginning" (Badiou, 2005, p. 64). Along the same lines, in a conversation dedicated to conceptualizing the relationship between dance and philosophy, French choreographer Mathilde Monnier tells her interlocutor, philosopher Jean-Luc Nancy: "I believe that this text [Nancy's] approaches dance like a the first movement of being, as if seeing and describing movement, is already seeing it as dance" (Monnier & Nancy, 2005, p. 14). For each of Badiou, Nancy, and Monnier, dance is like the primary movement of being, owing to which it is also a movement of *coming into* being: a movement that in itself is a creation. This thought is in line with Heidegger's way of conceptualizing the ontology of art in *The Origin (ursprung) of the Work of Art*. In this essay, Heidegger explores art in connection with its *Ursprung*, that is, in connection with its origin. For Heidegger, art is not about representation or *mimesis*. Rather, it is about a primordial (*Ur*) leap (*sprung*) into existence.[10] Art, just like *Dasein*, is capable of disclosing Being, and is therefore capable of being authentic or inauthentic. The connection between authentic movement and art is reflected in Whitehouse's experience:

> I think that we have separated the artist and therapy with no man's land in between. Eventually you will let go of the therapy and move through the whole thing that gets you ready for art and you will be an artist.
>
> (Frieder, 2007, p. 37)

Authentic movement captures the two senses of Heideggerian authenticity as a movement of creation that does not distinguish between therapy and art. Authentic movement is a way of disclosing one's own being by way of invention, given that this movement, as that which is closest to us and most intimate for us, is at the same time the farthest from us. Heidegger writes:

> Ontically, of course, Dasein is not only close to us—even that which is closest: we are it, each one us, we ourselves. In spite of this, or rather for just this reason, it is ontologically that which is farthest.

(§5, p. 36)

In DMT, the human being as *Dasein* discloses its potentiality-of-Being by way of movement. This could only be possible if movement was in the first place not merely a kinetic ability that we share with other types of beings, but a mode of Being, belonging uniquely to the kind of beings that we are. Since *Dasein* is such that he understands himself in his Being, the therapist plays an indispensable role in the process of opening up and creating a space of "ontological disclosure", giving the subject a free space to discover its innermost movement and authentic-Self, thereby transcending the understanding of herself as an inauthentic "they-self". This new self-understanding derives from the subject's own transformational progress in therapy. During this process, the patient becomes an "artist of movement" (rather than a dancer), like the eighteenth-century, Kantian figure of the Genius, the prototype of every artist, whose originality lies in inventing the rules of art rather than following them. Likewise, the discovery of authentic movement is an invention of a "rule" that is one's ownmost. This freedom is a moment of individuation, bringing us face to face with our potentiality-of-Being, a freedom "which has been released from the illusions of the 'they', and which is factical, certain of itself, and anxious" (§53, p. 311).

CONCLUSION

Philosophy and DMT come close in acknowledging that movement is a medium of authenticity. I should emphasize that this claim is not contextualized in the domain of art or the beautiful movement. Nevertheless, even if we did contextualize the claim in this way, this would be consistent with *Heidegger's thought that authentic movement is akin to a work of art insofar as both are events of the "unconcealment of Being".*

NOTES

1. This way of commencing is in the spirit of Thierry de Duve's opening of *Kant after Duchamp* (MIT Press, 1966), p. 3.
2. We see the distinction between ontic and ontological in the case of death. For example, being-towards-death is a mode of Being that is given to *Dasein* by virtue of the fact that it *is*, which is to say by virtue of its existence. It is therefore the object of study of an existential investigation. But death does not only have an ontological meaning; in its ontic meaning, we understand death as the termination of one's life (rather than being-towards-death as the manner in which our finitude shapes our life). Death in the ontic-biological sense is a property of organisms. Owing to this, death belongs properly to the domain of science and biology. For Heidegger, both the hard and social sciences, such as mathematics, physics, anthropology, and so on, address the ontic *because they are* concerned with the study of beings, *not* with their Being. For the purpose of this article, I use 'ontological' in the sense of that which pertains to *Dasein's* Being, and I use 'ontic' in the sense of all other characteristics of the human subject that do not pertain to its Being, but rather to its being (*Seiende*). The important point here is that, for Heidegger, the ontological is prior to the ontic, because *Dasein* first of all exists before it exists as X or Y. However, the ontological and the ontic are always connected: "For more on this distinction, see Heidegger, *Being and Time*, §1-§5.
3. For more on the modality of the "I can be" as a creative mode in a therapeutic setting, see also Wengrower Hilda (2016) The creative—artistic process in Dance/Movement Therapy. In S. Chaiklin & H.

Wengrower (Eds.), *The art and science of Dance/Movement Therapy* (2nd ed., p. 24). New York and London: Routledge.
4. According to Heidegger, as falling, "[E]veryday Being-towards-death is a constant fleeing in the face of death" (§51, p. 298). This fleeing is encouraged by "the They" who "provide a constant tranquilization about death" (p. 298). In *Dasein*'s public way of interpreting, "it is said that 'one dies', because everyone else and oneself can talk himself into saying that 'in no case is it I myself', for this one is *the 'nobody'*. (p. 297). For more on this point, see §51.
5. The connection between '*eigentlich*' (authentic, real) and *eigen* (own) is lost in translation. See translators' footnote 3 on *Being and Time* (§9, p. 68).
6. "We are ourselves the entities to be analysed. The Being of any such entity is *in each case mine*" (§9, p. 67).
7. *Parts outside parts*, in Latin literally means "parts outside parts". This is how Descartes describes the relation between body and mind, as things that exist alongside and exterior to each other, "side by side", as it were.
8. The full quote goes as follows: "Psyche is extended; knows nothing about it". See Freud, S. (2001/1938). "Findings, ideas, problems," in *The standard edition of the collected works of Freud*, vol. XXIII, Trans. J. Strachey. London: Vintage Press, pp. 299–300.
9. For a further elaboration of this point, with connection to improvisation and free association, see Wengrower (2016), p. 16.
10. This is a play on words for the German "*Ursprung*" (origin), which is pronounced in the same way as *Ur-Sprung*, meaning an original (*ur-*) leap (*sprung*).

REFERENCES

Badiou, A. (2005). *Handbook of inaesthetics* (A. Toscano, Trans.). Stanford, CA: Stanford University Press.
Bourdieu, P. (1990). *The logic of practice* (R. Nice, Trans.). Stanford, CA: Stanford University Press.
Carel, H. (2006). *Life and death in Freud and Heidegger*. Amsterdam and New York: Rodopi.
Carman, T. (2005). Authenticity. In H. L. Dreyfus & M. A. Wrathall (Eds.), *A companion to Heidegger*. Oxford: Blackwell Publishing.
Carman, T. (2015). Things fall apart: Heidegger on the constancy and finality of death. In D. McManus (Ed.), *Heidegger, authenticity and the self: Division two of being and time*. London and New York: Routledge.
Derrida, J. (1995). *The gift of death* (D. Willis, Trans.). Chicago: University of Chicago Press.
Frieder, S. (2007). Reflections on Mary Starks Whitehouse. In P. Pallaro (Ed.), *Authentic movement: Moving the body, moving the self, being moved: A collection of essays* (Vol. 2). London: Jessica Kingsley Publishers.
Heidegger, M. (1927/1962). *Being and time* (J. Macquarrie & E. Robinson, Trans.). San Francisco: Harper San Francisco.
King, M. (2001). *A guide to Heidegger's being and time*. Albany: State University of New York Press.
Lizardo, O. (2004). The cognitive origins of Bourdieu's habitus. *Journal for the Theory of Social Behaviour, 34*(4), 375–448.
Macann, C. (1992). Who is Dasein? Towards an ethics of authenticity. In C. Macann (Ed.), *Martin Heidegger: Critical assessments* (Vol. 4). London: Routledge.
McManus, D. (2014). Introduction. In D. McManus (Ed.), *Heidegger, authenticity and the self: Division two of being and time*. London and New York: Routledge.
Monnier, M., & Nancy, J.-L. (2005). *Allitérations: Conversation sur la danse*. Paris: Galilée.
Nancy, J.-L. (2008). *Corpus* (R. A. Rand, Trans.). New York: Fordham University Press.
Subin, A. D. (2015, September 19). Going Gaga for Ohad Naharin. *The New York Times*. Retrieved from www.nytimes.com
Wengrower, H. (2016). The creative-artistic process in dance/movement therapy. In S. Chaiklin & H. Wengrower (Eds.), *The art and science of dance/movement therapy* (2nd ed.). New York and London: Routledge.
Whitehouse, M. S. (1963/1999). Physical movement and personality. In P. Pallaro (Ed.), *Authentic movement: Essays by Mary Starks Whitehouse, Janet Adler and Joan Chodorow*. London: Jessica Kingsley Publishers.

CHAPTER 4

THE INVISIBLE OF THE DANCING BODY

Ruth Ronen

INTRODUCTION

How is the moving body experienced in dance by the observer? This question, which preoccupies in different ways dance theorists, historians of art, performance experts, and dance therapists, is posed and addressed in this chapter philosophically. In the present context, the philosophical approach means that we address the *a priori* conditions that make our visual *experience of bodies in dance* possible, even if these conditions may appear to counter common intuitions regarding the moving body. A common intuition would be that of assuming an immediacy regarding the moving body, since movement, unlike speech or intentional actions, appears not to require knowledge in order to be enacted, nor deciphering to be apprehended. This fundamental intuition regarding the primacy of movement and the immediate presence of the body as an object of experience, may also have to do with our apprehension of our own body as being "known immediately to everyone" (Schopenhauer, 1969, p. 100). For Schopenhauer the division of the world into will and representation commences from one's encounter with one's own body which attests to the force of will immediately present in the movement of the individual body.

However, despite this primary intuition regarding the immediacy of the moving body, this chapter will assess the presence of *a priori* assumptions regarding the body that condition the way the body is experienced. These assumptions vary according to the context in which the body is moving: in the theater, for instance, the moving body is assumed to be split between the body of the character it configures and the person of the actor. In the psychoanalytic clinic the body is taken as a reflection of the psyche (i.e., the body is symptomatic of the person, its psyche and pathologies, as having a headache due to stress); in social contexts the moving body is thought of in terms of a mediating site between the external social world and the person's needs. These are obviously generalizations that can be disputed, yet their importance lies in indicating that no body is immediately given as is: the body is always already given through prior assumptions determining the way the body *is* and is experienced.

In this chapter we aim to tackle and articulate the *a priori* principles that guide our encounter with the body moving in dance. By describing these principles as *a priori*, it is emphasized that the issue is not that of the *conventions of dance*. Rather, prior to conventions, there are conditions that determine the very visibility of the body in dance. To clarify the distinction between convention and *a priori* condition, let us consider an analogy from the theater. In (mostly realistic) theater, it is conventionally assumed that although the stage is open on one side to the hall and the audience, the missing fourth wall is there, completing the enclosure of the scene between four walls. Prior to this convention of theatrical presentation, an *a priori* principle that separates the scene on stage from the reality of the onlooker stipulates the visibility of a fourth wall in the first place. Without this ontological division given in the theatrical scene, the observer will not only fail to perceive the scene as taking place in the confines of a room, but may decide to jump on stage to rescue the heroine from an approaching train. In other words, we are concerned here with the ontological (related to the mode of being) and the phenomenological (related to the mode of experiencing) conditions which determine how a theatrical scene is apprehended. Once these conditions are determined, only then is it possible to experience the scene on stage as taking place in an enclosed space of a room (i.e., assume a fourth wall).

What is the *a priori* condition for experiencing the dancing body?

We claim that the *dancing body is a body to itself* and as such it is *a priori detached from external principles of unity* (whether unity is understood in terms of the body's own complete shape or function, or in terms of subjectivity, selfhood, purpose, or meaningfulness). It will be shown that *detachment* is an *invisible dimension of the body* (described as the body's mode of givenness), which yet conditions the dancing body's *visibility*.

The Dancing Body, Detached

The idea that dance exemplifies a gesture of *detachment* of the body draws on a remark made by the contemporary philosopher Jean-Luc Nancy.[1] Dance, he said, is a "gesture detached from its purpose, and hence a gesture of a body that goes nowhere apart from itself. . . . Dance is detachment much before and after being movement and a body in movement" (Ibid., p. 55). In dance, even before the body is engaged in movement, it is detached. Detached from what? Nancy appears to be qualifying detachment in the *a priori* terms of what the dancing body *is* to itself. At this juncture, being to itself, the dancing body is given as dissociated from any principle of unity (i.e., unity of a purpose, of a person, of an object).

Just as the idea of experiencing the dancing body according to a priori conditions seems to counter our intuitions regarding the immediacy of bodies, so the claim made by Nancy sounds radical in the sense that it runs counter to intuition. A dancing body is likely to be described as always already moving and as already associated with a composition, purpose, and meaning. This is a common intuition regarding dance even when the dance addresses a body *disengaging* itself from the purpose or meaning of dance. An exemplary case is *Bye*, by Mats Ek for the occasion of Sylvie Guillem's retirement from the stage, a choreography dedicated to the dancing body *disengaging* from the dancer's person, and from the aims of dance, thereby allowing the dancer, Guillem, to say "Bye" to the world of dance.[2] Counter to such holistic suppositions attached to the body in dance, Nancy claims the opposite: that prior to the way a body is seen dancing, it is already a *dancing-body* and hence detached from all these unifying attributes: *the dancing body is always already not a personal body, it is not unified by a purpose or meaning—it is, rather, to itself*. Detachment conditions the way the dancing body is experienced in its own terms, even if in the dance, in the final work, the body is engaged in a purposeful movement and participates in a dance composition.

Nancy's suggestion here points at the condition of experiencing a dancing body at a moment prior to the actual composition, prior to the body's involvement in the choreography. The philosopher here aims to define how the dancing body is actually given to us in the dance in terms *prior* to what usually directs our understanding of dance. The transformation of the body into a dancing body neither originates in the observer's way of looking nor in the dancer's competence or in the choreographical composition; rather *the body is in its mode of dancing* prior to the way it presents itself to the molding of the choreographer or to the consciousness of the observer, as will be explained in what follows.

If the *dancing* body is primarily given as detached, it exceeds or disrupts other ways of looking at moving bodies. While we are trained to associate bodies in movement to an organizing principle, whether in terms of the body itself (generally, the body has its own anatomical coherence), in terms of a semi-bodily principle (like identity), or in terms of a non-bodily principle (the unity of thought, the motivation to achieve a purpose, and so on), in dance the body is fundamentally disengaged from such considerations. The body in dance undergoes a primary shift of order that enables its particular movement. To start to grasp the meaning of the dancing body's detachment, let us look at the classical piece of contemporary dance by William Forsythe: *Solo*.[3] This piece, filmed in black and white, begins with the camera focusing on the moving feet of Forsythe dancing, and then moves on to the upper parts of the dancer's body; soon afterwards the dancer moves outside the illuminated ring into the darkness to reappear with his body again in a lighted zone of visibility, and so forth. Forsythe dances, and the question is what qualifies his body as a *dancing body*, rather than as a body generally engaged in movement. The detachment of the dancing body can be clarified by considering the series of *fragmenting gestures* Forsythe employs and their striking effect on the viewer. The idea of detachment means that these gestures of *fragmenting the body*, by the camera and by the movement inside and outside the lighted ring, are not experienced in relation to a *complete body*. Rather, the parts or separate organs of the body in dance, or the body which disappears from the stage, are unconditioned by a prior completeness of the body. Forsythe's body is *fragmented and experienced as such*, a fragmentation conditioned by the dancing body being *detached from an image of a unified, complete body*. The dancing body is *a priori* given as detached from any complete image of a body, from uninterrupted bodily presence, *from the idea of the unity of a body* (even if it may be—or not be—made complete by later movements of dance or the overall composition).

Detachment lies between the body itself and the spectacle (or image) of dance, as a condition for constituting *the dancing body*, thus allowing us to watch the dancer without assuming that his body is fundamentally complete yet dispersed by light and movement.

So the condition for experiencing a dancing body detaches it from a prior purpose, meaning or concept in terms of which a body is unified. And yet this detachment is *not a negative principle*. It does not simply negate certain criteria of coherence and unification. Detachment is a positive principle *asserting the terms of visibility of a dancing body*, terms that are simply different from those enacted when we observe a character on the stage of theater, or a person in our everyday surroundings or a body in an athletic competition. In Ohad Naharin's *Last Work*, the female dancer running at the background is dancing rather than jogging, even if she performs with the exceptional physical abilities demanded of an athlete doing long runs. Even if both dancer and athlete share body abilities, summoning up these abilities is a prior condition of unity that only defines the body of the athlete. When watching Naharin, however, the spectator assumes no athletic body abilities and may in fact be constantly anxious regarding the incessant run (will the dancer collapse? stop running? start dancing?). Hence the athlete's body is a priori unified and is bound to perform this unity when high-jumping, or running; no such condition of unity or purpose holds for the dancing body.

Let us schematize this notion of detachment regarding the dancing body (Figure 4.1):

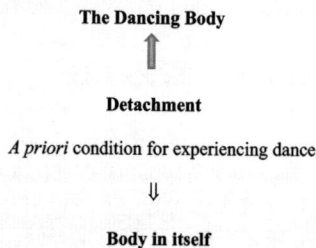

The Dancing Body

⬆

Detachment

A priori condition for experiencing dance

⇓

Body in itself

Figure 4.1 Detachment Splits the Dancing Body from the Body Itself

This scheme demonstrates that *detachment* is a prior condition mediating between the body in itself and the dancing body as we experience it. The dancing body as image, as spectacle of dance, is produced by what the body encounters as condition for becoming a dancing body, and this condition is detachment. Detachment *mediates* between the body in itself and the dancing body. To clarify this point, let us look at another classic example: Loïe Fuller's *serpentine dance*.[4] In what sense does Fuller, with her inventive veil dances, present the dancing body as detached?

> The veil is not only an artifice that enables one to imitate all sorts of forms. It also displays the potential of a body by hiding it. . . . The novelty of Loïe Fuller's art is not the simple charm of the sinuous. It is the invention of a new body.
>
> (Rancière, 2013, p. 96)

This description of Fuller's art by the contemporary philosopher Jacques Rancière appears in the context of his reference to aesthetic occurrences that blur the distinction between forms of life and forms of art. These are instances of what Rancière has named the aesthetic regime. Fuller's dance is part of an aesthetic regime (and pertains to Rancière's investigation of the notion of "aesthesis" in philosophical thought) because she exemplifies how art creates a new form which is transformative of reality itself (a transformation typical of the aesthetic regime). A transformation of reality is suggested by Fuller's use of veils in her dance, veils that do not function as props wrapping or disguising a pre-given body form. Rather, Fuller's *dancing body is composed, even made, of veils* and is not a body to which the forms created by veils are added. The dancing body put forward in Fuller's dance is already a veiled body, and it has thus changed its function and form and has been *transformed into a new body*, a dancing serpentine body made of veils. The spirals and swirls with which Fuller's veils create curved lines constitute a new body to which the organic, naturally shaped human form is no longer relevant. Fuller's dancing body is hence detached from the regular shape of a body, and this detachment is what enables Fuller to create a serpentine-like body shaped by veils as a new art form.

There is hence a condition that mediates between the body in itself and the dancing body, the latter being the result, the effect of detachment from a body's regular forms and functions.[5] Fuller presents a dancing body experienced as unconstrained by its physiological borders; her dancing body, detached from ordinary body forms, can construct its own limits through dancing. Experiencing the body of veils is conditioned by the absence of a prior idea of unity, which is what detachment amounts to: a condition *imposed* on the dancing body prior to its movement in dance and determining its modes of visibility.

Detachment can further explain on what grounds Alain Badiou can claim, regarding the dancing body, that it "does not express any kind of interiority . . . it is itself interiority" (Badiou, 2005, p. 64). The body in dance is anonymous, claims Badiou, it is never the body of a someone, it resists the idea of particular identity. Badiou articulates here in a similar manner (although for different purposes) the idea that the dancing body is not subject to the confines, but also to the coherence, of a person's identity. Even if the dancer appears with his/her idiosyncratic, singular way of performing, his/her dancing body is yet given *as disengaged* from any prior correlation with an inner world, a personal purpose, identity, or intention. The singularity of the dancing body is uncorrelated with an interiority, and this is, according to Badiou, a way of describing the status necessary for the body to participate in dance.

The Given Body, Invisible

Jean-Luc Marion, another contemporary philosopher working in the phenomenological tradition, has introduced the idea of *givenness* in order to indicate that any thing visually experienced is already subject to an originary condition that makes this visibility possible. The examples just given, indicating the possibility of a veiled body (Fuller's body outside its organic shape) or a body made of fragmented parts as in *Solo*, suggest that the body in dance is experienced by way of a unique *a priori* condition on the way it presents itself as visible. Marion names the condition that precedes our experience and determines it to be *the givenness of the phenomenon* and shows that givenness inserts a distorting interval between the thing in itself and the image produced by way of this condition.

In order to clarify the nature of the distortion involved, let us look at just one illuminating visual example from Marion and then complement it with an example from dance. Dürer's *Lamentation for Christ* (approx. 1500) (Marion, 2004, p. 7) describes a scene which is conveyed by employing perspective methods, and Marion shows how perspective mediates between the visible canvas and the effect of depth produced. The painting in itself is nothing but a meaningless surface covered with colored paint and it is what is called "perspective" that creates depth in the painted scene. But how does perspective mediate the painted canvas and the depth of the depicted scene?

This painting, as many in this "golden age" of perspective art, disguises and at the same time exposes the artificiality of geometrical perspective. But Marion does not describe the artificiality of perspective; rather, he indicates how perspective is essential for creating visibility. First, perspective is not something visually tangible per se, and it is by its *invisible* nature that it allows us to experience the diagonal arrangement of the figures on the canvas, the constant oblique rising of the composition from one line of human figures to the next, as a series of layers, that is, as depth. Perspective hence introduces an *irreal dimension* of the picture, producing visibility as depth (i.e., there is nothing "natural" or real-like in the construction of depth, and yet it is what makes the painting realistic). Lastly, Dürer blatantly exposes the *distorting* effect of perspective by leaving the personages of the patrons at the bottom of the canvas outside the perspective scheme (sized on a much smaller scale than the rest of the scene). Dürer "excludes them from perspective; the painting is only partially governed by the organizing principle of perspective, from which it is necessary to conclude that perspective itself is invisible" (Ibid., p. 8–9).

By stressing these aspects of the painting's terms of visibility, Marion succeeds in bringing out the fact that perspective is not tantamount to the arrangement on the canvas, but to a prior condition on visibility as such, a condition that allows the observer to "translate" this arrangement into depth. As such a condition, perspective is equivalent to the way we are led to observe the scene, to experience the painted canvas. Perspective in this spectacle of lament is an invisible condition on visibility that produces an effect of depth. Perspective inscribes in the picture something (depth) we cannot identify with any visible element in the painting.

In some places, Marion names the invisible thing that is the vehicle for crossing the flatness of a painting, what creates the depth of a painting—*anamorphosis* (Marion, 2004, p. 12).[6] This term that originates in visual language, indicates the transformation of form, a distortion that requires reconstruction according to adequate methods to become visible. The invisible, Marion shows, is a kind of anamorphosis exercised in every painting, and it could not be exercised if the painting did not "always already contradict the expectation of the gaze, or at least only satisfy it by still frustrating it" (Ibid., p. 41). The idea of anamorphosis indicates that only through a method that instructs us how a thing is given, can we experience the visibility of reality. "The more the invisible is increased, the more the visible is deepened" (Ibid., p. 5). The more perspective, the condition on visibility, is increased in the painting (as a combination of colors, shapes, light, and shadow), the more the depth of the scene becomes visible. Perspective, in between the visible object and the image viewed, is a condition of visibility which is itself *invisible, distorting, and irreal.*

The relation of perspective to depth in painting is similar to the relation of detachment to the dancing body, which will be illustrated here through the practice of group dance. Group dance is a powerful and peculiar practice of dance in which dancers move in a group in a more or less uniform manner. Sometimes the group decomposes into smaller clusters, and sometimes a dancer is separated from the group to dance a solo. Detachment can account for the way a single dancing body would be experienced in relation to the group and with the following example we will see that detachment of the single dancer from the unity of person, is assumed as a prior condition to group dance. Pina Bausch's *Rite of Spring* (1975)[7] can exemplify that group dance assumes the body of the dancer as an impersonal singularity. In this work, one of the intriguing scenes is that of selecting the chosen one to be sacrificed. The work as composed by Stravinsky and originally choreographed by Nijinsky, in fact, puts in a central place the scene of the young girl chosen as victim to then dance herself to death. However, the choosing of the one who among the ensemble of dancers will stand out to be sacrificed does not decompose the group *nor single out the sacrificed one as a victim.*

So the scene is intriguing both because it marks out one from among a group that dances-as-one and because the chosen one is part of the group (rather than its victimized/excluded member). Bausch sets up a version in which the distortive and haphazard gesture of selection is accentuated: it is not a dancer chosen to be sacrificed, but a process of choosing is enacted with a piece of red cloth, tossed away and around, time and again, until a dancer gives her consent to it, puts it on, as if half-aware, thus isolating herself from the others. With this gesture the invisible condition of dance is made visible through the evident fact that *the one chosen in dance is not personally chose*n as a victim nor is her choice due to an interior cause. The one who dances the victim remains a member of the group and only contingently marked out.

The invisible condition of dance is such that the disengagement of one body from a group of bodies cannot be related to the dancer herself, to something subjective that makes this dancer a candidate for sacrifice (while in drama for instance, the one to be sacrificed is chosen on the grounds of concrete traits—like being the daughter of the victorious commander or being the first-born of the ruler). The procedure of selection of the one from the group hence follows the invisible condition of dance according to which the singular body is not distinguished from others by way of personal or interior qualities. This idea of the singular dancing body-to-itself, is not confined to modern/contemporary dance. In the context of classical dance also, when a singular dancer is marked out for solo, the dancer's singularity is not "personal", nor "meaningful". Bausch's *Rite of Spring* appears to expose this fact.

The invisible condition which determines how a phenomenon is experienced is described by Marion as its *givenness*. This notion of givenness stresses that what makes a phenomenon visible is not imposed by the observer but is rather owing to the way the phenomenon imposes its reality (including the way we should orient ourselves with regard to it) on us. A thing is given in a certain way before it turns into an object for our perception and apprehension. There is a primary condition that determines the way we experience things, their givenness, which predicates neither the perceiver nor the perceived (object). Positively put, givenness is a kind of vanishing mediator between the two, yet it attributes priority to the object and to the way it imposes a mode of experiencing it. Givenness refers to the very hinge on which a thing is transformed into a visible final form and is irreducible to either a real object or to a consciousness.[8]

Givenness is a notion that aims to capture these terms that condition at an originary phase how we look at something and, as was articulated through the case of perspective, remain invisible. Marion proposes that while knowledge always traffics in images, its origin remains invisible. Hence, the thing we see, our referent, is in a sense always missing (we can see a cube from six different sides, but never actually *see* it) (Ibid., p. 54–5). Following this notion of *givenness as the invisible condition that produces a visible image*, we can now return to the visibility of the dancing body.

To grasp the idea of givenness in relation to the visibility of the body, we will start with an example outside dance:

> "About three years ago," I said, "I was bathing with a young man who at that time had a wonderful quality of physical grace. He was about sixteen years old; and since he had only vaguely attracted the attention of women, the first traces of vanity were barely discernible. It happened that we had both just seen the statue of the youth removing a splinter from his foot; (the cast of this sculpture is included in most German collections). As my young friend was drying himself, he put his foot on a stool; a glance at his reflection in a large mirror reminded him of the statue. He smiled and told me his discovery. In fact I had made the same discovery at that very moment, but to counter his vanity I laughed and replied that he was seeing ghosts. He blushed and lifted his foot a second time to show me. Of course, the experiment failed. Confused, he lifted his foot a third and fourth time; he lifted it possibly ten times in all and in vain. He was incapable of reproducing the gesture; in fact, the movement that he made had such an element of oddity that it was hard for me to repress my laughter.
>
> "From that day on, practically from the very moment, the young man was changed. Day after day he stood before a mirror, and one by one his charms fell away from him. An invisible and inconceivable pressure (like an iron net) seemed to confine the free flow of his gestures, and after a year had passed there remained not a trace of that loveliness that had so delighted everyone."
>
> (*On the Marionette Theater*, Heinrich von Kleist)

With this excerpt from Kleist, we can first question the fundamental intuition we have regarding the presence of the body as an immediate object of visual perception. Regardless of how we interpret the scene depicted, it undermines the possibility of knowing anything about the body in itself (i.e., the question of whether the boy's body is actually beautiful or graceless remains undecided). The difficulty seems to stem from the fact that the idea of the body is always and already mediated, *personalized*; that is, the body as imaged already assumes a person who regulates this image. But by exemplifying the disrupted relations of the person with the body, Kleist demonstrates the impossibility of personalizing the body, the resistance of the body to the unity of a person. And when the body is impersonalized, it is reduced to an assembly of body parts, to a mere combination of organs which the person cannot control.

The declining charm of the boy's body hence exemplifies the idea that the visibility of the body as object of perception is not a primary given because there is a prior condition on making the body a complete visible image, and here the condition is that of the unity of a person.

Kleist brings out very vividly the presence of this prior condition on the visibility of the body by pointing at something we habitually overlook: the irreducible distance between the visible body, that is, the body image, and what the body is in and to itself. We tend to bridge this distance with any principle of unification, like "person", that would turn the body into a visible thing. The body is hence visible because it is already returning to our gaze as personalized.

In questioning the straightforward relation of body to person, Kleist does not only indicate a possible disruption between the body and the person (that a beautiful body can be inhabited by a despaired soul that will gradually dim this beauty) but undermines our very assumption that the person or individual can consolidate the identity of the body. What the body reflects is not the unity of a person, as this unity is disintegrated by the power of the other's (narrator's) gaze, or by the unsteadiness of the person. Kleist, in other words, made apparent that the visibility of the body is neither maintained by the person nor by the other's gaze—these rather distort (anamorphize) the reality of the body. The image of the body made visible by Kleist is of a body resistant to unity.

What is exemplified here can also be claimed regarding the dancing body: the originary condition on the visibility of the dancing body is that the body in dance is not given as a unity. This condition, itself invisible, is exposed in dance where the relation of the body to the unity assumed by singular identity or by a person, is questioned. Our claim is that the dancing body is conditioned by detachment in the sense that the dancing body permanently maintains an irreducible distance between the single body in dance and any organizing/unifying principle (in terms of person or purpose). *The dancing body is the spectacle that resists such a unification, and this resistance to the unity of person, or of purpose, is what constitutes its visibility as a dancing body.*

The example from Kleist shows how control over one's body can be lost, even reversed (the body rises against its "owner") or severely disrupted; hence we come across the fact that it was the unity of a person that had stipulated the givenness of the body. Once this condition (of the unity of a person) is removed, the givenness of the body must assume other conditions, and we need alternative terms for grasping the body's singularity. This idea exemplified here, that a body is neither immediate nor unified, is the body that the art of dance relies on.

So the body is given as visible on condition of a prior principle and since the principle of the unity of a person is so automatically and widely applied, we tend to apply it also to dance (Kleist's is an illustration of how this automatism can be disrupted in contexts other than dance). *Our claim is that dance is permanently detached from the unifying condition of a person or purpose and creates its effects through the disruption of the body's relation to principles of unity.*

Let us briefly look at another case of disruption, as seized by Nietzsche in *The Gay Science*, to further support our attempt to disengage the body image from the conditions of its visibility. Here Nietzsche describes the sick person, who has lost control over the body due to illness and surrenders body and soul to science. But what does "surrendering the body" mean in this context? Nietzsche maintains that in case that person is a philosopher "the unconscious disguise of physiological needs under the cloaks of the objective, ideal, purely spiritual goes to frightening length" (Nietzsche, 1974, p. 34). In other words, the philosophical temperament is bound to interpret the reality of the sick body in a philosophical way (rather than flatly surrendering the body to medicine). As in the case Kleist presents, in this example, too, the moment when one appears to lose control over one's body is *a moment that exposes the body phenomenon as already determined by an originary condition of visibility.* The body of the philosopher is given through ideal assumptions regarding the uselessness of the body. The ideal assumptions of the philosopher *pre-determine that the ailments of the philosopher's body would not affect the philosopher's mind.* The philosopher solves the loss of control over the personal body by assuming a body that is already alien to thought, a burden on spirit, and hence belongs to a separate reality than the reality of thought. Note that here also, philosophical tradition has offered diverse explanations of the limited control of one's body, explanations that made the body a non-issue for philosophy; but whatever the philosophical explanation to excluding the body, it complies with the philosophical condition posed on the visibility of the body. According to this condition, the body of the philosopher is already evacuated, devoid of philosophical spirit. In other words, the general condition which defines the givenness of the philosophical body is that of the *evacuation of the body of spirit (or reason)*, a condition that holds from Descartes until a late stage in the history of philosophy (signaled by the advent of phenomenological thought).

If the body of the philosopher is un-inhabited by the philosopher (because this body tends to fall ill, Nietzsche suggests), and hence hardly has exteriority, the body of the dancer on stage *has no interiority.* So while phenomenologically the body appears as visible in both cases, it is the distorting condition of givenness, that makes the body visible in a specific way.

The Dancing Body, Anamorphosized

We have now seen that an image of the body is always the product of distortion. Whether the image presents a harmonious correlation between body and interior mind, a disturbed association between body and person (Kleist), or an alienation between body and thought (Nietzsche), the image of the body is always anamorphosized, distorted by a condition of visibility. Again, while conventions (of culture, of an art) affect the way a condition of visibility is enacted, we have come across attempts to name the very condition itself, as in Nietzsche and the philosophical body (the philosopher's body is evacuated from the philosopher's mind), or in Kleist and the body given to aesthetic contemplation (a body harmonized/controlled by a person).

In attempting to articulate the fundamental givenness of the dancing body, the notion of *detachment* was suggested after Nancy to name the condition of visibility of the body in dance. The dancing body is given as detached from any principle of unity (in terms of person, purpose or meaning), as body-to-itself, whatever the choreography aims to achieve. When watching Forsythe's *Solo*, the body is given as detached from any notion of completeness, which is why we experience its visual fragmentation differently than we would experience the shadow of a body or the sight of just mincing steps on the stage of a theater.

Let us return to the notion of detachment and attempt to develop further its *affirmative* dimension. Detachment may seem counterintuitive to dance experts, since, as mentioned in the beginning of this chapter, we tend to approach the dancing body as having a kind of immediacy. Especially in what pertains to certain trends in contemporary dance, the dancing body appears to be specifically unmediated by symbolic and social meanings, resistant to mythologies and conventions, a body the observer encounters in its unmediated, even abstract being. We must therefore go a step further in articulating the *anamorphic condition* of the body given to-itself, and reconcile the alleged detachment of the dancing body with the idea of immediacy.

The history of dance delineates a gradual movement outside thematized forms and symbolic patterns and toward a growing immediacy and direct presence of the dancing body. The dancing body *per se* appears to move to the foreground, as described by Nancy regarding the revolutionary presence of Nijinski on the scene of modern dance:

> [A] body finds itself there knotted to itself and torn from itself, thrown, flung in a frenzy . . . where it will touch at the same time at its most intimate possibility and at its limit, its disarticulation or its dispossession as a body complete, integrated, present and reacting.
>
> (Monnier & Nancy, 2005, p. 70)

Nijinski's dance, according to Nancy, exposes and touches the most intimate place of the being of a body, a place where there is nothing but body (which is the reason why the solo dance is considered "an emblem of modernity in dance" [Ibid.]). Nancy, even if as a philosopher and not as an expert of dance, acknowledges the center or central place on stage which the body has come to occupy with Nijinski: as a body knotted to nothing other than itself, Nijinski dances solos that mark a moment in the course of emancipating dance from ballet, where by this emancipation the dancer can find new grounds for reviving fantastic mythologies and replay cult scenes.

But how should we understand the place of immediacy where the body has turned into an intimate presence? Does modern dance enable the spectator to directly encounter the dancing body's drives and its impulse to perform, as exemplified in the body's spasmatic movement? Is a dancing body, when uninterrupted by symbolic and social meanings, given *directly* to the spectator's gaze? Following the logic of our investigation, this is evidently not a convincing option,[9] but how can we reconcile detachment with the idea of an immediate encounter with the body?

The solution that follows from our approach is that experiencing the body at its most intimate place, is itself a *condition of visibility* set up by modernism in dance. Immediacy, in other words, is a mode of conditioning, of anamorphosizing the body as given. In fact, Nancy's account of Nijinski clearly resembles what we have defined as the prior condition on the visibility of any dancing body: a singular body, knotted to itself, a body alone, moving toward its intimacy, yet devoid of a pre-given unity, completeness, or integration: it is to be made complete by dancing.

Granted that modern dance, at certain phases of its development, aims to touch the kernel of the body's intimacy, we can further say that modernist solos enact the very condition of the dancing body's visibility. The solo dance of a Forsythe is hence the exemplary demonstration of detachment: it produces a spectacle of a body denuded of concrete signification, a body immediately present as imposing an utmost bodily intimacy. The modernist agenda indeed introduces a way of implementing the condition of detachment already given in every dancing body (the body in dance is a body that "goes nowhere apart from itself", as Nancy in the quotation opening this chapter, states). In other words, the immediacy of a body-to-itself substantiates the condition of detachment from principles of unity, such as the unity of a person, a detachment which we have come to associate with the dancing body in general.

To conclude, in the context of modernism, the solo dance, says Nancy, has taken the challenge of dance, "concentrating on a single body (*un seul corps*) and on a body alone (*un corps seul*)—at the limit, without music—on a body delivered unto itself, unto its wordless nudity, a charging of a meaningless sense, of a spasm of sense" (Monnier & Nancy, 2005, p. 71). While outside dance the body is anamorphised as an image of unity (of person, meaning, or purpose), in dance the body is detached from unity and is given as image of a body-to-itself. The solo dance exposes this originary condition for experiencing the dancing body as a body-to-itself, devoid of unifying principles, similarly to the way Kleist's young

The (solo) dancing body

Image (spectacle) of a sole body, a body-to-itself

⇓

Detachment

Impersonal singularity

⇓

Body in itself

Assemblage of parts

Figure 4.2 Detachment Produces a Body-to-Itself

boy alienated from his body exposes the originary condition for experiencing the body as an image of one's self, of one's person. The dancing body in modernist solos is experienced as a body-to-itself, detached from conventions, symbolism, coherent themes, that have nourished dance for many centuries. These have also camouflaged, for long periods in the history of dance, the dancing body's givenness and its particular modes of transforming/distorting the body.

The dancing body, detached from principles of unity and coherence, appears as anonymous, resistant to the idea of person or to its unifying force, and also resistant to being characterized through personal difference (as being of a certain sex, class, and so on). The intimately present body, encountered in the modernist solo dance as a body-to-itself, hence exposes the detachment through which any dancing body is given, a detachment that always mediates the body in itself with the spectacle of the body. We can now reconcile the dancing body's givenness as detached, with the singularity of its intimate and immediate presence as a (solo) dancing body (Figure 4.2).

NOTES

1. In conversations held electronically between himself and the choreographer Mathilde Monnier during 2003–2004 that were later published in book form. All translations from this collection are mine.
2. For a short excerpt, see: https://www.youtube.com/watch?v=4cH_rUklsY0.
3. www.youtube.com/watch?v=hDTu7jF_EwY.
4. www.youtube.com/watch?v=8zkXb4aWVZs.
5. Similar ideas regarding the detachment of the dancing body from the regular body shape and body unity are performed and articulated widely in the dance world. I came across a very similar idea to the one enacted by Fuller in a program dedicated to the Nederlands Dans Theater and the choreographer Medhi Walerski. The choreographer gave the following instructions to his dancers: "You must tease the music, move with it, play with it, reach the limit of music. *Because in dance, what you feel is the air in between the dancers*" [my transcript and emphasis].

   Here is another expression of the idea that the limit of the dancing body is not the one given by physiology, by the body in itself, but these limits are reconstituted in dance where the body is mediated by detachment.
6. In *Being Given: Toward a Phenomenology of Givenness*, Marion describes *Anamorphosis* as an essential characteristic of givenness. See p. 123ff.
7. https://www.youtube.com/watch?v=NOTjyCM3Ou4.
8. See Marion (2004, p. 12).

9.   In order to illustrate the paradox of immediacy involved here, we can mention in this context Jérôme Bel's work *Shirtology*, which presents the dancer removing an absurd number of shirts off his body, one after another, to appear eventually with the "shirt" of his naked torso (a shirt with a pattern of its own), which is a way of demonstrating the irreality of the idea of immediate encounter with a body. www.youtube.com/watch?v=wJErLyEGJ8E.

REFERENCES

Badiou, A. (2005). *Handbook of inaesthetics* (A. Toscano, Trans.). Stanford, CA: Stanford University Press.

Marion, J. L. (2004). *The crossing of the visible* (J. K. A. Smith, Trans.). Stanford, CA: Stanford University Press.

Monnier, M., & Nancy, J. L. (2005). *Allitérations: Conversations sur la danse*. Paris: Éditions Galilée.

Nietzsche, F. (1974). *The gay science* (W. Kaufmann, Trans.). New York, NY: Random House.

Rancière, J. (2013). *Aesthesis scenes from the aesthetic regime of art* (Z. Paul, Trans.). London and New York: Verso.

Schopenhauer, A. (1969). *The world as will and representation* (E. F. J. Payne, Trans., Vol. 1). New York: Dover Publications.

Part II

RESEARCH

CHAPTER 5

THE SIGNIFICANCE OF DANCE IN DANCE MOVEMENT THERAPY

An International Online Survey with DMT Novices

Iris Bräuninger and Ulf-Dietrich Reips

INTRODUCTION

Dance movement therapy (DMT) and dance are connected in a one-way dependency: without dance there would not be DMT. Levy (1992) talks about the pioneers of dance movement therapy who all had a strong dance background. For example, Marian Chace had received her dance training with the Denishawn company. Her dance knowledge in folk and ethnic dance and structure likely influenced her practice in using a circle formation and its potential for social interaction among participants. Chace stated that "dance is communication and this fulfills a basic human need" (Levy, 1992, p. 24). Another DMT pioneer, Blanche Evan, was a dancer, choreographer and performer who had been influenced by Birch Larson and "natural dance" (Levy, 1992). Evan used expressive improvisational dance, Spanish and ethnic dance, dance improvisation, and in-depth improvisation. She "stressed dance as the art form which utilizes the most direct and complete connection to the psyche" (Levy, 1992, p. 35). For Evan, apparently, dance improvisation was especially important, as it "is the complete welding of oneself, as you are at the moment with your theme in the terms of dance" (Levy, 1992, p. 40). Mary Whitehouse, a dance movement therapist from the West Coast, had received her dance training at the Mary Wigman School in Dresden, Germany, and was influenced by Martha Graham. Trudi Schoop, a Swiss mime living on the West Coast of the United States, had her first dance recital at the age of 16 at the Schauspielhaus (the main local theatre) in Zurich, Switzerland. Schoop definitely was a DMT pioneer to many of the second generation of dance movement therapists and had made a big impact on DMT in Germany and Switzerland. The German DMT pioneer Fe Reichelt was a master student of Mary Wigman and continues to dance in her nineties (Hillhauser, 2015). Wally Kaechele, also a German DMT pioneer, started off with a dance school for couple dance in the 1950s before developing toward DMT. These few pioneers just named seem to have used their professional dance background to pave the way for the development and foundation of DMT in many countries. DMT pioneers in the UK, however, came from health and education backgrounds, although some had a background in Laban movement (Association for Dance Movement Psychotherapy UK, ADMP UK, 2018). Rudolph von Laban influenced DMT all over the world and especially in Europe with the Laban Movement Analysis (LMA).

Three major themes may come to mind when thinking about DMT's relation to dance. Throughout history, dance has played an important role as a healing activity. Furthermore, dance has always been an art form for expressing one's thoughts, emotions, dreams, and conflicts through the body and creative choreographies. Finally, dance has a therapeutic effect that reduces anxiousness, channels aggression, supports social interaction, and fosters transformation (Biasutti, 2013; Bräuninger, 2014a, 2014b; Hanna, 1995; Levy, 1992).

DMT has arisen from dance, and the power of dance has consciously been used as an important and specific tool in DMT. Dance has been *the* basis and core for the foundation of DMT. The following sections explore the three dance aspects and their relation to DMT.

DANCE AS A HEALING ACTIVITY

The use of dance as a catharsis and therapeutic remedy has been described as one of the very early functions of dance (Levy, 1992). Thus dance (Levy, 1992) and ritual dance (Shannon, 1993) have always been healing activities, which have been deeply rooted in human societies. Throughout history, peoples have expressed themselves by moving together in a common rhythm and sharing their emotions by moving together with others (Schmais & White, 1986). Hanna (1995) offered an explanation for dance as a healing activity:

> Dance in the healing process appears to involve the possibility of a person gaining a sense of control in at least these four ways: (1) possession dance, (2) mastery of movement, (3) escape or diversion from stress and pain through a change in emotion, states of consciousness, and/or physical capability, and (4) confronting stressors to work through ways of handling their effects.
>
> (Hanna, 1995, p. 329)

DANCE AS AN ART FORM

Different dance techniques represent important roots of DMT (Bräuninger, 2014a; Capello, 2007; Cruz, 2012; Stromsted, 2009). Moreover, dance composition, choreography (Bräuninger, 2009 2014b; Stromsted, 2009; Willke, 2007) and stage presentation (Allegranti, 2009; Victoria, 2012) have their space in DMT sessions. Dance improvisation has been described as "a spontaneous, creative and non-planned movement characterized by the expression of emotions and body feelings" (Biasutti, 2013, p. 126). Dance improvisation has remained an important technique used in DMT (Bräuninger, 2014a; Meekums, 2002; Wengrower, 2009), which allows the expression of unconscious feelings and states, a process that could be compared to free association in a psychodynamic therapy (Bräuninger, 2014a).

DANCE AS A THERAPEUTIC ACTIVITY

In 1959 Rudolf von Laban promoted the educational and therapeutic value of dance (Laban, 1959). It exceeds the scope of this chapter to give a thorough overview of the evidence of the therapeutic value of dance, but recent systematic reviews on the effect of dance on health-related issues from 2017 to August 2018 shall be covered here. Dance interventions seem to be feasible for the improvement of balance and gait in adults with neurological conditions other than Parkinson's disease (Patterson, Wong, Prout, & Brooks, 2018). They also seem to foster motor parameters and functional mobility in Parkinson's patients (dos Santos Delabary, Komeroski, Monteiro, Costa, & Haas, 2017) and quality of life in patients in cancer care (Rudolph, Schmidt, Wozniak, Kubin, Ruetters, & Huebner, 2018). Furthermore, dance may strengthen and increase the range of motion in upper limbs in women with breast cancer (Boing, Rafael, de Oliveira Braga, de Moraes, Sperandio, & de Azevedo Guimarães, 2017). Dance interventions are also improving various physical health outcome measures in adults compared to other forms of physical activity (Fong Yan et al., 2018). However, DMT interventions seem not to reduce falls in older people but may improve their fear of falling (Veronese, Maggi, Schofield, & Stubbs, 2017).

As outlined earlier, the pioneers described that their dance roots were crucial to the development and the practice of DMT. The profession was established in some countries a few decades ago and in other countries a few years ago. Meanwhile, the role of DMT is widespread and has been categorized with regard to health care as preventive, curative, rehabilitative, and promotional DMT[1] (Bräuninger & Bacigalupe, 2017). Even though these categories focus on health care, they overlap with DMT in educational settings.

The first author's research showed that dance interventions in DMT are still used and demonstrated promising results: one finding of an RCT (Randomized Controlled Trial) with regard to the improvement of quality of life through DMT (Bräuninger, 2012) revealed that *dance techniques* used by therapists "correlated positively to the improvement of *daily life* in the short term. In particular, *Improvisation (with body contact)* was associated with an improvement of *Somatization*" (Bräuninger, 2014a, p. 449). The international Internet-based survey undertaken with practitioners (N=113) on DMT with the elderly mentioned nine practitioners who stressed the importance of certain dance interventions: They should be used in order to foster participation in elderly people who otherwise may suffer from dependency and feeling they are a burden to others. Those dance interventions included the following: "Choreographing a group dance builds up community, learning simple steps and movement sequences in a circle or folk dance offers successful experiences, . . . Improvisation provides a satisfying feeling about one's own activity" (Bräuninger, 2014b, p. 145).

Despite these testimonies of the value of the dance in DMT, we were wondering if the meaning of dance in DMT may be dwindling and if the importance and the presence of subjects such as psychotherapy, medical science, and neuroscience may increase in importance at the expense of the dance. For this project, we therefore were interested in the question of whether dance would still be crucial to DMT novices nowadays and whether DMT novices would value the importance of our dance heritage.

PROCEDURE AND PARTICIPANTS

Online Survey, and Data Collection with DMT Novices

Online Survey

We created an online survey (see Appendix 1) in order to find out how DMT novices evaluate the importance of dance for DMT. The survey contained questions regarding demographic data (gender, age), country of birth and country of study, level of DMT studies, and end of DMT training (three options: a. "I have just finished recently or less than 12 months ago", b. "I will finish approximately in the following 6 to 12 months", c. "I finished more than one year ago". Participants who checked a or b were considered novices, participants who checked c were considered experts and were used as a control group to the novices. The designation in "novices" and "experts" was chosen in order to differentiate professional beginners with no or little DMT experience from therapists with professional experience). For the following seven questions (q), a 7-point Likert scale (from zero point "very inaccurate" to six points "very accurate") was provided to the participants to answer the items:

q1: To have a strong dance background is important in dance movement therapy.

q2: To have a professional dance background is important in dance movement therapy.

q3: During my DMT training, we learn how to integrate dance as an intervention.

q4: As a future dance movement therapist, I feel prepared to integrate dance interventions.

q5: My personal dance background is very strong.

q6: In the future, I plan to use non-dance based techniques and interventions.

q7: Non-dance based techniques and interventions are more relevant to DMT than dance.

The online survey was created with WEXTOR (http://wextor.eu, Reips & Neuhaus, 2002), a service provided by the iScience group at University of Konstanz to create and run Internet-based experiments and surveys. WEXTOR follows best principles of methodologies for online research and automatically implements many related procedures (see, e.g., Reips, 2010, 2012).

We searched the websites of the American Dance Therapy Associations (ADTA) and the European Association for Dance Therapy (EADMT) for acknowledged DMT training institutions, DMT associations, and potential multiplicators who could distribute the online survey to DMT novices. Additionally, we searched online for DMT programs and professional DMT training institutions that we assumed would offer high-quality DMT training, ideally on a master's level. We then created a set of addressees to which we planned to send the online survey; we hoped the recipients would want to collaborate and invite their students and former students to take the survey. Before sending off the email message with the link to the survey, we approached two experienced professional international dance movement therapists. They agreed to examine the online survey test version. The survey was revised incorporating their feedback. In total, we approached 55 email contacts of training institutions and DMT associations from 23 countries.[2] Thus, international study participants were recruited through national institutions, through two mailing lists (German Dance Movement Therapy Association BTD & European Dance Movement Therapy Association EADMT), and various other multiplicators such as heads of DMT master programs and DMT institutions. We sent two types of email letters with the online survey:[3] (1) one type of email letter was sent to two mailing lists (one to the EADMT, the other to the German dance movement therapy association BTD. For the email letter, please see Appendix 2; (2) the second type of email letter was sent to the heads of DMT master's programs and DMT institutions; for the email letter to the multiplicators, please see Appendix 3. No reminder was sent and data was analyzed ten weeks later.

We planned on extracting country-specific answers in order to evaluate whether national differences would exist.

RESULTS

The first page of the online survey was accessed 87 times following the recruitment described earlier. With the analyses conducted, we included all cases except for 21, because they indicated in the seriousness check (see e.g., Reips, 2009 and Appendix 1) that they would not participate seriously, either by actively selecting "just look" or not responding to the check item. We also did not include another six cases where participants had skipped one or more of the first six items. Of the remaining 60 who participated in the survey (a) 40 reported to be *novices* who had recently finished their training less than 12 months ago or who would finish approximately in the following 6 to 12 months, and (b) 20 reported to be dance movement therapists whom we call *experts* and who finished their DMT training more than a year ago.

DEMOGRAPHICS

Demographic information reported by the participants with regard to their age, sex, country of birth, country of study, and type of DMT program attended is presented in Table 5.1.

Table 5.1 Demographics

		Total	Novice (<1 year)	Experts (>1 year)
Reported sex	Male	0	0	0
	Female	60	40	16
	No Answer	0	0	0
Reported age	Mean	33.57	32.44	36.15
	SD	10.21	9.45	12.27
	Minimum	20	20	20
	Maximum	60	60	55
	No answer	4	1	3
Reported country of birth	Belgium	1	1	0
	Canada	5	5	0
	Colombia	2	1	0
	Denmark	1	0	1
	Germany	12	7	5
	Greece	3	3	0
	Iran	1	1	0
	Israel	8	5	3
	Italy	4	2	2
	Kyrgyzstan	1	0	1
	Latvia	1	1	0
	Mexico	1	0	1
	Netherlands	4	4	0
	Norway	1	0	1
	Occupied Palestinian Territory, Occupied	1	1	0
	Portugal	1	1	0
	Romania	1	1	0
	Russian Federation	1	0	0
	Slovenia	1	0	0
	Switzerland	2	2	0
	Spain	4	2	2
	Turkey	2	2	0
	United States	1	1	0
	No answer	1	0	0
Reported Country of Study	Canada	5	5	0
	Colombia	1	0	0
	Denmark	1	0	1
	Germany	14	9	5
	Greece	2	2	0
	Israel	6	4	2
	Italy	3	1	2
	Latvia	1	1	0
	Netherlands	9	7	1
	Spain	14	11	3
	United Kingdom	1	0	1
	United States	1	0	1
	No answer	2	0	0
Type of Program (multiple selection possible)	University program (postgraduate or MA/MS)	37	23	13
	Non-university program	20	16	3
	No answer	3	0	0
	No answer	3	0	0

All 60 participants reported to be female, with a mean age of 33.6 years (SD = 11.2). Mean reported age for novices was almost four years younger (mean age of 32.4, SD = 9.5) than for experts (mean age of 36.2, SD = 12.3), even though the same range between 20 and 60 was reported in both groups. Participants reported 23 countries of birth and 12 countries of studies (no answers = 2). When asked about the type of DMT program attended, nearly two-thirds reported to come from a university program (postgraduate or MA/MS) (n = 37) and one-third from non-university programs (n = 20) (no answers = 3).

Dance in DMT: Comparison Between DMT Novices and Experts

We further compared type of programs: Answers by those having been educated in a university program (postgraduate or MA/MS) versus those in a non-university program did not differ statistically on q2, q4–q7. However, for q1, novices answered 3.05 on average (with a 95% confidence interval of ± .51), while experts responded with a mean of 3.90 (with a 95% confidence interval of ± .68), resulting in a significant difference, $t(55) = -2.03$, $p < .0.05$. For q3, those from a university program answered 3.92 on average, while those from a non-university program responded almost a point on the scale higher, with a mean of 4.80 (both groups with a 95% confidence interval of ± .54), resulting in a significant effect, $t(55) = -2.15$, $p < .0.05$. Thus, overall, those from a non-university program rated higher on "To have a strong dance background is important in dance movement therapy," and on "During my DMT training, we learn how to integrate dance as an intervention." One has to take into account that the significant result in one of the two cases statistically may have been caused by chance.

The following section compares the novices with the experts in DMT. For an overview of answers per questions q1–q7, see Table 5.2. Due to the wide range of countries and the small number of cases from each country, we cannot specify whether national differences exist.

Importance of Strong Dance Background to DMT (q1: To Have a Strong Dance Background Is Important in Dance Movement*)*

The great majority of the 40 novices who answered the question agreed that a strong dance background is important or very important to DMT. The distribution included the whole

Table 5.2 Answers per Questions q1–q7

Descriptives

	chk35g	q1	q2	q3	q4	q5	q6	q7
N	exp	16	16	15	15	14	14	14
	nov	40	40	40	40	40	40	39
Missing	exp	0	0	1	1	2	2	2
	nov	0	0	0	0	0	0	1
Mean	exp	3.19	1.44	4.40	3.93	3.79	4.36	2.86
	nov	3.48	2.13	4.28	4.25	3.70	3.80	1.77
Median	exp	3.00	1.00	4	4	4.00	5.00	3.00
	nov	4.00	2.00	5.00	4.00	4.00	4.00	2
Minimum	exp	1	0	2	1	0	0	1
	nov	0	0	1	2	1	0	0
Maximum	exp	6	5	6	6	6	6	6
	nov	6	6	6	6	6	6	6

range of answers from 0 to 6. In the opinion of the experts (n = 16), a strong dance background only plays a medium importance (see Figure 5.1).

Importance of Professional Dance Background to DMT (q2: To Have a Professional Dance Background Is Important in Dance Movement Therapy)

The distribution of answers in the novices included the whole range of answers from 0 to 6, whereas none of the experts thought that a professional dance background would be very important to DMT. Of the 40 novices, the great majority answered that a professional dance background is not important or less important to DMT, but seven indicated that it would be important. The experts, on the other hand, mostly stated that a professional dance background is not at all or of very little importance (see Figure 5.2).

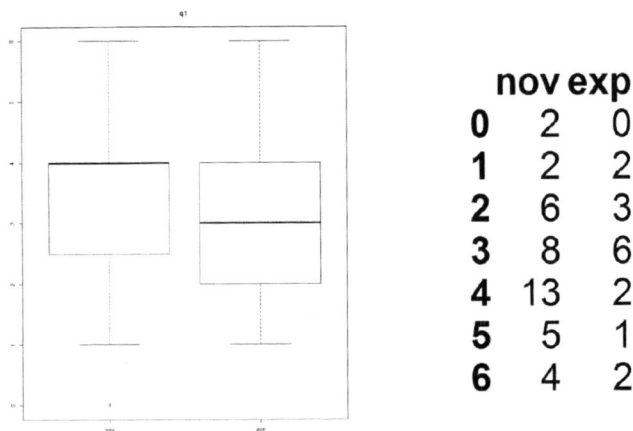

nov	exp
0	2	0
1	2	2
2	6	3
3	8	6
4	13	2
5	5	1
6	4	2

Figure 5.1 Novices' (nov) and Experts' (exp) Opinion on Strong Dance Background to DMT

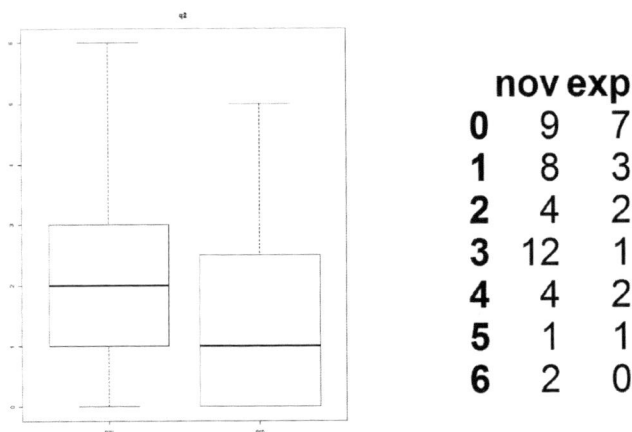

nov	exp
0	9	7
1	8	3
2	4	2
3	12	1
4	4	2
5	1	1
6	2	0

Figure 5.2 Novices' and Experts' Opinions on Importance of Professional Dance Background to DMT

Integration of Dance Interventions During DMT Training (q3: During My DMT Training, We Learn How to Integrate Dance as an Intervention*)*

Novices gave an average of five points and experts four points; both are above the middle of the scale, which means that both groups on average felt that during their DMT training, they learned how to integrate dance as an intervention. About two-thirds of novices (n = 28, from 40) and experts (n = 11, from 15) stated that it is quite accurate or very accurate that dance interventions had been integrated during their DMT training. The distribution in both groups, however, is quite wide: in novices from one to six and in experts from two to six (see Figure 5.3).

Integration of Dance Interventions in the Future (q4: As a Future Dance Movement Therapist, I Feel Prepared to Integrate Dance Interventions*)*

Both novices and experts have an average of four points, which is above the middle. The distribution of answer options in novices is much wider than in experts. Most novices and experts agreed that they would feel prepared to integrate dance interventions in the future. The great majority of both groups think that they would feel prepared to integrate dance interventions (see Figure 5.4).

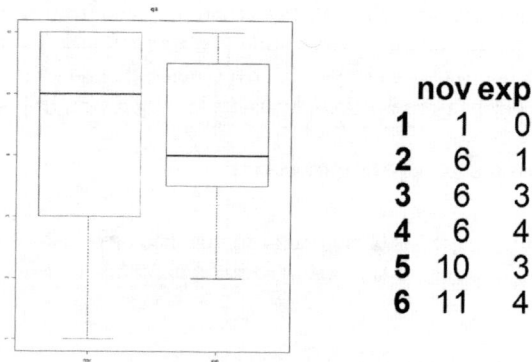

	nov	exp
1	1	0
2	6	1
3	6	3
4	6	4
5	10	3
6	11	4

Figure 5.3 Novices' and Experts' Opinions on Integration of Dance Training During DMT Training (Option 0 Not Displayed, as It Was Used By None of the Participants)

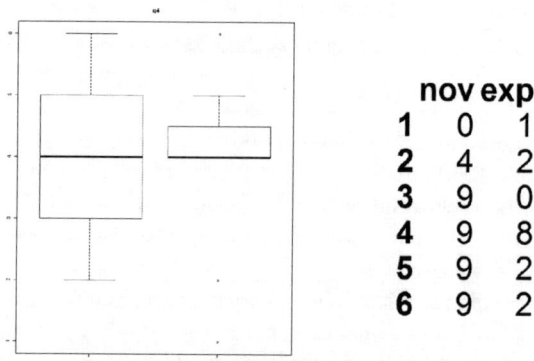

	nov	exp
1	0	1
2	4	2
3	9	0
4	9	8
5	9	2
6	9	2

Figure 5.4 Novices' and Experts' Opinions Integrating Dance Interventions in the Future

Strong Personal Dance Background (q5: My Personal Dance Background Is Very Strong*)*

Both novices and experts here indicated an average of four points. Two thirds (27 of 40) of novices stated that it is accurate or very accurate that they would have a strong personal dance background; among the experts eight out of 14 made that statement. Two experts stated that it would be very inaccurate to say that they have any personal dance background. The distribution of answers both in novices and experts is quite scattered, and experts' answers covered the full range between 0 and 6. Thus, it is a reality that most, but by far not all, respondents have a dance background and that this is true for both those who have entered the field some time ago or only recently (see Figure 5.5).

Non-Dance Based Techniques and Interventions (q6: In the Future, I Plan to Use Non-Dance Based Techniques and Interventions*)*

Here the average in novices is four points and in experts five points. About two-thirds of novices and experts stated that it would be quite accurate to very accurate that they would plan to use non-dance based techniques and interventions in the future (see Figure 5.6).

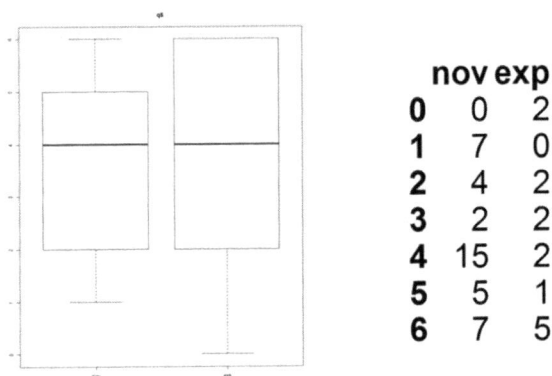

	nov	exp
0	0	2
1	7	0
2	4	2
3	2	2
4	15	2
5	5	1
6	7	5

Figure 5.5 Novices' and Experts' Personal Strong Dance Background

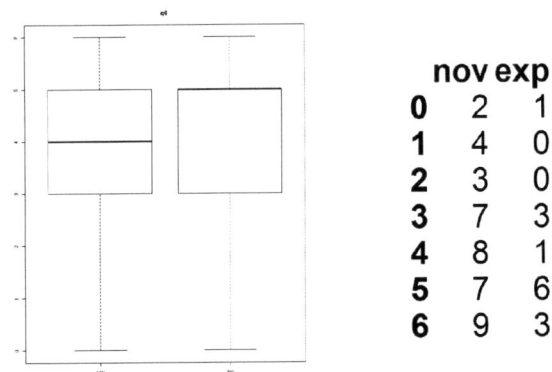

	nov	exp
0	2	1
1	4	0
2	3	0
3	7	3
4	8	1
5	7	6
6	9	3

Figure 5.6 Novices' and Experts' Opinions on Future Use of Non-Dance Based Techniques and Interventions

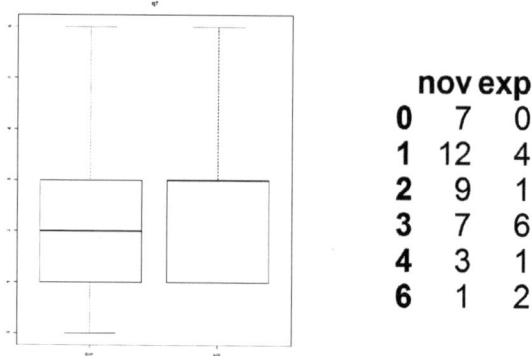

	nov	exp
0	7	0
1	12	4
2	9	1
3	7	6
4	3	1
6	1	2

Figure 5.7 Novices' and Experts' Opinions on Non-Dance Based Techniques and Interventions to DMT (Note That Option 5 on the Answer Scale Was Not Chosen by Novices or Experts)

Relevance of Non-Dance Based Techniques and Interventions to DMT (q7: Non-Dance Based Techniques and Interventions Are More Relevant to DMT Than Dance*)*

Non-dance based techniques and interventions seem to play a minor role both for novices and experts: With an average of about two points in novices and about three points in experts, respectively; see Figure 5.7.

In summary, four main findings can be highlighted: (1) On average, novices tended to evaluate the importance of a strong background in dance, a professional background in dance, and the integration of dance into the DMT training higher in comparison to the experts (q1, q2, q3). (2) On average, experts evaluated the relevance of non-dance based techniques and interventions to DMT higher than novices (q6, q7). (3) The highest agreement between novices and experts and within each group existed with regard to integrating dance interventions in the future (q4). (4) When asked about their strong personal dance background, the average in both novices and experts was four points, but the distribution in both groups was the widest compared to the other questions (q5).

DISCUSSION

This survey aimed to find out how dance movement therapy novices nowadays would evaluate the importance of dance for their profession and their work: Is dance still as crucial to them as it was to the pioneers or is DMT becoming more of movement therapy with a minor role of the dance in it? We looked at the novices' answers and compared them with experts' answers. Furthermore, we compared their answers to DMT pioneers' dance background and suggested implications for the influence and relevance of dance on the DMT profession.

The DMT pioneers came from a professional dance background; many had performed with professional companies, and some, such as Trudi Schoop, had their own performance groups. A strong personal dance background was natural to the DMT pioneers. The pioneers' development from dancers to dance therapists was a process, as they began to use dance in a therapeutic way in order to support personal well-being and communication in others. The pioneers described their personal dance heritage as being crucial to the development and the practice of DMT (Levy, 1992). Many of them took the dance into institutions and started to experiment with how they could adapt their dance knowledge to the new environment and to clients' needs and how the potential of dance could foster health in a clinical environment (for example, Trudi Schoop and Marian Chace). Other pioneers such as Mary Whitehouse introduced the healing aspects of movement and dance in their classes and linked the dance, the body, and creativity with soul and psychology. The new competencies eventually entered into private practice and influenced the way of approaching and working with clients. Those processes gradually created the rise of a new profession, which we now know as dance movement therapy.

Over the years and decades, the DMT field has been constantly developing and has become more professional in the sense that structured training courses have been set up and programs have been offered by trained dance movement therapists who fulfilled the standards defined by their national DMT associations. National associations were established in many countries and have constantly undergone developmental improvements and professionalization. International associations, such as the European Association of Dance Movement Therapy (EADMT, 2018), were created that set standards for national dance movement therapy associations and their training courses, which permit practitioners to be eligible for full professional membership.

These positive and valuable developments have increased DMT's visibility as an interdisciplinary field. Nevertheless, it remains to be asked whether *the dance* in DMT may suffer because of the need and pressure for "professionalizing" DMT. The wish and the pressure to include modules and subjects into the DMT curriculum from related fields such as psychotherapy, medical, social, and behavioral sciences seems to have grown, while the importance of integrating dance-related modules into the DMT training seems to have shrunk or vanished over the years.

When asked about participants' strong personal dance background, the average in both novices and experts stated that a strong personal dance background was more than important to them (4 points on a scale from 0= very inaccurate to 6= very accurate). The distribution of answers within this question was in both groups the widest compared to all the other questions (q5), and it was bigger in experts than in novices. Thus, not all agreed that a strong personal dance background would be important to DMT, and a minority of dance movement therapists, especially experts, even thought that a personal dance background would not be that important to DMT. However, novices evaluated the importance of a personal and professional background in dance and the integration of dance into the DMT training on average one point higher in comparison to experts (q1, q2, q3). On the other hand, both groups evaluated a professional dance background as not so important (q2). These answers seem to differ from the pioneers' attitudes to whom their dance heritage had been important and who had a strong personal and professional dance background. Thus, the dance background and especially a professional one, plays a more minor role to dance movement therapists nowadays than at the beginning of the profession's rise. But has our dance heritage itself become less important to both dance movement therapy novices and experts? Novices interestingly considered the importance of dance higher than experts. It could be hypothesized that the relevance of dance seems to fade away over time as practitioners gain more experience in dance movement therapy practice and perhaps because they grow older. On the other hand, both groups answered that they would intend to integrate dance interventions in the future (q4), and the distribution in that particular answer was the smallest compared to all questions, indicating agreement among the respondents. Other studies showed that dance interventions remain an integrated part of DMT sessions but also other non-dance based interventions would be used (Bräuninger, 2014a, 2014b).

Perceived effectiveness of a mix of dance interventions and other interventions also seems to be reflected in the following finding: experts evaluated non-dance based techniques and interventions higher than novices (q6), and experts seemed to be more likely to include other interventions into DMT (q7). For novices, dance interventions were more important than for experts. This may indicate that in becoming experts, therapists may move on and feel more open towards non-dance interventions and may move away from dance. Possibly, this tendency is an effect of many novices entering DMT from dance. With expertise and experience, a therapist might feel the need and necessity to expand their tools and intervention repertoire in order to fulfill clients' needs. Additionally, dance may set out limitations with certain client groups or may put restraints on the (aging) therapist when working with specific client groups. For example, when working with clients with multiple special needs, non-dance based techniques may offer alternative options to address physical and psychological issues.

Limitations

For methodological reasons, the online survey was distributed exclusively in English, and every participant received the same survey. Knowledge of English was mandatory in order to participate in the survey. This consequently may have excluded dance movement therapists with a limited or no understanding of English.

Our group of experts had entered the field earlier than the group of novices. However, one should keep in mind that some of them may have entered the field relatively recently and thus may be more like advanced novices than long-time experts in DMT.

CONCLUSION

It seems that dance interventions are still important to dance movement therapists nowadays, and more so to novices than to experts. On the other hand, the dance in DMT seems to be less important in the 21st century compared to the last century and the role of dance has changed over time compared to the early days of DMT. Dance has become less important and non-dance interventions are integrated in DMT. When entering the field of DMT, students nowadays may have a dancer's background, but they don't have to have a professional dance background and may come from other professional fields. The answers of novices and new professionals (whom we called experts in this survey) reflect the numerous backgrounds in DMT. Does dance continue to be crucial in DMT or is the heritage of dance in DMT endangered? Yes and no: Dance movement therapists who enter the field still value dance in DMT. With more experience dance movement therapists then introduce other interventions, however. Thus, dance alone apparently can't fully satisfy and describe what is done in DMT. Our findings show a similar picture in various countries.

DIRECTIONS FOR FURTHER INVESTIGATION

Future research may ask the present questions of dance movement therapists at a later stage of their career.

ACKNOWLEDGMENTS

We thank Laura Höhner for assisting with the preparation of the WEXTOR-based survey and the descriptive statistics.

NOTES

1. Promotional DMT does relate to people without clinical problems. It

   aims to improve health and resilience, and promotes physical, psychological, and spiritual wellbeing. It is participatory, interdisciplinary, and integrative. Interventions promote self-regulated health behaviour and a healthy lifestyle. . . . It is provided in private practice, as well as in schools, hospitals, communities, and workplaces on an individual, group, organizational, and public health level.
   (Bräuninger & Bacigalupe, 2017, p. 736)

2. Argentina, Australia, Austria, Canada, China, Czech Republic, Finland, France, Germany, Greece, India, Israel, Italy, Korea, Japan, Latvia, The Netherlands, Poland, Russia, Spain, Switzerland, UK, USA.
3. By end of May 2018.

REFERENCES

Allegranti, B. (2009). Embodied performances of sexuality and gender: A femi-nist approach to dance movement psychotherapy and performance practice. *Body, Movement and Dance in Psychotherapy*, *4*, 17–31. doi:10.1080/17432970802682340

Association for Dance Movement Psychotherapy UK (ADMP UK). (2018). About us. *History*. Retrieved from https://admp.org.uk/about-us/history/

Biasutti, M. (2013). Improvisation in dance education: Teacher views. *Research in Dance Education*, *14*(2), 120–140. doi:10.1080/14647893.2012.761193

Boing, L., Rafael, A. D., de Oliveira Braga, H., de Moraes, A. D. J. P., Sperandio, F. F., & de Azevedo Guimarães, A. C. (2017). Dance as treatment therapy in breast cancer patients: A systematic review. *Revista Brasileira de Atividade Física & Saúde*, *22*, 319–331. doi:10.12820/rbafs.v.22n4p319-331

Bräuninger, I. (2009). *Tanztherapie: Verbesserung der Lebensqualität und Stressbewältigung* [Dance movement therapy: Improvement of quality of life and stress management] (Vol. 21). Weinheim: Beltz.

Bräuninger, I. (2012). The efficacy of dance movement therapy group on improvement of quality of life: A randomized controlled trial. *The Arts in Psychotherapy*, *39*(4), 296–303. doi:10.1016/j.aip.2012.03.008

Bräuninger, I. (2014a). Specific dance movement therapy interventions: Which are successful? An intervention and correlation study. *The Arts in Psychotherapy*, *41*, 445–457. doi:10.1016/j.aip.2014.08.002

Bräuninger, I. (2014b). Dance movement therapy with the elderly: An international internet-based survey undertaken with practitioners. *Body, Movement and Dance in Psychotherapy*, *9*(3), 138–153. doi:10.1080/174 32979.2014.914977

Bräuninger, I., & Bacigalupe, G. (2017). Dance movement therapy in health care: Should we dance across the ward floor? In S. Lycouris, V. Karkou, & S. Oliver (Eds.), *The Oxford handbook for dance and wellbeing* (pp. 729–734). Oxford: Oxford University Press.

Capello, P. P. (2007). Dance as our source in dance/movement therapy education and practice. *American Journal of Dance Therapy*, *29*, 37–50. doi:10.1007/s10465-006-9025-0

Cruz, R. F. (2012). Introduction to Marian Chace foundation lecture: October 21, 2011. *American Journal of Dance Therapy*, *34*, 3–5. doi:10.1007/s10465-012-9124-z

dos Santos Delabary, M., Komeroski, I. G., Monteiro, E. P., Costa, R. R., & Haas, A. N. (2017). Effects of dance practice on functional mobility, motor symptoms and quality of life in people with Parkinson's disease: A systematic review with meta-analysis. *Aging Clinical and Experimental Research*, *30*, 727–735. doi:10.1007/s40520-017-0836-2

European Association of Dance Movement Therapy (EADMT). (2018). Retrieved from http://eadmt. com/?action=article&id=36

Fong Yan, A., Cobley, S., Chan, C., Pappas, E., Nicholson, L. L., Ward, R. E., . . . Hiller, C. E. (2018). The effectiveness of dance interventions on physical health outcomes compared to other forms of physical activity: A systematic review and meta-analysis. *Sports Medicine*, *48*, 933–951. doi:10.1007/ s40279-017-0853-5

Hanna, J. L. (1995). The power of dance: Health and healing. *The Journal of Alternative and Complementary Medicine*, *1*, 323–331. doi:10.1089/acm.1995.1.323

Hillhauser, R. (2015). *Erlebte Geschichten mit Fe Reichelt* [Erlebte Geschichten mit Fe Reichelt]. Retrieved from www1.wdr.de/radio/wdr5/sendungen/erlebtegeschichten/fe-reichelt-100.html

Laban, R. (1959, May). The educational and therapeutic value of dance. *Laban Art of Movement Guild Magazine*, 22(Special commemorative number), 18–21.

Levy, F. J. (1992). *Dance Movement Therapy: A healing art* (Rev. ed.). Reston: National Dance Association, American Alliance. American Alliance for Health, Physical Education, Recreation and Dance, NDAAAH-PERD, ISBN 0-88314-531-6.

Meekums, B. (2002). *Dance Movement Therapy: A creative psychotherapeutic approach*. London: Sage Publications.

Patterson, K. K., Wong, J. S., Prout, E. C., & Brooks, D. (2018). Dance for the rehabilitation of balance and gait in adults with neurological conditions other than Parkinson's disease: A systematic review. *Heliyon, 4*, e00584. doi:10.1016/j.heliyon.2018.e00584

Reips, U.-D. (2009). Internet experiments: Methods, guidelines, metadata. *Human Vision and Electronic Imaging XIV, Proc. SPIE., 7240*(1), 724008.

Reips, U.-D. (2010). Design and formatting in internet-based research. In S. Gosling & J. Johnson (Eds.), *Advanced methods for conducting online behavioral research* (pp. 29–43). Washington, DC: American Psychological Association.

Reips, U.-D. (2012). Using the internet to collect data. In H. Cooper, P. M. Camic, R. Gonzalez, D. L. Long, A. Panter, D. Rindskopf, & K. J. Sher (Eds.), *APA handbook of research methods in psychology, Vol 2: Research designs: Quantitative, qualitative, neuropsychological, and biological* (pp. 291–310). Washington, DC: American Psychological Association. doi:10.1037/13620-017

Reips, U.-D., & Neuhaus, C. (2002). WEXTOR: A web-based tool for generating and visualizing experimental designs and procedures. *Behavior Research Methods, Instruments, & Computers, 34*, 234–240.

Rudolph, I., Schmidt, T., Wozniak, T., Kubin, T., Ruetters, D., & Huebner, J. (2018). Ballroom dancing as physical activity for patients with cancer: A systematic review and report of a pilot project. *Journal of Cancer Research and Clinical Oncology, 144*, 759–770. doi:10.1007/s00432-018-2606-8

Schmais, C., & White, E. Q. (1986). Introduction to dance therapy. *American Journal of Dance Therapy, 9*, 23–30. doi:10.1007/BF02274236

Shannon, L. (1993, October). *Living ritual dance: Dreaming the past, dancing the future*. Paper presented at the American Dance Therapy Association 28th Annual Conference Proceedings, Atlanta, Georgia.

Stromsted, T. (2009). Authentic movement: A dance with the divine. *Body, Movement and Dance in Psychotherapy, 4*, 201–213. doi:10.1080/17432970902913942

Veronese, N., Maggi, S., Schofield, P., & Stubbs, B. (2017). Dance movement therapy and falls prevention. *Maturitas, 102*, 1–5. doi:10.1016/j.maturitas.2017.05.004

Victoria, H. K. (2012). Creating dances to transform inner states: A choreographic model in dance/movement therapy. *Body, Movement and Dance in Psychotherapy, 7*, 167–183. doi:10.1080/17432979.2011.619577

Wengrower, H. (2009). The creative-artistic process in dance/movement therapy. In S. Chaiklin, & H. Wengrower (Eds.), *The art and science of dance/movement therapy: Life is dance* (pp. 13–32). New York, NY: Routledge.

Willke, E. (2007). *Tanztherapie: Theoretische Kontexte und Grundlagen der Intervention*. Bern: Hans Huber.

APPENDIX 1

THE SIGNIFICANCE OF DANCE IN DANCE MOVEMENT THERAPY (DMT): INTERNATIONAL ONLINE SURVEY WITH DMT NOVICES

Dear dance movement therapy novice,

Thank you for your interest in participating in this International Online Survey conducted by Iris Bräuninger at the University of Applied Sciences of Special Needs Education, Zurich. The aim of this survey is to learn how dance movement therapy (DMT) novices assess the significance of dance for their work in dance movement therapy (DMT).

To fill out the survey will take approximately 10 minutes. Your answers will be confidential and your identity cannot be traced. The survey will not contain information that will personally identify you. The results of this survey will be used for research purposes only and may be published. Your participation in this survey is voluntary and you may withdraw at any time. If you participate in this International Online Survey, you agree that the results can be used for publication.

ELECTRONIC CONSENT FORM: Please click your choice:

Clicking on the "agree" button below indicates that:

- you have read the information provided above
- your participation is voluntarily
- you are 18 years of age or older

○ AGREE
○ DISAGREE

Let's move it . . . .

NEXT

Age

Gender

I originally come from (please name your country of birth): _____

I study in (please name the country): _____

NEXT

I study DMT (please select)

☐ as a DMT student at a University program (postgraduate or MA/MS)

☐ as a DMT student at a non-University program

My DMT training (please select)

☐ I have just finished recently or less than 6 months ago

☐ I will finish approximately in the following 6 to 12 months

☐ I finished more than one year ago

To have a strong dance background is important in dance movement therapy

Very inaccurate

Very accurate

NEXT

To have a professional dance background is important in dance movement therapy

Very inaccurate

Very accurate

During my DMT training, we learn how to integrate dance as an intervention

Very inaccurate

Very accurate

NEXT

As a future dance movement therapist, I feel prepared to integrate dance interventions

Very inaccurate

Very accurate

My personal dance background is very strong

Very inaccurate

Very accurate

NEXT

In the future, I plan to use non-dance based techniques and interventions

Very inaccurate

Very accurate

Non-dance based techniques and interventions are more relevant to DMT than dance

Very inaccurate

Very accurate

NEXT

THANK YOU

Thank you for participating in this survey.

Warm regards,
Iris Bräuninger

APPENDIX 2

The following text was sent to the following two mailing lists (BTD, EADMT) with the link http://wextor.org:8080/danceth/dmtsurvey/?qu=instx:

listserve@eadmt.com (European DMT Association listserve) and

mailingliste@btd-tanztherapie.de (German DMT Association listserve)

"Dear DMT head of DMT departments and training institutions,
Please forgive me for writing in English. I am interested in how dance movement therapy novices evaluate the importance of dance for our profession. May I kindly ask you to distribute the following Email to your DMT students? Thereby you support an International Research Project on the topic of DMT and Dance.
Importantly, please distribute the link as it is below, without change.
Thank you in advance.
Warm regards,
Iris

"Dear dance movement therapy novice,
My name is Iris Bräuninger and I would like to invite you to participate in an International Online Survey. The aim of this survey is to learn how you assess the significance of dance for your work. Filling out the survey will take approximately 5–10 minutes. Your answers will be confidential and your identity cannot be traced. The survey will not contain information that will personally identify you. The results of this survey will be used for research purposes only and may be published. Your participation in this survey is voluntary and you may withdraw at any time. If you participate in this International Online Survey, you agree that the results can be used for publication.
To participate in the International online survey with DMT novices please click to:

http://wextor.org:8080/danceth/dmtsurvey/?qu=instx

Thank you very much.
Sincerely yours,
Iris Bräuninger
University of Applied Sciences of Special Needs Education, Zurich
iris.braeuninger@hfh.ch

APPENDIX 3

The second type of Email letter was sent to the heads of DMT master programs and DMT institutions: The multiplicators have been addressed with the following Email letter (addresses of international multiplicators see the following) and the following link: http://wextor.org:8080/danceth/dmtsurvey/?qu=instx

"Dear DMT head of DMT departments and training institutions,

Please forgive me for writing in English. I am interested in how dance movement therapy novices evaluate the importance of dance for our profession. May I kindly ask you to distribute the following Email to your DMT students? Thereby you support an International Research Project on the topic of DMT and Dance.
Importantly, please distribute the link as it is below, without change.
Thank you in advance.
Warm regards,
Iris

Dear dance movement therapy novice,
My name is Iris Bräuninger and I would like to invite you to participate in an International Online Survey. The aim of this survey is to learn how you assess the significance of dance for your work. Filling out the survey will take approximately 5–10 minutes. Your answers will be confidential and your identity cannot be traced. The survey will not contain information that will personally identify you. The results of this survey will be used for research purposes only and may be published. Your participation in this survey is voluntary and you may withdraw at any time. If you participate in this International Online Survey, you agree that the results can be used for publication.
To participate in the International online survey with DMT novices please go to:

http://wextor.org:8080/danceth/dmtsurvey/?qu=instx

Thank you very much.
Sincerely yours,
Iris Bräuninger
University of Applied Sciences of Special Needs Education, Zurich
iris.braeuninger@hfh.ch"

CHAPTER 6

A WAY TO EMBODIMENT THROUGH AESTHETIC RELATIONSHIP
Transformational Body Tracings

Zeynep Çatay and Marcia Plevin

THE METHODOLOGY OF TRANSFORMATIONAL BODY TRACINGS

Various uses of the body outline have been common in arts therapies. They have been used for exploration of the body image (Della Cagnoletta, 2010), or for building a narrative for the sense of self where one can represent various social, cultural influences and traumatic experiences (Jager, Tewson, Ludlow, & Boydell, 2016). Body outline is also used with children widely to support the development of the sense of self and affect regulation (e.g., Steinhardt, 1985). Medical art therapy is another field where body mapping is used extensively, mostly where difficult sensations and pain in the body can be expressed and processed (Luzzatto, Sereno, & Capps, 2003).

Our use of the body outline differs from these methods in several ways. While most of the commonly used body drawing methods call for representations of the body image or bodily experience, the Transformational Body Tracing (TBT) is directed at capturing the immediacy of the bodily experience and its transformation over time.

What follows is a description of the way TBT can be implemented in a workshop or training seminar. At the beginning of the process the movers are asked to lie down on a large piece of paper and the contours of their body are outlined. These outlines are then hung on the wall at the eye level of the mover and remain there for the duration of the work. After movers are guided through movement experientials, they are invited to meet their TBT. They are asked to stay closely connected to their just lived-in-body experiences while bringing them onto the TBT, expressing what they are aware of in their bodies at that time. We have chosen to provide three types of art materials for this process, namely, markers with large heads, oil and chalk pastels. After filling in their TBTs, movers also have a time to do reflective writing on both their movement process and their body outlines. The process of going between movement and filling in the TBT continues throughout the seminar or the session. Over time, the TBTs become fuller, more saturated and keep being transformed. At various points movers can also be instructed to observe their TBTs and transfer what they perceive back to their bodies through moving in response to their outlines. This basic methodology can be adapted according to the context, the population worked with and the goals. It can be used in an educational setting, to support development of dance therapy students or it may be used in clinical settings (see Photo 6.1). For an example of TBT being used with a clinical population see Karadayi, 2017.

The TBT has been experimented with and used since 1993 within the Creative Movement, a method called the Garcia-Plevin training program, that began in Rome and has since been taught in various parts of the world. This chapter is based on an investigation of the TBT as used in an educational setting with students of the Creative Movement – Garcia-Plevin method. Although the basic form had been employed with variations in different settings, the current formulation of the methodology was spelled out and the name "Transformational Body Tracings" was coined by Marcia Plevin in the context of this investigation.

The student group for the Creative Movement class comprised psychologists, counselors, educators or artists who wanted to learn this method so they could integrate it into their work or for personal development. TBTs were used in intensive three-day or five-day seminars. Students' reflection papers about their process were thematically analyzed to inquire into the phenomenology of this experience. In addition, TBTs were photographed and catalogued digitally so that their development could be documented. In order to identify the appearance of different body elements on the TBTs, these catalogued images were examined by the authors. The common elements that became evident in the body outlines, the use of color, line quality and so on, were noted. The transformation in the use of these elements and how they connected with each other were also examined.

ON EMBODIMENT

The term embodiment is mainly rooted in the research literature of embodied cognition, which highlighted the vital connections between physically acting on the world and knowing it. In this view, the body is not seen as a passive processor of information. Its active engagement with the world surrounding us is a crucial aspect of the dynamic processes that bring forth perception and cognition (Varela, Thompson, & Rosch, 1991). What we perceive affects the way we move and how we move affects the way we feel, perceive and come to know the world, hence forming a feedback loop (Koch & Fuchs, 2011). The philosophical roots of the concept are generally tied to Merleau-Ponty's (1962 [1945]) vision of the physical and phenomenological body and the importance of the experienced, lived-in-body as the connection point of agency and subjectivity. Through moving and acting on the world we become aware of and actualize our agency.

The importance of the concept of embodiment is supported today by multiple lines of research demonstrating the inseparable ties between bodily experience and development of various psychological faculties such as affect, cognition and interpersonal processes. In developmental psychology, many studies demonstrate that the earliest body-based experiences form the nucleus in the organization of the self and implicit memories (Schore, 2003; Beebe & Lachmann, 2014; Stern, 1985). The Kestenberg Movement Profile also provides us with a refined understanding of how rhythmic and spatial elements of movement and interaction are connected to development (Kestenberg-Amighi, Loman, Lewis, & Sossin, 1999). Hence many forms of psychotherapy today try to find ways to tap into the layers of information that are stored in the body and to reach an understanding of self that is embodied.

Dance/Movement Therapy provides a wealth of methods to tap into the body wisdom, understand the interconnections between affect, memory, intersubjective experience and bodily experience while also engaging the creative, expressive capacities. A number of authors have pointed out that the latest developments in neuroscience provide the area of dance therapy with new concepts and tools to refine our understanding of how this process works (Payne, 2017; Homann, 2010).

Linking dance therapy with the literature on embodiment research, Koch and Fuchs (2011) have actually proposed to define dance therapy as one of the "embodied arts therapies." As the authors remind us, the body is the only object that can perceive itself from inside and outside (p. 276). It is the point of integration and reorganization of varied sensory data. Our body can move in the space and also feel the experience of moving. If we pay enough attention and bring awareness into it, it can also become aware of the subtleties of how the movement is lived-in the body. This phenomenological information in turn gives birth to the impulse for the next movement. Going back and forth between these two modes of expression and impression, engaging the circular feedback loop, leads to an ever growing state of integration of the sense of self as an active subjectivity (Koch & Fuchs, 2011).

The use of Transformational Body Tracings is in fact a detailed form of engaging this feedback loop while also integrating a visual medium (Garcia, Plevin, & Macagno, 2011 [2006]). We have observed that it leads to a more embodied sense of being in the body while also leading to growth and transformation. The way we will refer to embodiment in this chapter is as a desired state of being present in the body where movement is accompanied with increasing levels of awareness. It can be defined as an achieved state of growing consciousness into the connections between the moving/sensing body and various layers of self. We believe that exploring different stages in the use of TBT and what happens for the mover at the phenomenological, symbolic and neuropsychological levels provides us with insight into how this process grows.

MULTIPLE CONTAINERS

Bringing together different layers of self necessitates a reliable container. Winnicott (1965) was one of the major psychoanalysts who enabled us to understand the importance of the containing function of the parent for the child and the therapist for the patient. In this work there were many containers that functioned at different levels. Drawing of the TBT itself, where the body boundaries are outlined with the help of another group member, can become a containing experience from the beginning. One mover's description of her body outline being drawn is a good example:

> I let my body lie comfortably on the paper. My body outline being drawn felt like an experience of being contained. I felt myself relaxed, peaceful and contained.

When the body outlines are hung on the walls of the studio, they encircle the space in a way that holds the movers (see Photo 6.2). They mark the boundaries of the space where deepening levels of movement work is to take place. The nonjudgmental attitude of the teachers/therapists, the encouragement of play and the group process also create the trust necessary for the mover to experiment. A reciprocal nurturing field slowly establishes itself between the TBT and the mover, and among the group of movers through moving together, encountering each others' TBTs in the studio and verbally sharing their experiences during the day. One participant particularly spoke to the sense of safety in the group that allowed her to express playfulness:

> The last group exercise which included lots of play and physical contact brought joy and was reflected as a pink contour surrounding my body on my TBT. When I think about how grateful I was towards this safe space and the group which let me play freely, I interpret that pink outline as the womb, containing and safe.

With the ongoing accumulation of movement experiences, written reflections and body memories, the TBT in fact becomes a container for the body sense and the whole person. At the end, it helps the mover understand how one's body provides containment and support for the self so that it can become a body that one can truly inhabit.

STARTING AT THE SENSORY LEVEL

We believe that an essential aspect of how TBT enhances embodiment is that coloring the TBT anchors the movers at the level of sensations in the body before moving up to the level of meaning.

After an experiential that may focus on a certain movement quality or a certain body connection, the mover is asked to go to her TBT that has been hanging on the wall and transfer the sensations she has in her body onto the TBT. Some movers first stand facing their TBT and wait, while others rush immediately over and start coloring with clear intent. Slowly, the blank TBTs start filling up with various colors and lines sometimes filling a specific area, sometimes connecting a body area with another with a very specific line quality. One starts to see circles, zigzags, lines that concentrate in the center or zoom out from the center with a sense of force.

The same body area, the left arm, for example, may be colored with three different colors in different parts, which could reflect distinct sensations of warmth, pain or deadness. Sensations can be powerful but are also elusive. They appear in the moment and can disappear swiftly. Translating the body sensations onto the TBT helps the mover maintain her attention and seek for ways to discern body sensations.

The action of putting the colors on is also sensorial and reengages the same neuromuscular pathways as movement. While the movers color body parts on the life-sized TBT, the sensations that are in their body memory are rekindled. The kinesthetic sense is still awake but is integrated into a visual expression. The colors can be applied with different degrees of force. The particular line formations also have a certain strength, energy and so on. In a way, the movers keep dancing with colors. However, the dance keeps transforming and finding more definition and form.

The importance of tuning into the sensory-level of experience has been gaining much recognition in various domains of psychology and psychotherapy. Daniel Stern (1985) wrote extensively about how the basic aspects of our experiences are represented at a sensorial level through the integration of common elements in multisensorial input. Researchers such as Beebe and Lachmann (2014) showed that the intensity, rhythm, spatial form and affective tone of early interactions mold our way of engaging with the world and our experience of the self. According to Stern (2010), these elements coalesce to form the "vitality affects" which color and form our experience. Consequently, he suggests focusing on the sensorial elements of experience (such as the sense of rising versus sinking in the chest; sense of being blocked versus flowing, and so on) in psychotherapy as a way to tap into the not yet symbolized intricacies of implicit knowledge of being in the world and in relationships.

The process of filling in the TBT also provides a way to anchor the person at the sensory/perceptive level. What often transpires on the TBT reflects the immediacy of the experience and is not based on a preconceived representation of the body-image. As the mover maps the felt sensations in different parts of her body on a unifying piece of paper, she begins to see the contrasts and continuities in her experience and works towards an integration. What follows is how one mover describes her experience of coloring the TBT and what it meant to her.

After the first movement experience, it gave me a feeling of clarity and fluidity to start coloring the TBT. I always felt that TBT was a great helper to uncover the meaning of my experience.

First, I used the orange color to express the aliveness of the feet, the connection with the ground and the energy flow. I made the contours of the feet, legs and hips clear with orange color. Focusing on the breath and the movement synchronized with the breath, created a sense of centering and connection within me. . . . With the effect of breathing and then being in contact with the power of the core, the center became well-defined in the form of a green circle. The center's power linked both up and down through the spine. I used the dark blue rings, spreading towards the sides of the body as an expression of opening and comfort in the upper body. The effect of this on the shoulders was expressed in orange and flame like forms. In addition to all of this, I still felt the uneasiness of being seen. I expressed it with a yellow band on my eyes. I chose yellow, which is a color that I like and gives me energy because it was a restraint that was increasingly relieved in time. . . . . . After coloring the TBT, I felt that my experiences came to an integration in the mind, emotion and body dimension. This gave me a ground for clarity and adaptation.

(see Photo 6.3)

This mover's narrative exemplifies how the visual, sensorial and kinesthetic functions become integrated through coloring the TBT. While expressing the inner experience in color and form on the paper, the mover also comes to experience a growing sense of integration and grounding in her body.

The choice of colors while coloring the TBT is described by the movers as a significant process but one that relies on intuition rather than deliberate decision making. It follows from the immediacy of the lived-in experience. The sensations that resonate in the body connect with particular colors for the specific mover. Looking back at the TBT, the mover can define their meaning for her. The following quotation by a participant elucidates her experience with colors eloquently:

Coloring the TBT helped me solidify the sensations, the connections in my body; to define what was yet not fully defined in my bodily consciousness. The fact that this process was not verbal but happened through color and imagery allowed me to experience it as a completely personal language, a field of expression that did not rely on concepts.

EMERGENCE OF THE BODY SENSE

In order to study how TBTs evolved, we examined their photographs taken at different points in time. Analyses of 54 photographs belonging to 13 different TBTs allowed us to identify common elements that appeared on the paper and seemed to be important markers in the evolving of the body sense.

One of the most significant elements was the image of *center*. This could appear around the heart place or the belly area. The sense of the center was represented by captivating images sometimes in circular forms, sometimes extending out into the space or at times involving specific symbols such as the heart. Another element was *body connections* that appeared between different centers or the center and the periphery. The color and quality of the lines used to express these connections revealed different degrees of felt sense of strength and integration.

In some TBTs, images of sensation in the *peripheries* emerged early on, seeming to provide a port of connection with one's body. Especially feet and hands were often colored with bright colors emanating a sense of aliveness. *Grounding* was another important element that emerged in the process. The connection of the feet to the space below was worked on with a variety of colors, usually expressing a deepening of the sensation.

One of the most significant elements was *body boundaries* appearing at different points in the process. Some movers began with a clear delineation of the boundaries, while others reinforced the boundaries much later in the process. The use of different colors and line quality allowed for fine distinctions in different parts of body boundary.

Space within the body and *space around the body* also became important elements in the TBTs. Differential coloring of the left and right body halves or upper and lower body articulated contrasting sensations in these areas. In some TBTs these colorings converged at some point, expressing the integration the mover had attained.

Overall, there seemed to be a process of emergence, development and integration of the body sense in the TBTs. Tracking the appearance of these different elements and how they related to each other provided a sense of the particular pathway to embodiment the mover carved out. As an example, one could walk through the images of one mover's TBT with Photos 6.4, 6.5, 6.6 and 6.7.

WHAT HAPPENS WHILE LOOKING BACK AT THE TBT?

An important component of the process of filling out TBTs is stepping back and looking at them. This appears to be a rich experience at various levels. The mover's first encounter with her TBT is actually when it is first put up on the wall in its empty state. This is described as an experience that brings up elements of surprise and sometimes discomfort, as it triggers self-criticism. One mover describes quite poignantly all the feelings that are evoked by facing her empty TBT:

> The first look at my body outline gives me a feeling of the first encounter with myself. . . . At the same time it feels like the quiet before the storm. Makes you feel the unknown of what it will turn into, what it will give birth to with that form and the empty space that surrounds the outline inside and outside.

Despite the discomfort of the unknown what also stood out in students' accounts were feelings of curiosity and acceptance with the knowledge that the TBT was going to be transformed. The element of transforming the body outlines allows it to be seen as a tool for change and not a fixed entity.

When the mover steps back and looks at her partially colored in TBT we believe that the process of resonating with one's movement experience expands to a new level. This is a point where the mover switches from actively expressing her experience with color and form on the TBT to stepping back, looking at it and taking it in. Koch and Fuchs (2011) identify the process of going between the expressive and impressive functions as the central element in the development of embodiment. Each element feeds into the other, expanding on the enactive capacity of the mover as someone who actively shapes her/his experience and environment while at the same time responding to it.

Recent publications in neuroscience enable us to appreciate how the process of perceiving an image is a bodily one. As Damasio (1999) had pointed out, the brain's response to imagery is as if it is really experienced. Vision is a multimodal capacity; it engages multiple brain regions such as sensory, olfactory, memory, emotion-related networks, not just the visual cortex.

Therefore, the experience of viewing an image and particularly our life-sized body out-line engages our capacity to resonate at different levels of the brain. It is in fact a process that likely engages the mirror neuron system. Research on mirror neurons since the 1990s has demonstrated that the corresponding sensorimotor networks in our brains become activated while we observe someone else move or display an affective expression, while we imagine doing a movement, or even at the sight of an object that suggests movement (Gallese, Fadiga, Fogassi, & Rizzolatti, 1996). Hence, perception is an embodied phenomenon, which seems to be a crucial part of our capacities for empathy. Heimann, Umiltà, and Gallese (2013) point to a number of studies that suggest that a similar process is in action when we look at printed letters, scribbles or graphic images. While looking at these images, which suggest a distinct hand movement, the viewer's motor representation of their hand becomes activated. Similar responses were observed in reaction to viewing art work that included dynamic brushstrokes (Sbriscia-Fioretti, Berchio, Freedberg, Gallese, & Umiltà, 2013). Gallese (2005) coined the term "embodied simulation" to explain these processes where the viewer is able to under-stand the intention of the other through reconstructing the same experience in her bodily experience. In fact, Gallese postulates that the internal experience triggered by artwork is more intense than real-life experiences due to an increased effect of embodied simulation. He states that while viewing art work, being immersed in it, we can distance from the exter-nal world and do not need to attend to its demands. This positioning allows for deployment of more simulative energies, a process he names "liberated embodied simulation".

Hence, looking back at one's own colored TBT with its particular strokes and colors is likely to expand one's bodily resonance process. It is also significant that the image of the body that is reflected back to the mover through the TBT is in a transformed visual form, as will be exemplified in the next excerpt. The colors, lines and sometimes specific imagery that appear on the TBT evoke their own affective resonances in the mover. As it becomes evident in the following quote, the TBT reflects back not only the resonance of the actual movement but also the potential for movement. It awakens different senses in hidden corners of the body and kindles new capacities. The creative and aesthetic process helps put on paper the possibility of an awakened sense of self and new potentials as elucidated so poignantly by this participant's reflection:

> The first piece I put on my TBT were light pink circles that spiraled around each other in the very center of my body. . . . They appeared easily, feeling soft and strong. Like a stone being dropped into the water. Pink fell into my body, it expands into the peripheries of my whole body. . . . Deep inside me a green snake appears. It leaves a feminine energy everywhere it touches.

> Every time I encounter my TBT I witness it becoming more alive. The pink circles already started rotating around themselves and into every direction. I feel the vibrations very strongly. But I can't discern the source. Is it coming from me/my body or from the body that is hanging on the wall across from me?

MULTIMODAL NATURE OF THE PROCESS

Transitioning from movement to coloring in the TBT brings the visual art element into the mover's process. The importance of moving from one modality to another in the expres-sive process has been delineated by Knill and his colleagues' *Crytallization Theory* (Knill, Barba, & Fuchs, 1995). The authors underline the fact that imagination is multimodal. An image can have representation in many different modalities, and moving from one form of expression to another keeps the image alive and three-dimensional. This process of transferring allows different aspects of the internal experience to unfold and its meaning to become crystallized. The use of TBT in an educational or therapeutic setting allows for various levels of multimodal transfer. After going from the process of movement to coloring the TBT, the participant can go back to moving in response to the TBT or to writing in prose or poetry. In every step, a new aspect of the experience is revealed to the mover. New connections can be built among the parts of the body as well as among the body and the emotional and the relational world. What is significant is that as the mover engages in further exploration through movement or writing, the TBT is present in the room, hanging on the wall with all its colors and forms. In a way, it keeps the body alive and visible in the room, always grounding the meaning one arrives at, at the bodily level. The following quotation exemplifies one participant's process of reaching integration through her work with movement and TBT:

> We had experienced the dance of the right and left halves of the body. I was experiencing movement and mobility on my right side, while my left side all the time wanted to make 90 or 180 degree turns and resisted moving forward, in a polarity with the other side. This created a sense of limitation and being stuck in me. It was kind of a dilemma like "I can, I cannot". I expressed this on the TBT with the circular forms on the left side and with a pink mold covering the left foot. After we completed the dance that integrated the right and the left sides, this feeling of being stuck began to disappear and all of my body became more mobilized. I drew this on the TBT as a red line connecting my right and left palms. That day and the following day, when I remembered this limiting sensation and started to feel unpleasant, seeing my TBT really helped me, through reminding me this integration through the hands.

THE PROCESS OF AESTHETIC DIALOGUE

Over time, a dialogue seems to unfold between the moving body and the body that appears on the paper. The sensations of flow, aliveness as well as pain or being stuck come to awareness and find expression on the paper through a creative and aesthetic medium. Going back and engaging with the image in turn allows the body to find a way of integration.

This process of engaging with the image and continuing to explore it and responding to it is in fact akin to what McNiff (1992) describes as the process of "Aesthetic Dialogue". McNiff proposes treating an image as having semi-independent reality. This approach involves seeing the image not as something that can be "interpreted" but almost as an animated thing that can offer support and guidance. This can be achieved through adapting an attitude of "receiving" the image and engaging with it in a dialogue. This dialogue involves a real openness, where the meaning is not presumed but emerges in the process. It also involves a sensitivity to the aesthetic elements that become evident in the artistic expression. According to McNiff and his colleagues (1992), it is this sensitivity to the aesthetic elements that moves the dialogue further and allows for crystallization. According to Knill et al. (1995), the aesthetic element allows us to approach painful material without mobilizing our anxiety and defenses. Staying in the creative realm invites one to maintain an aesthetic sensitivity where the senses are engaged and alive and can be present to what appears. In fact, this effect is supported by findings from neuropsychology of aesthetics. As demonstrated by Di Dio et al. (2016) while viewing artwork, our interoceptive neural network is stimulated. When we are aesthetically moved by an artwork, we also want to stay attuned to it, to look at it more, which increases access to memory (Tschacher et.al., 2012). It can be said that when our aesthetic sense is stimulated, we become more present to ourselves and to that which we are viewing. It opens up space inside for deeper processing.

In arts therapies, the aesthetic element emerges from the authenticity of expression and the high sensitivity to experience rather than any skill (Knill, Levine, & Levine, 2005). Being true to oneself and letting the inner experience find full expression are the key elements of aesthetics in arts therapies. The impact seems to be one that feeds into the experience of bodymind (Koch, 2017). Research in neuroscience also supports that the aesthetic element triggers the primary reward systems in the brain and stimulates pleasure and bonding with the piece of art even when the content may be unpleasant (Hanich, Wagner, Shah, Jacobsen, & Menninghaus, 2014). Hence, it supports the motivation and commitment to one's process that is needed for deep exploration.

In this work, as the movers' engagement with their TBTs deepened, they often reported encountering new, unexpected imagery that appeared on the TBT. One mover describes her process:

> After exploring the left and right body halves in movement I go back to my TBT. I add a pink wing to the right side of my body while deep purple iron bars appear on the left side. I am surprised. Butterflies and a cage together in the same body!

Sometimes the new imagery that emerges out of the dialogue is received with joy as a precious gift that seals in the newly found sense of cohesion. At other times it can lead to a striking and difficult encounter with an aspect of oneself that was not in one's consciousness as evidenced by the reflection below by a participant:

> Through the process, I added spirals on the drawing and began coloring the whole body. . . . Later I realized that I hadn't drawn anything on my face. My whole body and even my hair was full of colors yet my face was plain white. Realizing this fact was striking; whiteness in my face was pure, clean but also frozen and vacuous.

TBT AS A PARTNER IN DIALOGUE

When the TBT is first drawn and hung up on the wall, movers have a lot of reactions to it. At first it looks raw and empty, and as such it can bring up surprise or discomfort. Over time, as the creative and aesthetic process deepens, a strong connection develops. Many movers described their TBT as a "mirror", a resource for getting to know oneself. However, this was not just a passive, inanimate mirror; it was described as a "multi-dimensional mirror".

Many movers described it almost as an animated being, an independent entity with connections to one's self. In fact, the boundaries between oneself and the TBT could become blurred. One mover described her experience as "I don't know if it was my mirror or my shadow. Reflecting many bodies inside my body."

Another mover described her TBT as "It is both me and a product of me. Something that I worked on little by little, I waited for, I cultivated and I discovered."

Many movers also described the development of an affective bond with their TBT as their process unfolded as exemplified by the following quotation:

> I could not take my eyes off my TBT. I wanted to look at it all the time. It was as if the more I looked the more we got to know each other, our connection became deeper, more intimate. It was as if my TBT was gaining a personality, becoming animated. As I was walking to the studio in the mornings, I found myself wondering how it was, how it had spent the night.

It seemed that the process of coming to own one's TBT with openness and affection paralleled accepting oneself and owning one's process of growing embodiment. The bond that was created with one's TBT secured one's commitment to the process.

The fact that the TBT accompanied the movers throughout their process seemed to lead them to feel contained and held in their experience. Many movers talked about feeling "seen" or "heard" due to its presence, which then "opened up space inside of them" to see themselves better. It was obvious that the TBT became an important support, a partner and a figure of guidance in one's process. Some students also reflected on the *intimate dialogue* that began between their bodies and the TBT. In this dialogue the TBT was depicted as an active partner, "speaking" to them or "making them move". The dialogue that emerged seemed to be happening beneath the level of consciousness:

> The TBT moved me. There appeared an intimate space between us and in that interactive field the movements were borne. It was really as if it talked to me. I felt that it commanded to that which was still inhibited, that could not yet dare to move.

THE TIME FACTOR

Completion of a TBT is like a journey that happens over time. The past, present and future possibilities of a mover seem to converge within the visual diary of the TBT. The realization of this journey is marked by one mover's remark:

> It was exciting to draw the outlines of my body at the beginning of the process, it feels like the excitement of a new trip.

The changes that become salient in the mover's body sense over time appear as different layers on the TBT. The resulting image conveys multidimensionality, and the transforming aspects of time can be seen and noted. Some movers stated that seeing the TBT hanging on the wall throughout the movement experience helped integrate and take note of the changes that had happened in their body sense. The following reflection by a participant is an example of this sense of change over time:

> Seeing my body outline while moving revived the previous stages of my work in my memory. . . . When I stopped and looked at my TBT, I reflected on where I was and where I was headed towards.

The multilayered character of the TBT allowed for past and future to be integrated with the present moment. These elements were also reflected in the writings of the movers. Many of the reflective writings about the TBTs included body memories or an aspired new sense of being in the world.

In our use of the TBT in this Creative Movement training we also asked the students to compare the TBTs they created in the first and last seminars of the training year. Many students commented on the increased sense of integration, flexibility, fluidity and the sense of grounding they noticed in their second TBT. They could also track how certain elements that appeared in the first TBT had evolved to a fuller shape in the second TBT. One participant carefully tracks these changes:

> When I compared my first TBT with the last one, I noticed a significant transformation. The red color which I thought signified my life force had moved from the hands to my center. In the final TBT my body space had expanded. I noticed a widening both to my roots and to my

periphery. I noticed that the lines were more circular and in spirals in the second one, which I thought expressed the strengthening of my body integration. The distinction between the outside and the inside of my body space was also more significant. It looked like my boundaries were clearer.

Some students expressed the transformation they noticed in developmental terms, "It seemed as if the first one grew older and wiser and became the second one."

CONCLUSION

In this chapter we explain the use of full-body outline for enhancing embodiment. As a result of using the TBT in a training seminar, cataloguing the photos of the emerging figures and reading the reflection papers of the students, we have recognized that the processes for the growth of embodiment are facilitated by this tool. When the full-body outline is embedded within the improvisational movement experience, the life-size drawing process allows for an integration of the kinesthetic and the visual/symbolic modes of expression. Also life-size expression of the body sensations through use of color, line quality and intensity leads to further differentiation and definition. It creates a feedback loop where the visual information feeds into the kinesthetic experience. The quotation that follows from a mover explains how her process of moving, coloring and reflecting on those actions strengthened each of them and culminated in the deepening of her sense of being in her body. Her following description captures the circular nature of the process:

> As I worked on my TBT, expressing the sensations that were evoked in me during movement carried me to the next step. The process built on itself, each step supporting and complementing the other. As the process deepened, it exposed a wound deeper inside. And through the exposure, it also opened up space for it to heal. At the end, it all became integrated both in the movement and in the drawing. Now I can feel myself move in a more fluid and clear way with my whole body.

What distinguishes the TBT is that it is a developing process where transformation in the body sense becomes evident. The resulting images have a multilayered quality and emanate a fuller sense of integration. New connections within the body and to the outside world appear on the TBTs and are evidenced by students' reflection papers. We found that the TBT functions both as a visual embodied diary and a container for the mover's experience. At the same time it allows them to engage in a creative, aesthetic dialogue. This chapter is based on the description of TBT in a training setting, but modifications of this methodology can also be implemented in clinical settings to stimulate, capture and reinforce the growth of embodied consciousness.

REFERENCES

Beebe, B., & Lachmann, F. M. (2014). *The origins of attachment: Infant research and adult treatment*. London: Routledge.

Damasio, A. (1999). *The feeling of what happens: Body and mind in the making of consciousness*. San Diego: Harcourt Press.

Della Cagnoletta, M. (2010). *Arte Terapia: la prospettiva dinamica* [Art therapy: The psychodynamic approach]. Roma: Carocci.

Di Dio, C., Ardizzi, M., Massaro, D., Di Cesare, G., Gilli, G., Marcheti, A., & Gallese, V. (2016). Human, nature, dynamism: The effects of content and movement perception on brain activations during aesthetics judgment of representational paintings. *Frontiers in Human Neuoscience, 9*. doi:http://dx.doi.org.libproxy.newschool.edu/10.3389/fnhum.2015.00705

Fuchs, T., & Koch, S. (2014). Embodied affectivity: On moving and being moved. *Frontiers in Psychology, 5*(508), 1–12. doi:10.3389/fpsyg.2014.00508

Gallese, V. (2005). Embodied simulation: From neurons to phenomenal experience. *Phenomenology and the Cognitive Sciences, 4*, 23–48.

Gallese, V., Fadiga, L., Fogassi, L., & Rizzolatti, G. (1996). Action recognition in the premotor cortex. *Brain, 119*, 593–609.

Garcia, M., Plevin, I. M., & Macagno, P. (2011 [2006]). *Creative movement and dance*. Rome: Gremese.

Hanich, J., Wagner, V., Shah, M., Jacobsen, T., & Menninghaus, W. (2014). Why we like to watch sad films: The pleasure of being moved in aesthetic experiences. *Psychology of Aesthetics, Creativity, and the Arts, 8*(2), 130–143. http://dx.doi.org/10.1037/a0035690

Heimann, K., Umiltà, M. A., & Gallese, V. (2013). How the motor-cortex distinguishes among letters, unknown symbols and scribbles: A high density EEG study. *Neuropsychologia, 51*, 2833–2840. doi:10.1016/j.neuropsychologia.2013.07.014

Homann, K. B. (2010). Embodied concepts of neurobiology in dance/movement therapy practice. *American Journal of Dance Therapy, 32*(2), 80–99.

Jager, A., Tewson, A., Ludlow, B., & Boydell, K. (2016). Embodied ways of storying the self: A systematic review of body-mapping. *Forum: Qualitative Social Research, 17*(2). Retrieved from http://openresearch.ocadu.ca/id/eprint/1206/

Karadayi, G. (2017). *Transformational body tracings in creative movement & Dance Movement Therapy: A qualitative comparison of an educational and a psychiatric group* (Unpublished master's project). Istanbul Bilgi University, Istanbul, Turkey.

Kestenberg-Amighi, J., Loman, S., Lewis, P., & Sossin, K. M. (1999). *The meaning of movement: Developmental and clinical perspectives of the Kestenberg Movement Profile*. Amsterdam: Gordon and Breach.

Knill, P., Barba, H. N., & Fuchs, M. N. (1995). *Minstrels of soul: Intermodal expressive therapy*. Toronto, Ontario: Palmerstone Press.

Knill, P., Levine, S., & Levine, E. (2005). *Principles and practices of expressive arts therapy*. London: Jessica Kingsley Publishers.

Koch, S. (2017). Arts and health: Acive factors and a theory framework of embodied aesthetics. *The Arts in Psychotherapy, 54*, 85–91. doi:10.1016/j.aip.2017.02.002

Koch, S., & Fuchs, T. (2011). Embodied arts therapies. *The Arts in Psychotherapy, 38*, 276–280. doi:10.1016/j.aip.2011.08.007

Luzzatto, P., Sereno, V., & Capps, R. (2003). A communication tool for cancer patients with pain: The art therapy technique of the body-outline. *Palliative and Supportive Care, 1*, 135–142. doi:10.1017/S1478951503030177

Mcniff, S. (1992). *Art as medicine*. Boston, MA: Shambhala Publications.

Merleau-Ponty, M. (1962 [1945]). *Phenomenology of perception*. London: Routledge.

Payne, H. (2017). The psycho-neurology of embodiment with examples from authentic movement and laban movement analysis. *American Journal of Dance Therapy, 39*, 63–178. doi:10.1007/s10465-017-9256-2

Sbriscia-Fioretti, B., Berchio, C., Freedberg, D., Gallese, V., & Umiltà, M. A. (2013). ERP modulation during observation of abstract paintings by Franz Kline. *PLoS One, 8*(10), e75241.

Schore, A. N. (2003). *Affect dysregulation and disorders of the self*. New York, NY: W.W. Norton & Company Ltd.

Steinhardt, L. (1985). Freedom within boundaries: Body outline drawings in art therapy with children. *The Arts in Psychotherapy, 12*(1), 25–34. http://dx.doi.org/10.1016/0197-4556(85)90005-X

Stern, D. N. (1985). *The interpersonal world of the infant*. New York, NY: Basic Books.

Stern, D. N. (2010). *Forms of vitality: Exploring dynamic experience in psychology and the arts*. Oxford: Oxford University Press.

Tschacher, W., Greenwood, S., Kirchberg, V., Wintzerith, S., van der Berg, K., & Tröndle, M. (2012). Physiological correlates of aesthetic perception of artworks in a museum. *Psychology of Aesthetics, Creativity, and the Arts, 6*(1), 96–103. http://dx.doi.org/10.1037/a0023845

Varela, F., Thompson, E., & Rosch, E. (1991). *The embodied mind*. Cambridge, MA: MIT Press.

Winnicott, D. (1965). *The maturational processes and the facilitating environment: Studies in the theory of emotional development* (pp. 1–276). The International Psycho-Analytical Library, Vol. 64. London: The Hogarth Press and the Institute of Psycho-Analysis.

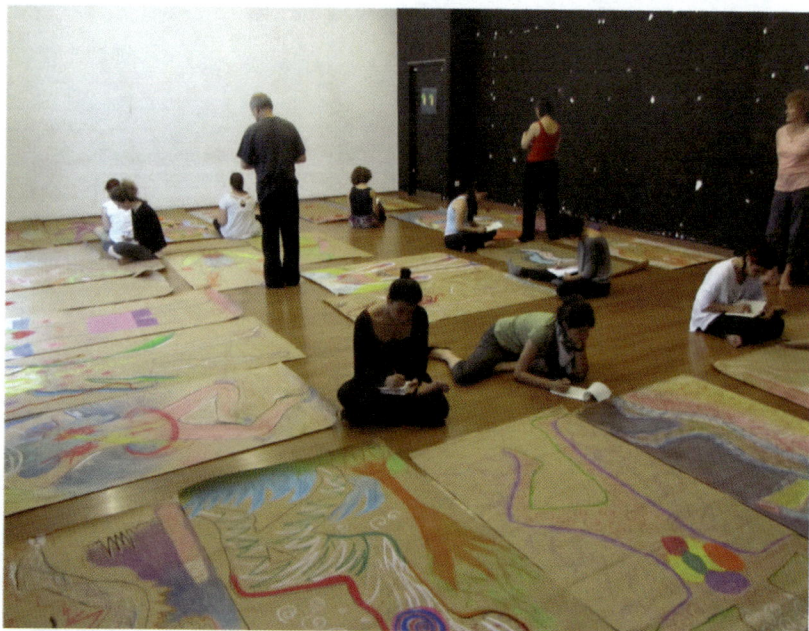

Photo 6.1 Movers doing reflective writing on their completed Transformational Body Tracings

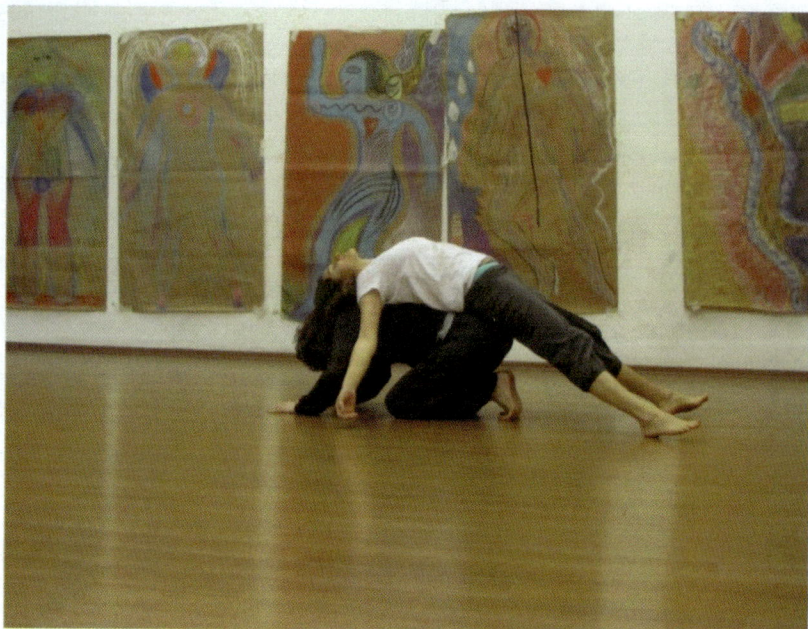

Photo 6.2 Movers in the studio surrounded by Transformational Body Tracings

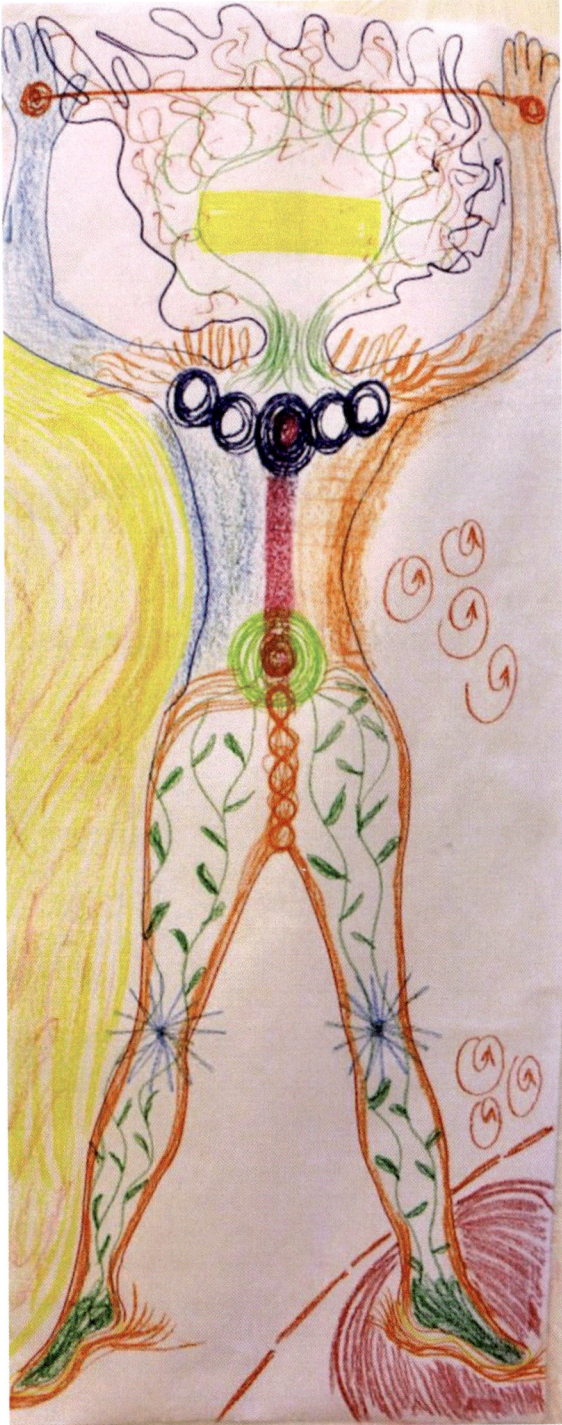

Photo 6.3 A Completed Transformational Body Tracing

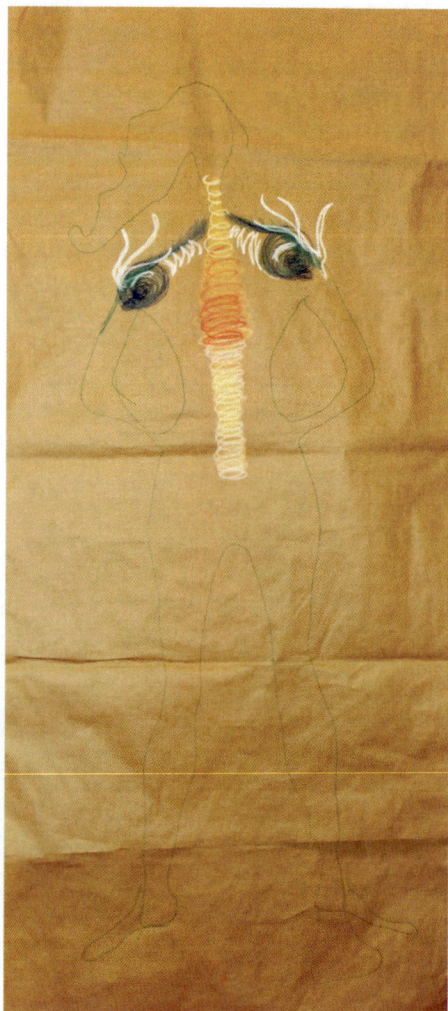

Photo 6.4 Evolution of a Transformational Body Tracing

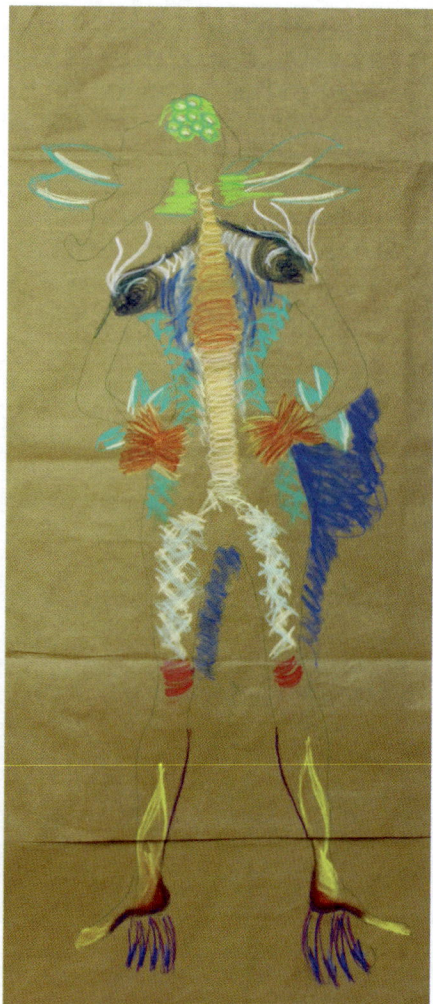

Photo 6.5 Evolution of a Transformational Body Tracing

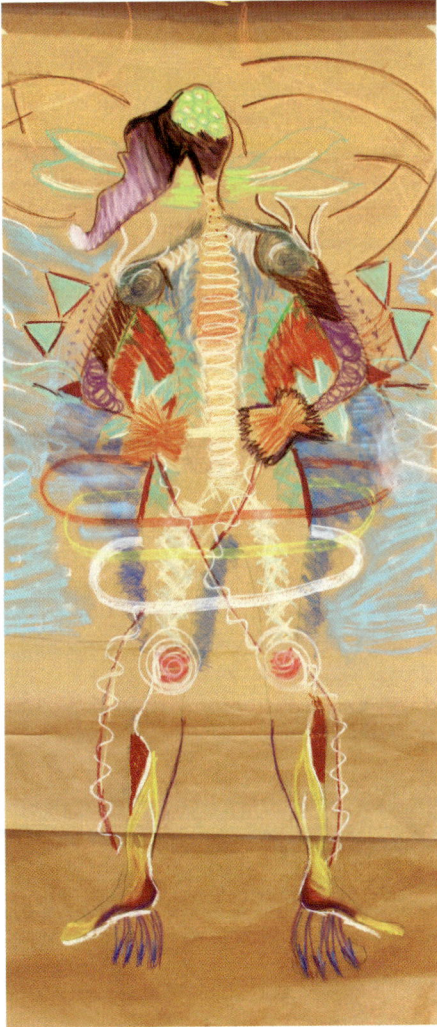

Photo 6.6 Evolution of a Transformational Body Tracing

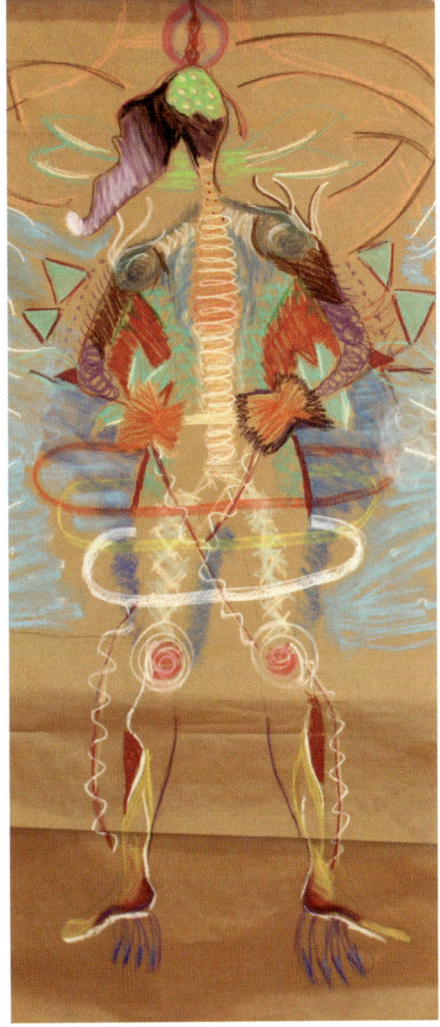

Photo 6.7 Evolution of a Transformational Body Tracing

CHAPTER 7

"BEING MOVED" AS A THERAPEUTIC FACTOR OF DANCE MOVEMENT THERAPY

Sabine C. Koch

INTRODUCTION

"I was moved to tears, when I saw her dance to that song." We are often moved by artwork, movies, songs, music, dance, drama, or poetry. No matter which sensory channel the stimuli that move us take, art can bring us to experience things deeply, touch us at the core, and make us feel the essence of the human condition. Recent research from the fields of psychology and aesthetics has contributed to the development of a theory of *being moved* as an emotion (Zickfeld, Seibt, Schubert, & Fiske, 2019; Menninghaus et al., 2015). In DMT, we can support the client to experience this emotion through encouraging awareness to motion and interoception, and we can use it in the healing process. We can encourage the client to follow the resulting action tendency of *being moved* and turn it into outer movement, into authentic expression that can catalyze inner tensions and distress into constructive actions for emotion regulation, balance, and well-being. Such expression of *being moved* can also help in creating interactional resonance,[1] bonding, personal and relational development, insight, and closure. Creative arts therapists (CATs) employ both moving and *being moved* in the service of restoring health. *Being moved* is an overall concept of DMT and CATs, and it is a necessary part of the healing process.

In this chapter, I want to stress that *being moved* and moving are part of one circular process (Fuchs & Koch, 2014; Koch, 2017), and consider how the mechanism of *being moved* is tied into the healing process. We are supposedly engaged in the circular process of *moving* and *being moved* at several occasions throughout our day (see Caldwell, 2018). *Being moved* is presumably one of the most important active factors or clinical mechanisms of dance movement therapy.[2] While *being moved* is part of the affective and the aesthetic experience as assumed in CATs (Koch, 2017) and in dance movement therapy (Adler, 2002; LaBarre, 2005; Pallaro, 2000, 2007), it is also an emerging concept in social psychology (cf. Seibt et al., 2017; Zickfeld et al., 2019), as well as aesthetics research (Menninghaus et al., 2015). The chapter introduces recent concepts of the neighbor disciplines of psychology and cognitive sciences and relates them to concepts of *being moved* in DMT. It further compiles active factors of DMT that have been empirically investigated in this research group in the appendix.

BEING MOVED IN DMT

DMT theory and practice. Within DMT, *being moved* is understood as a core element of the method of Authentic Movement (AM; Pallaro, 2000, 2007), a practice developed by Mary Whitehouse and Janet Adler (2002). AM consists in a mover, normally working with closed eyes and without music, waiting for a movement impulse to emerge from the body, and then following that impulse with a curious attitude of where it moves and what else emerges in conjunction with it. The mover is accompanied by a witness, who sits and lets herself be moved by the mover (and later on shares and reflects her experiences in a dialogue with the mover). The resulting movement (at the interface of moving and being moved) is understood as free association of mostly unconscious material on the body level, which can then be used to map out the symbolic world and to advance the therapeutic processes of the client (Pallaro, 2000). The witness's experience is one of being moved in the meaning of the special emotion introduced in this chapter.

In the *Chace method* (Sandel, Chaiklin, & Lohn, 1993), DMT also works with moving and being moved. Participants are letting themselves be moved by the others, part of the group or the entire group, when entering into mirroring in movement. By using kinesthetic empathy and the ability to synchronize, participants built relationships. These capacities allow us to be moved. A shared group rhythm can facilitate the experience (Sandel et al., 1993), and the therapist holds the individual's and group's experience of being moved. While in AM being moved comes from within, in Chace it also comes from without in a situation of a receptive state to impulses from the music and from others.

Frances LaBarre (2005), a psychoanalyst, dancer, and developmental researcher, aimed at connecting scholarly work on dance and nonverbal communication on one hand, and psychoanalytic research on the other hand. She points out how "acting out" is assumed to occur in all patients in psychoanalysis (pathology-orientation), and suggests using this concept to employ enactment methods (from the creative arts therapies with their resource-orientation) to structure and advance the therapeutic process to the maximum benefit of the client. Clients, enacting aspects of their problems, cause attunement and embodied resonance in the therapist (being moved), which can then fruitfully be used in the therapeutic process. During training, therapists learn to attune with the patient and to be aware of their embodied resonance (or embodied countertransference; see Pallaro, 2007).

Fuchs and Koch (2014) detail how emotions are directly related to bodily changes (body feedback effects; Koch 2014) and thus result from the circular process of moving and being moved (Fuchs & Koch, 2014). Caldwell (2018) details how every therapeutic process consists of sensing, breathing, moving, and relating with multiple feedback loops using our ability of embodied resonance within, between, and among us: moving and being moved. Therapy in general can take forward steps when the inner impulse of *being moved* is carried to an outer expression and followed mindfully. Embarking on this journey, requires attention to the authority of the body and can lead the patient to solutions, coping, action completion, and closure (Caldwell, 2018).

Also, there is yet another very concrete way of *being moved* relevant to DMT: in addition to the present description of *being moved* by one's own active movements and inner impulses, there is the passively being moved, for example, in the context of a sculpture or marionette game, or simply in massage, where one person manipulates the other's body. This form of being moved has an important relation to being able to yield, to trust, and to give oneself into another's hands, which can be crucial issues for some clients. This form of being moved is not addressed in this chapter and would in fact require its own chapter.

Experiences From Empirical Projects

In the context of a research project proposal on active factors of arts therapies for palliative care patients, we planned to measure their *aesthetic experience* before, while, and after CAT sessions. We created a scale of 12 items to measure active factors of creative arts therapies (see Appendix A), one item being "*I feel moved/touched*". Next to the scale, we planned to ask clients regularly for changes on the item: *How much beauty do you experience?* (from 1, no beauty, to 10, extreme beauty), we envisioned working with a nice-to-touch wooden scale, where they could just push a lever to the level of experienced beauty in case talking was difficult. Correlational analysis of preliminary data from a student sample revealed that *experienced beauty* was related to *being moved* ($r = .57$), and both were confirmed as part of one meaning dimension by a factor analysis of the eight items. At present, both aspects can thus be understood as an operationalization of the aesthetic experience.

In another project, DMT students provided DMT to the most impaired patients in a care home context (many with late-stage dementia) who were no longer able to leave their rooms or their beds and in most cases did not talk or even react. The general goal of the intervention was to provide an aesthetic experience and a pleasurable interaction to promote well-being for these patients. The idea was to provide "receptive DMT", with some of our DMT students taking turns in dancing for the care home residents (one at a time in their room), and some other DMT students (one at a time) observing the changes in participants' attention, affect, sparks in their eyes, and moist/teary eyes. These observational measures rely a good deal on our human capacity for intersubjective resonance (subjectivity needs to be debated; "objective measures" versus use of human resonance to assess, for example, the degree of being moved of a palliative care patient; but this is another debate). Here *being moved* was an outcome, operationalized by the observation of gaze (for attention), affect, and teary eyes. This conceptualizes **being moved as a visible expression of the aesthetic experience** but still does not account for other form of expression of the same feeling, or for participants who are keeping the experience of *being moved* inside, without any outward expressive signs thus not being a sufficient condition.

BEING MOVED IN COGNITIVE SCIENCES, PSYCHOLOGY, AND AESTHETICS RESEARCH

Being moved as an emotion has long been overlooked and was recently rediscovered and empirically investigated with physiological operationalizations such as tears and goosebumps (Menninghaus et al., 2015). It was also investigated across 15 different countries where its components were mapped by the research group of Seibt, Schubert, Zickfeld and Fiske who introduced *kama muta* (Sanskrit for "moved by love") as a technical term for the emotion of *being moved*. They chose the term, since definitions and connotations of the concept varied considerably across different cultures, and in a few cultures the term "being moved" did not exist (Seibt, Schubert, Zickfeld, & Fiske, 2017; Zickfeld et al., 2018).

In their 2019 review paper on *being moved*, (Zickfeld et al., 2019) provide an excellent overview of the theory, empirical research, and components of the construct. They suggest that *being moved*, also often termed *being touched*, typically (but not always) refers to a distinct and potent emotion that results in social bonding, often includes tears, piloerection, chills, or a warm feeling in the chest, and is often described as pleasurable, sometimes as a mixed emotion.

About the linguistic properties of the concept they write:

> "Etymologically, *moved* derives from Latin *moveō* via French *émouvoir*. Interestingly, the word *emotion* derives from the same Proto-Indo-European root (as do *motive* and *motion*). One could therefore think, as Claparede (1930) did, that *being moved* might represent a kind of proto-emotion. Analyses of linguistic properties within the German language have identified that *moved* is related to similar lexemes indicating some kind of passive action (Kuehnast, Wagner, Wassiliwizky, Jacobsen, & Menninghaus, 2014; Menninghaus et al., 2015). English lexemes such as *moved*, *touched*, and *stirred* are based on the same metaphors of passive displacement or

contact that a number of other languages use to denote more or less the same emotion (e.g., Mandarin *gǎn dòng*, literally, 'to feel movement'; Fiske, Schubert, & Seibt, 2017)."

Historically, the concept of *being moved* was first described by McDougall (1919), who called it "the tender emotion", and by Claparede (1930), who termed it *être ému*. Nico Frijda (2007) refers to a category of emotions he called *being moved*. He argues that these "ambiguous" experiences (Frijda, 2001) are aesthetic emotions that "grip the body." (Zickfeld et al., 2019).

Zickfeld et al. (2017) claim that the construct contains *empathy* as one of its subcomponents. Kama Muta (Seibt et al., 2017) further includes an attachment component: "It motivates affective devotion and moral commitment to communal relationships" (Zickfeld et al., 2019, p. 5). In a recent national survey, about 51% of adults from the United States reported *being moved* by media or something on the internet at least several times a week (Zickfeld et al., 2019).

BEING MOVED AS A PHYSIOLOGICAL REACTION ACROSS CULTURES

Being Moved as a Physiological Reaction

Darwin (1872) and James (1890) describe tears based on tender feelings. While almost all researchers have described tears or moist eyes as a common aspect of *being moved* (see Zickfeld et al., 2019), Menninghaus et al. (2015) add goosebumps as a second characteristic and argue that the mix of tears and goosebumps ("goosetears") is a sufficient physiological operationalization of being moved. Piloerection has been successfully measured with cameras (e.g., Wassiliwizky, Koelsch, Wagner, Jacobsen, & Menninghaus, 2017). Note that both parts of the operationalization of goosetears depend on subjective judgment from embodied resonance. Musical chills are a related important psychophysiological correlate of *being moved* (e.g., Panksepp, 1995; Sumpf, Jentschke, & Koelsch, 2015). Warmth in the chest is another often described experience (e.g., Seibt et al., 2017; Tan & Frijda, 1999).

Being Moved Across Cultures

In order to measure self-reported *being moved*, Seibt et al. (2017) asked people to write down an episode involving positive tears (for an enumeration of other methods suited to elicit being moved, see Zickfeld et al., 2019, pp. 13/14). The findings of Seibt et al. (2017), resulting from cultural comparisons carried out as a comprehensive test across the United States, Norway, China, Portugal, and Israel, show very similar patterns of self-reports regarding being moved cross-culturally.

Evidence from the meta-analysis of 42 studies by Seibt, Schubert, Zickfeld, Zhu, et al. (2017) and Zickfeld et al. (2018, 2017) with 7084 participants from all over the world showed a medium to large correlation of $r = .47$ [.43, .51] for the relationship between tears and *being moved* (Cohen 1988 classified correlations of $r = .1, .3, .5$ as small, medium, and large, respectively). All this research is based on self-report; no objective measure of tears has been used in the context of *being moved* so far (Zickfeld et al., 2019). Results from the meta-analysis yielded a small-to-medium correlation of $r = .35$ [.31, .39] for the relationship between self-report of chills or goosebumps and *being moved*, where there is also initial evidence from psycho-physiological studies, measuring piloerection (Wassiliwizky, Koelsch, et al., 2017).

They further detected a medium correlation of $r = .50$ [.46, .54] between felt warmth (in the chest) and *being moved* (Zickfeld et al., 2019). While Seibt et al. (2017) speculate that it may be the combination of all three sensations that uniquely indicates *being moved* (Schubert et al., 2016; Seibt et al., 2017), there are reports of *being moved* without any of the three characteristics (Zickfeld et al., 2019). In any case, it can be assumed both sympathetic and parasympathetic systems are activated during the experience of *being moved* (for a more extensive review and the connections to neuroscience, see Koelsch et al., 2015 and Zickfeld et al., 2019).

Nonverbal Indicators of Being Moved

Based on interviews, participant observation, and literature reviews, Fiske and colleagues (2017) found that kama muta experiences can include taking a deep breath, experiences of buoyancy (feeling light, floating), and/or exhilaration (feeling refreshed, energized, optimistic) that may endure after the experience. In addition, increases in heart rate, respiration rate, and skin conductance may occur along with reported chills during experiences that people may describe as *being moved*. Nonverbal expressions of *being moved*, other than the autonomous reactions reported (tears, goosebumps, chills, or warmth) have not been systematically described yet. Fiske et al. (2017) describe that there is no distinct facial expression for *kama muta*; instead they propose that *kama muta* sometimes includes putting one or both palms on the chest, and adding an exclamation such as "Ahhhh!". However, to date no defined method exists for an observer to identify the instance or degree of *being moved* (Zickfeld et al., 2019).

BEING MOVED AS AN (AESTHETIC) EMOTION

Being Moved as an Emotion

Some researchers recently have conceptualized "being moved" as a distinct emotion (Cova & Deonna, 2014; Menninghaus et al., 2015; Tan, 2009; Zickfeld et al., 2018). The experience has been categorized as purely positive (Cova & Deonna, 2014; Seibt et al., 2017), occurring with mixed affect (Frijda, 2007; Menninghaus et al., 2015), and even as primarily negative (Bartsch, Kalch, & Oliver, 2014).

From an arts therapies perspective, an unfolding explanation for this positive and negative mixed conceptualization (Zickfeld et al., 2019) of *being moved* could reside in the fact that as an active factor it *actually arises from problem actualization* (Grawe, Donati, & Bernauer, 1994), which is an important common factor of psychotherapy. *Problem actualization* refers to the phenomenon of reexperiencing the problem on the sensory level and in detail. There is empirical evidence that if I do not experience the problem in the therapy session, I will not be able to find efficient possibilities to deal with it or solve it. We can assume that the problem, question, or feeling that constitutes a present challenge for a client (developmental task; striving for closure) is working inside the client for the entire time, and there is an organismic need to solve it (e.g., feeling lost or lonely after a separation). In therapy, the problem needs to be sensorially actualized. A song, for example, can actualize an issue that is inside of a person and create a feeling of an inner-outer resonance (as for example described in Reik's famous "The haunting melody"; Reik, 1953). Such a form of aesthetic resonance (see Lange, Hartmann, Eberhard-Kaechele, & Koch, 2020) can make the person feel understood, consolidate the person, and at the same time potentially transform the problem (often by providing metaphors as a joint anchoring "object" for the therapist and the patient).

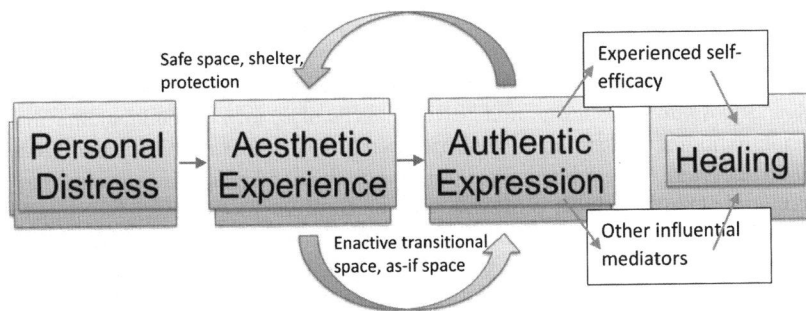

Figure 7.1 Process Stages of Being Moved in the Context of Arts Therapies

Note. Being moved takes place in the middle two components and their circular relation. In DMT, the expression often comes before the aesthetic experience and is dialectically intertwined with it (Koch, 2017); both aesthetic experience and authentic expression support and create experiences of self-efficacy (Bandura, 1977), strength, control, effectiveness, resources, and empowerment) as another important active factor feeding into health and healing. While self-efficacy is directly connected to moving (motor control effects; also in making music, and across the arts), the relationship of self-efficacy and being moved needs more investigation and specification.

The aesthetic experience may, in a second step, also inspire a person to actively express a question or begin to envision an emerging solution and thereby make use of it for further understanding and continuing growth to the topic. One can start with a reflection of it in music, movement, or art, and from there use the enactive transitional space or as-if space (Koch, 2017) to transform it and to arrive at insights and workable solutions (see Figure 7.1).

Art has the particular quality to unite opposites, constituting one of the reasons why it has the potential for integration and healing ("beyond polarity" view; e.g., Koch & Fischman 2011). In the same vein, psychological research shows that positive and negative affect are not opposite poles on one dimension: they are often distinct aspects of an experience and thus need to be measured separately (such as with the Positive Negative Affect Scale (PANAS) by Watson, Clark, & Tellegen 1988). In this respect, Frijda (2001) states that *being moved* includes "joy with a melancholy overtone" or "sadness with a not unpleasant tone". Similarly, Menninghaus et al. (2015) divide *being moved* into two different aspects: one with joy as the main component, another with sadness.

Being Moved as an Aesthetic Emotion

Interestingly, Menninghaus, who argues for a distinct emotion theory, is an aesthetics researcher. He and his colleagues (2015) state that *being moved* is often caused by significant relationship events or aesthetic stimuli. In their *Distancing-Embracing* Model (Menninghaus, Wagner, Hanich, et al., 2017), they assume that *being moved* helps integrate negative affect into positive states in art reception.

Research on *being moved* brings together embodiment (see Seibt et al., 2017; Zickfeld et al., 2018), attachment (see Feniger-Schaal, Hart, Lotan, Koren-Karie, & Noy, 2018), moral (see Sheets-Johnstone, 1999), and aesthetics research in a rich and holistic theoretical support for what creative arts therapies claim to do. Yet CATs and particularly DMT are enactive modalities: they use active art-making as their intervention method. It is thus interesting to see what the psychological approach to *being moved* says about actions.

BEING MOVED LEADS TO APPROACH ACTION TENDENCIES

Being Moved Causes Action Tendencies

Zickfeld et al. (2019) assume the following components of emotions: (1) an appraisal pattern/elicitor, (2) bodily reactions, (3) a feeling or affect (valence and arousal), (4) action tendency or motivation, and (5) expression and labels (facial or verbal; Scherer, 2005). Points (4) and (5) are clearly related to action, and the expressive side, which Zickfeld et al. (2019) further outline as *being moved* basically causes approach tendencies in persons affected (see Table 7.1). For us as creative arts therapists, the *action side* is particularly interesting, for there is a general void of theory and empirical work on the action side in psychology and the cognitive sciences (see Koch, 2017). Our active creative modalities that prepare patients to stand in the world, bond, and take action are in need of a good theory model on the active art-making side, such as the role of movement/dance and nonverbal expression for health.

Table 7.1 Action Tendencies From *Being Moved*

Label of Concept	Action Tendency	Domains	Reference
(Moral) Elevation	Approach	Affiliation, love, moral, action, altruism	Thomson and Siegel (2016), Pohling and Diessner (2016)
Empathic Concern	Approach	Empathy-altruism hypothesis, altruism, relieving other's need	Batson (2010), Batson (1991)
Being Moved (Cova & Deonna)	Reorganization of hierarchy of values and priorities	Altruism/prosocial	Cova and Deonna (2014)
Being Moved (Menninghaus)	Approach	Bonding, altruism, aesthetic, promoting bonds	Menninghaus et al. (2015)
Being Moved (Bartsch)	Insight	Satisfy meaning-related needs, personal growth	Bartsch et al. (2014)
Being Moved (Tan)	Approach	Bonding, signaling significance	Tan (2009)
Kama Muta	Approach	Sustaining, engaging in relation	Fiske et al. (2017)

Source: Adapted From Zickfeld et al., 2019.

Note. Action tendencies are what a person is physiologically and cognitively prone and/or primed to do; *Approach* action tendencies involve sequences of responding with positive evaluation and moving towards a stimulus, or bringing the stimulus in the direction of one's own body (such as in appetitive behavior; as opposed to avoidance or withdrawal-tendencies; Cacioppo et al., 1993; Kafka, 1950; Koch, 2014). *Being moved* causes approach action tendencies, which can be used toward therapeutic goals in CATs.

Implications for Arts Therapies

Social psychologists found that *being moved* may reduce stereotypes and prejudice, and increase altruistic and helping behavior (Schnall et al., 2010), humanization of outgroups, and interpersonal closeness (Oliver et al., 2015). This aspect may be particularly important for *the therapist*, particularly for keeping up the therapist's motivation and restorative resources. On the other hand, and more relevant to the client, *being moved* may also be related to insight, meaning, and personal growth (Bartsch et al., 2014; Oliver & Bartsch, 2011; see also research on *peak experiences* often described as "deeply moving": e.g., Maslow, 1970). Zickfeld et al. (2019) point out the potential of the concept to contribute to clinical areas among others:

> The study of the concept that is often referred to as *being moved* may help inform a number of research areas. . . . It also seems to play a major role in the appreciation and enjoyment of arts, psychotherapy, support groups, addiction-recovery groups, marketing, politics, and religion. There is much promising ground to explore.
>
> (Zickfeld et al., 2019, p. 33)

There is no clear consensus on what evokes *being moved* (Zickfeld et al., 2019). Because it corresponds to one's own situation and the questions and open loops (Fuchs, 2008) in one's own system, it may be caused by *a match of inner and outer*, a significant relation of one's own situation and the environmental stimuli in a given situation (and thus would presuppose interoception and introspection). Artistic stimuli are particularly suited to address the ambiguity of feelings and situations. However, the experience of beauty can only be actively used for health if the therapist offers space and time to explore and enact it through movement. No matter which modality is used in creative arts therapies, we offer space and materials for the clients to come to an experience of *being moved*. Creative arts therapists try to "meet the clients where they are" to jointly find ways to transform their situation in the manner appropriate for them to move forward. Mirroring is a way into this joint search (Sandel et al., 1993). Mirroring has been recently related to attachment by Feniger-Schaal et al. (2018), who found that the degree of mirroring in movement corresponded to attachment styles (Bowlby, 1969), with securely attached persons using freer mirroring, this relates to the concept of being *moved by love*, discussed later in the chapter. Next to social and moral emotions, we propose that *being moved* has consequences for and a function in healing (see Figures 7.1 and 7.2). The process may be the following: Being moved → action tendency → unfolding action → self-efficacy → healing (see Figure 7.1). In this way, the process is based on *being moved by love* in a more receptive mode, and develops into *being moved by love* ideally in an active mode (compare Maturana & Varela, 1987). The therapist can help facilitate the transition from action tendency into action.

BEING MOVED IN THE MODEL OF EMBODIED AESTHETICS

The Model

The model of embodied aesthetics helps to explain how and what works in creative arts therapies. It is based on the model of embodied affectivity (Fuchs & Koch, 2014). The model of embodied aesthetics was conceived because cognitive sciences models on aesthetics were all concerned exclusively with the perceptive side of the aesthetic experience (Koch, 2017). Cognitive science models are thus only of partial use for disciplines that work with active art-making, such as all CATs and particularly DMT, where there are no receptive techniques explicitly described

Receptive

Aesthetic Perception
Affection, Judgment
(to be moved, to evaluate)

Beauty
Body-Mind-Unity

Imagination
Emergence

Impression

| B O D Y | Embodied **Person** Bodily resonance | F E E D B A C K | | Environment **Art** Aesthetic affordances |

Test Acting
Creation

Play, Creativity
Improvisation,
Nonverbal
Communication

Ritual,
Metaphor

Expression

**Art-Making
Aesthetic Action**
E-Motion, Realization of Ideas
(to move, to conceptualize)

Active

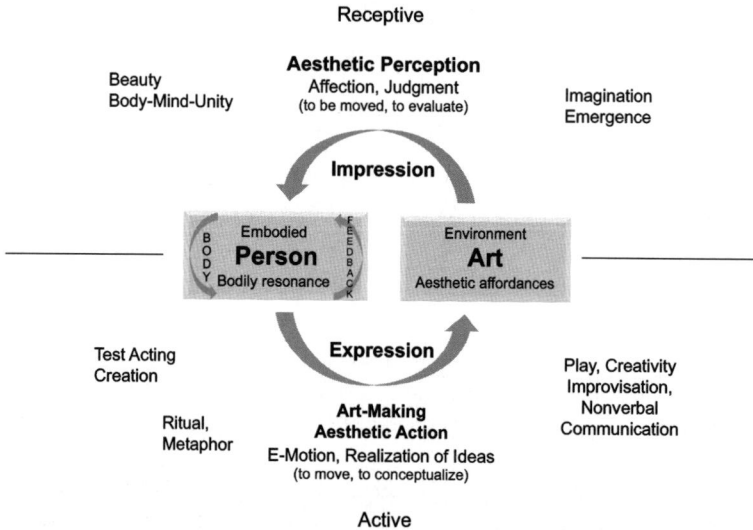

Figure 7.2 Model of Embodied Aesthetics
Source: Koch, 2017.

yet. It thus was necessary to model the active art-making side in addition to the receptive side of the aesthetic experience (see Figure 7.2). The active side strengthens the clients' self-efficacy.

The core of the model is the ongoing process of impression (being moved: the working on affect, and being affected, the sensory side) and expression (moving: the moving out from the body and expressing, the motor side). Impression is inner movement, expression is outer movement, and in fact the body is at the same time subject and object, active and passive (Merleau-Ponty, 1962), moving and being moved (Sheets-Johnstone, 1999; Fuchs & Koch, 2014; LaBarre, 2005).[3] In creative arts therapies, the persons creating art are expressing some meaning related to their thinking and feeling, and this expression is feeding back into their thinking and feeling. There is a circularity in the process of art-making with a constant interchange between expression and impression, moving and being moved, closely related to how emotion and affect create a circle in the model of embodied affectivity (Fuchs & Koch, 2014). Figure 7.2 shows this assumed process and displays major active factors of CATs that now can be anchored in the model of embodied aesthetics, either on the active (moving) side or on the receptive (sensing) side of the circular process.

In the model of embodied aesthetics, *being moved* is conceptualized as (a) the ground for other more distinct emotions (in dialectic relation with *moving*), and (b) the intertwined counterpart (receptive or sensory side) to moving and emoting as the circular dynamic of the model. Here, *being moved* is in a broad sense conceptualized as "being affected". The therapy process is based on the dialectics of moving and *being moved* in order to initiate the desired change (Caldwell, 2018; Fuchs & Koch, 2014; Koch, 2017).

In dance movement therapy, this dialectic is particularly pure insofar as it is not mediated by music, art object, or text, it is the moving body—"naked" in its emoting and being affected—that speaks. Movement is also particularly volatile in that it changes from moment to moment and after each moment is gone. In our research lab, we have started to investigate active factors of DMT, with first empirical results available (see Appendix B).

Implications for Future Research

With respect to future research on *being moved*, it would be interesting to measure the being moved concept with the *Kama Muta scale* of Seibt, Schubert, Zickfeld, and Fiske, plus a broader conceptualized *being affected* concept (Fuchs & Koch, 2014; LaBarre, 2005). This would help to specify the relation of the *being moved* concept of psychology and aesthetics research with the broader (and healing-related) perspective in dance movement therapy and CATs. Furthermore, the connection of *being moved* and self-efficacy and the necessary steps in between as hypothesized earlier (see Figure 7.1) need to be investigated in future research.

From the list of aspects implied in *being moved*—empathic, altruistic, helping, moral behavior—one can assume that *being moved* not only is important for the client but is particularly so for the therapist, in being a source of the therapist's professional motivation. It would thus make sense to examine the degree to which the therapist reaches the therapeutic goals with the clients, based on the active factor of *being moved* as a personal and professional resource. This would call for mediation-analysis of *being moved* as a mediator of the therapist's effect on reaching the therapeutic goals. It is the therapists' resource and capacity to be moved by their own art modality (here dance), and their ability to constructively use this *being moved*, which drives the therapeutic process further. For example, by using *aesthetic answering* as an arts-based method (Lange et al., 2020). An example for this technique would be: every time a client talks about her *hopeless search*, the therapists may spontaneously think of the song "I still haven't found what I am looking for." In the next therapy session, the therapist could bring the song and suggest to move to it and see what develops. In addition, the therapist may hand a printout of the song lyrics to the client to go into resonance with the text between sessions and possibly bring her own aesthetic answer back. . . . *Being moved* is a basis of aesthetic resonance and can constructively drive the therapy process.

CONCLUSIONS

In this chapter, *being moved* has been described as a major active factor of DMT, and a recent emotion concept in social psychology, intercultural studies, and aesthetics research. While the concept of *being moved* from the theories in psychology and cognitive sciences is slightly narrower (focused on a specific emotion encompassing positively evaluated bodily resonance), DMT/CAT theorizing includes all possible ways of being affected, with an evaluative abstinence and in application is focused on its use in the context of healing. The attachment aspect of the concept of *being moved* is particularly interesting with regard to health and healing, and has not explicitly been addressed in the theories on being moved. Attachment is a driving force of human motivation with a profound impact on health. It is a relevant factor in any field of therapy, in the work with mental health patients as well as with those affected by medical illnesses.

A second major concept of enactive healing environments is the experienced self-efficacy of the clients which is connected to the active art-making side. Self-efficacy beliefs are strengthened in the resource-oriented active art-making modalities of CATs and DMT. The crucial point for our clients, as pointed out throughout the chapter, is to carry the *being moved* into action (authentic expression), to find access to the bodily correlates and work with them, until integration, action completion,[4] mastery, and closure are reached. This is possible in movement per se, on the nonverbal level, which is a chance for many clients who's preference is not to work with words or who cannot work with words. This is the beauty of all CATs.

For DMT, research on *being moved* brings preliminary good news: The process of *being moved* by movement presumably connects experiencing beauty with the strengthening of self-efficacy. The patients learn that they can create the conditions that let them be moved and make them experience beauty and in this way can contribute to their own health and healing.

NOTES

1. Resonance: e.g., synchronizing with another person on one or more levels.
2. Next to being an active factor of DMT and CATs, *being moved* can also be a treatment goal, e.g., for clients with depression, autism, schizophrenia, dementia, or psychopathy.
3. This "ambiguity" is owed to the fact the body is the only object in the world that we perceive both from the inside and the outside.
4. Symbolic self-completion in the arts medium is an important active factor worth investigation in future studies.

REFERENCES

Adler, J. (2002). *Offering from the conscious body: The discipline of authentic movement.* Rochester, Vermont: Inner Traditions.

Bandura, A. (1977). Self-efficacy: Toward a unifying theory of behavioral change. *Psychological Review, 84*(2), 191–215.

Bartsch, A., Kalch, A., & Oliver, M. B. (2014). Moved to think: The role of emotional media experiences in stimulating reflective thoughts. *Journal of Media Psychology, 26*(3), 125–140. https://doi.org/10.1027/1864-1105/a000118

Batson, C. D. (1991). *The altruism question: Toward a social-psychological answer.* Hillsdale, NJ: Erlbaum.

Batson, C. D. (2010). Empathy-induced altruistic motivation. In M. E. Mikulincer & P. R. Shaver (Eds.), *Prosocial motives, emotions, and behavior: The better angels of our nature* (pp. 15–34). Washington, DC, US: American Psychological Association.

Bowlby, J. (1969). *Attachment & loss: Volume I: Attachment.* New York, NY: Basic Books.

Cacioppo, J. T., Priester, J. R., & Berntson, G. G. (1993). Rudimentary determinants of attitudes: II. Arm flexion and extension have differential effects on attitudes. *Journal of Personality and Social Psychology, 65*(1), 5–17. http://dx.doi.org/10.1037/0022-3514.65.1.5

Caldwell, C. (2016). The moving cycle: A second generation dance/movement therapy form. *American Journal of Dance Therapy, 38*, 245–258. doi:10.1007/s10465-016-9220-6

Caldwell, C. (2018). *Bodyfulness: Somatic practices for presence, empowerment, and waking up in this life.* Boulder, CO: Shambhala Publications.

Claparede, E. (1930). L'emotion "pure" [The "pure" emotion]. *Extrait des Archives de Psychologie, 22*, 333–347.

Cohen, J. (1988). *Statistical power analysis for the behavioral sciences.* Hillsdale, NJ: Erlbaum.

Cova, F., & Deonna, J. A. (2014). Being moved. *Philosophical Studies, 169*(3), 447–466. https://doi.org/10.1007/s11098-013-0192-9

Darwin, C. (1872). *The expression of the emotions in man and animals.* London, UK: John Murray.

Feniger-Schaal, R., Hart, Y., Lotan, N., Koren-Karie, N., & Noy, L. (2018). The body speaks: Using the mirror game to link attachment and non-verbal behavior. *Frontiers in Psychology, 9*, 1560. doi:10.3389/fpsyg.2018.01560

Fiske, A. P., Schubert, T. W., & Seibt, B. (2017). "'Kama muta'" or "being moved by love": A bootstrapping approach to the ontology and epistemology of an emotion. In J. Cassaniti & U. Menon (Eds.), *Universalism without uniformity: Explorations in mind and culture* (pp. 79–100). Chicago: University of Chicago Press.

Frijda, N. H. (2001). Foreword. In A. J. J. M. Vingerhoets & R. R. Cornelius (Eds.), *Adult crying: A biopsychosocial approach* (Vol. 3, pp. XII–XVIII). Hove, UK: Brunner-Routledge.

Frijda, N. H. (2007). *The laws of emotion.* Mahwah, NJ: Lawrence Erlbaum Associates Publishers. Retrieved from http://psycnet.apa.org/psycinfo/2006-11796-000

Fuchs, T. (2008). *Das Gehirn—ein Beziehungsorgan. Eine phänomenologisch-ökologische Konzeption* [The brain, a relational organ: A phenomenological-ecological conception]. Stuttgart: Kohlhammer.

Fuchs, T., & Koch, S. C. (2014). Embodied affectivity: On moving and being moved. *Frontiers in Psychology, 5*, 508. Retrieved from www.frontiersin.org/articles/10.3389/fpsyg.2014.00508/full

Grawe, K., Donati, R., & Bernauer, F. (1994). *Psychotherapie im Wandel. Von der Konfession zur Profession* [Psychotherapy in transition: From confession to profession]. Göttingen: Hogrefe.

Hahnefeld, R., & Koch, S. C. (2017). Glück im Herz und in den Beinen. Wirkung und Wirkfaktoren des Swingtanzes. *Zeitschrift für Sportpsychologie (2017)*, *24*, 77–82. https://doi.org/10.1026/1612-5010/a000194.

James, W. (1890). *The principles of psychology*. Cambridge, MA: Harvard University Press.

Kafka, G. (1950). Über Uraffekte. *Acta Psychologica, 7*, 256–278. doi:10.1016/0001-6918(50)90018-7

Kestenberg, J. S., & Sossin, K M. (1973/1979). *The role of movement patterns in development, Vol. 1*. New York: Dance Notation Bureau Press.

Koch, S. C. (2011). *Embodiment. Der Einfluss von Eigenbewegung auf Affekt, Einstellung und Kognition* [Embodiment: The influence of self-propelled motion on affect, attitudes and cognition]. Berlin: Logos.

Koch, S. C. (2014). Rhythm is it: Effects of dynamic body feedback on affect and attitudes. *Frontiers in Psychology, 5*, 537. doi:10.3389/fpsyg.2014.00537

Koch, S. C., Mergheim, K., Raeke, J., Machado, C. B., Riegner, E., Nolden, J., . . . & Hillecke, T. K. (2016). The embodied self in Parkinson's Disease: Feasibility of a single tango intervention for assessing changes in psychological health outcomes and aesthetic experience. *Frontiers in neuroscience, 10*, 287.

Koch, S. C. (2017). Arts and health: Active factors and a theory framework of embodied aesthetics. *Arts in Psychotherapy, 54*, 88–98.

Koch, S. C., & Fischman, D. (2011). Embodied enactive Dance Movement Therapy. *American Journal of Dance Therapy, 33*(1), 57–72.

Koch, S. C., Mehl, L., Sobanski, E., Sieber, M., & Fuchs, T. (2015). Fixing the mirrors. A feasibility study of the effects of dance movement therapy on young adults with autism spectrum disorder. *Autism, 19*(3), 338–350. doi: 10.1177/1362361314522353.

Koch, S. C., Morlinghaus, K., & Fuchs, T. (2007). The joy dance. Effects of a single dance intervention on patients with depression. *Arts in Psychotherapy, 34*, 340–349. doi: 10.1016/j.aip.2007.07.001

Koelsch, S., Jacobs, A. M., Menninghaus, W., Liebal, K., Klann-Delius, G., von Scheve, C., & Gebauer, G. (2015). The quartet theory of human emotions: An integrative and neurofunctional model. *Physics of Life Reviews, 13*, 1–27.

Kuehnast, M., Wagner, V., Wassiliwizky, E., Jacobsen, T., & Menninghaus, W. (2014). Being moved: Linguistic representation and conceptual structure. *Frontiers in Psychology, 5*. https://doi.org/10.3389/fpsyg.2014.01242

LaBarre, F. (2005). *On moving and being moved: Nonverbal behavior in clinical practice*. Hillsdale, NJ: The Analytic Press.

Lange, G., Hartmann, N., Eberhard-Kaechele, M., & Koch, S. C. (2020). Aesthetic answering: A method of embodied analysis and arts-based research in the context of creative arts therapies. In J. Tantia (Ed.), *Embodied research methods*. New York: Routledge.

Lange, G., Leonhart, R., Gruber, H., & Koch, S. C. (2018). The effect of active creation on psychological health: A feasibility study on (therapeutic) mechanisms. *Behavioral Sciences Journal, 8*(2), 25, doi: 10.3390/bs8020025.

Maslow, A. (1970). *Religions, values, and peak-experiences*. New York, NY: Viking.

Maturana, H. R., & Varela, F. J. (1987). *The tree of knowledge: The biological roots of human understanding*. Boston, MA: Shambhala Publications.

McDougall, W. (1919). *An introduction to social psychology*. Boston: John W. Luce & Co.

Menninghaus, W., Wagner, V., Hanich, J., Wassiliwizky, E., Jacobsen, T., & Koelsch, S. (2017). The distancing-embracing model of the enjoyment of negative emotions in art reception. *Behavioral and Brain Sciences, 40*. https://doi.org/10.1017/S0140525X17000309

Menninghaus, W., Wagner, V., Hanich, J., Wassiliwizky, E., Kuehnast, M., & Jacobsen, T. (2015). Towards a psychological construct of being moved. *PLoS One, 10*(6), e0128451.

Merleau-Ponty, M. (1962). *The phenomenology of perception*. New York, NY: Routledge.

Oliver, M. B., & Bartsch, A. (2011). Appreciation of entertainment: The importance of meaningfulness via virtue and wisdom. *Journal of Media Psychology, 23*(1), 29–33. https://doi.org/10.1027/1864-1105/a000029

Oliver, M. B., Kim, K., Hoewe, J., Chung, M.-Y., Ash, E., Woolley, J. K., & Shade, D. D. (2015). Media-induced elevation as a means of enhancing feelings of intergroup connectedness: Media-induced elevation. *Journal of Social Issues, 71*(1), 106–122. https://doi.org/10.1111/josi.12099Pallaro, P. (2000). *Authentic movement: Essays by Mary Starks Whitehouse, Janet Adler and Joan Chodorow* (2nd ed.). London: Jessica Kingsley.

Pallaro, P. (2007). *Authentic movement: Moving the body, moving the self, being moved*. London: Jessica Kingsley.

Panksepp, J. (1995). The emotional sources of "chills" induced by music. *Music Perception: An Interdisciplinary Journal, 13*(2), 171–207. https://doi.org/10.2307/40285693

Pohling, R., & Diessner, R. (2016). Moral elevation and moral beauty: A review of the empirical literature. *Review of General Psychology, 20*(4), 412–425.

Reik, T. (1953). *The haunting melody: Psychoanalytic experiences in life and music*. Oxford: Farrar, Straus & Young.

Sandel, S., Chaiklin, S., & Lohn, A. (1993). *Foundations of dance/movement therapy: The life and work of Marian Chace*. Columbia, Maryland: The Marian Chace Memorial Fund.

Scherer, K. R. (2005). What are emotions? And how can they be measured? *Social Science Information, 44*(4), 695–729. https://doi.org/10.1177/0539018405058216

Schnall, S., Roper, J., & Fessler, D. M. (2010). Elevation leads to altruistic behavior. *Psychological Science, 21*, 315–320.

Schubert, T. W., Zickfeld, J. H., Seibt, B., & Fiske, A. P. (2016). Moment-to-moment changes in being moved match changes in perceived closeness, weeping, goosebumps, and warmth: Time series analyses. *Cognition and Emotion*. https://doi.org/10.1080/02699931.2016.1268998

Seibt, B., Schubert, T. W., Zickfeld, J. H., & Fiske, A. P. (2017). Interpersonal closeness and morality predict feelings of being moved. *Emotion, 17*(3), 389–394. https://doi.org/10.1037/emo0000271

Seibt, B., Schubert, T. W., Zickfeld, J. H., Zhu, L., Arriaga, P., Simao, C., . . . Fiske, A. P. (2017). Kama Muta: Similar emotional responses to touching videos across the US, Norway, China, Israel, and Portugal. *Journal of Cross-Cultural Psychology*. https://doi.org/10.1177/0022022117746240

Sheets-Johnstone, M. (1999). *The primacy of movement*. Philadelphia: John Benjamins.

Sumpf, M., Jentschke, S., & Koelsch, S. (2015). Effects of aesthetic chills on a cardiac signature of emotionality. *PLoS One, 10*(6). https://doi.org/10.1371/journal. pone.0130117

Tan, E. S. (2009). Being moved. In D. Sander & K. R. Scherer (Eds.), *Companion to emotion and the affective sciences* (p. 74). Oxford, UK: Oxford University Press.

Tan, E. S., & Frijda, N. H. (1999). Sentiment in film viewing. In C. Plantinga & G. M. Smith (Eds.), *Passionate views: Film, cognition and emotion* (pp. 48–64). Baltimore, MD: John Hopkins University Press.

Thomson, A. L., & Siegel, J. T. (2016). Elevation: A review of scholarship on a moral and other-praising emotion. *The Journal of Positive Psychology, 12*(6), 628–638. https://doi.org/10.1080/17439760.2016.1269184

Wassiliwizky, E., Koelsch, S., Wagner, V., Jacobsen, T., & Menninghaus, W. (2017). The emotional power of poetry: Neural circuitry, psychophysiology, compositional principles. *Social Cognitive and Affective Neuroscience, 12*(8), 1229–1240.

Watson, D., Clark, L. A., & Tellegen, A. (1988). Development and validation of brief measures of positive and negative affect: The PANAS scales. *Journal of Personality and Social Psychology, 54*(6), 1063–1070. http://dx.doi.org/10.1037/0022-3514.54.6.1063

Wiedenhofer, S., & Koch, S. C. (2016). Active factors in dance therapy: Specifying effects of non-goal-orientation in movement on health. *Arts in Psychotherapy, 52*, 10–23.

Wiedenhofer, S., Wagner, K., Hofinger, S., & Koch, S. C. (2017). Active factors in dance therapy: Health effects of non-goal-orientation in movement. *American Journal of Dance Therapy, 39*(1), 113–125.

Zickfeld, J. H., Schubert, T. W., Seibt, B., Blomster, J. K., Arriaga, P., Basabe, N., & Fiske, A. P. (2018). Kama Muta: Conceptualizing and measuring the experience of being moved across 19 nations and 15 languages. *Emotion*. https://doi.org/10.1037/emo0000450

Zickfeld, J. H., Schubert, T. W., Seibt, B., & Fiske, A. P. (2017). Empathic concern is part of a more general communal emotion. *Frontiers in Psychology, 8*. doi:10.3389/fpsyg.2017.00723

Zickfeld, J. H., Seibt, B., Schubert, T. W., & Fiske, A. P. (2019). Moving through the literature: What is the emotion often denoted being moved. *Emotion Review, 2*. doi:10.1177/1754073918820126

APPENDIX A

Table A1 Active Factors of Creative Arts Therapies Scale (extension of Koch et al., 2016; EAS-Scale into AF-CATs-Scale); Preliminary Version

	If you think back to the last 60 mins What did you do? I did: _____	Not at all					Very much
1	How happy have you been?	1	2	3	4	5	6
2	How much beauty did you experience?	1	2	3	4	5	6
3	How much were you able to let go?	1	2	3	4	5	6
4	How well (authentically) were you able to express your emotions?	1	2	3	4	5	6
5	How strong was your experience of *flow* (= the absorption in an activity)?	1	2	3	4	5	6
6	How much did you come to an experience of integration/closure?	1	2	3	4	5	6
7	How strongly were you moved (i.e., internally moved/touched)?	1	2	3	4	5	6
8	How well could you dive into the sensory medium?	1	2	3	4	5	6
9	How strongly did you experience aspects of creation?	1	2	3	4	5	6
10	How much lightness/playfulness did you experience?	1	2	3	4	5	6
11	To which degree did you feel at one with yourself (body-mind unity)?	1	2	3	4	5	6
12	To which degree did you feel at one with the others (unity with others)?	1	2	3	4	5	6
13	To which degree did you feel at one with the arts medium (e.g., music)?	1	2	3	4	5	6
14	How much growth did you experience in/through the artistic medium?	1	2	3	4	5	6
15	How much were you able to express yourself symbolically in the medium?	1	2	3	4	5	6
16	How strongly did you experience mastery of what you were doing?	1	2	3	4	5	6
17	How important was the relationship with the therapist?	1	2	3	4	5	6
18	To what degree did you feel seen?	1	2	3	4	5	6
20	How well were you able to work on important questions for yourself?	1	2	3	4	5	6
21	How comfortable did you feel with the facilitator?	1	2	3	4	5	6
22	How important were other things? Which ones?:	1	2	3	4	5	6

Note. Items 1–15 form the core items of the Active Factors of Creative Arts Therapies-scale (AF-CATs-Scale); the other items refer to important related constructs (e.g., self-efficacy; relation with therapist/facilitator, etc.). The scale is a development on the base of the EAS-Scale (Embodied Aesthetics Scale developed for Parkinson's patients; see Koch et al., 2016).

APPENDIX B

Table A2 Overview of Active Factors of Dance Movement Therapy, Empirically Investigated by the Research Group of Koch et al.

	Active Factor/ Mechanisims and Instruments	**S**	**Authors**	**Results**
1	Aesthetic Experience, Embodied Aesthetics Scale (EAS)	E	Koch et al. (2016)	The enactive aesthetic experience increased after a one-hour session of Tango for Parkinson Patients (clinical study, Parkinson's Disease)
2	Aesthetic Experience (M), *Embodied Aesthetics Scale*	M	Bodingbauer, unpubl.	The aesthetic experience was a significant mediator in Chace sessions as well as in Authentic Movement sessions led by the same DMT/dancer/researcher. Self-efficacy particularly increased after the therapist witnessed the client (versus active participation) (E)
3	Active Creation (all CATs), *Experience of Creation Scale (ECS)*	M A	Lange, Leonhart, Gruber, and Koch (2018)	The ECS-scale, consisting of the experience of freedom, creativity, control and efficacy, mediated the effect of active creation on self-efficacy and well-being
4	Non-Goal-Directedness (of Dance), *Body Self-Efficacy Scale (BSE)*	E E	Wiedenhofer and Koch (2016); Wiedenhofer, Wagner, Hofinger, and Koch (2017)	The non-goal-directedness of movement (free improvisation) had a significant effect on stress reduction, body self-efficacy, and well-being
5	Experienced Unity with Music/Partner	U	Hahnefeld and Koch (2017)	No effect found (uncontrolled within-group design)
6	Being Mirrored (+Mirroring) in Movement, *BES-Scale* et al.	E	Koch, Mehl, Sobanski, Sieber, and Fuchs (2015)	Mirroring had a positive effect on body awareness well-being, social competence, and self-other-distinction (clinical study, Autism Spectrum Disorder)
7	Bouncing Rhythm (Jumping; Kestenberg & Sossin, 1973/1979) *HIS-Scale*	E E U	Koch, Morlinghaus, and Fuchs (2007) Hahnefeld and Koch (2017)	Bouncing caused a decrease of depressed affect, and an increase of experienced vitality, positive affect, and joy (clinical study; depression); bouncing caused an increase in happiness after swing dance (subclinical sample)
8	Movement Qualities *(indulgent versus fighting) MBAS-Scale*	E	Koch (2014)	Indulgent movement qualities cause more positive affect, fighting movement qualities more negative affect
9	Movement Shapes *(Approach versus Avoidance) MBAS-Scale*	E	Koch (2014); (see Cacioppo et al., 1993)	Approach toward own body caused more positive affect and attitudes; avoidance movements away from own body caused more negative affect and attitudes

Note. S=study type; E=experimental control group design; M=mediation analysis design (with control group); U=within-group design without control group (uncontrolled); A=arts-based research; CATs=creative arts therapies, EAS and ECS-Scales were used as operationalization of mediators/active factors of Embodied Aesthetics (EAS) and Experience of Creation (ECS).

CHAPTER 8

WORDING THE COMPLEXITY OF DANCE MOVEMENT THERAPY

A Scoping Review on How Dance Movement Therapists
Describe Their Clinical Practice

Rosemarie Samaritter and Marja Cantell

INTRODUCTION

The beneficial role of creative arts therapies, such as dance movement therapy (DMT), in the field of somatic and psychosocial well-being is increasingly recognized. From recent meta-analyses, there is also valuable research evidence of the effectiveness of DMT in health-related psychological problems (Ritter & Low, 1996; Koch, Kunz, Lykou, & Cruz, 2014; Strassel, Cherkin, Steuten, Sherman, & Vrijhoef 2011), depression (Mala, Karkou, & Meekums, 2012), dementia (Karkou & Meekums, 2014) and medical problems (Bradt, Goodill, & Dileo, 2011). Despite the promising findings, art therapies are under great pressure to show their evidence through academic research (Slayton, D'Archer, & Kaplan, 2010). A complication in the development of evidence-based recommendations for DMT for various somatic and psychosocial problems is that many DMT studies have methodological limitations. Studies often lack a clear description and integration of the DMT interventions applied (Baars et al., 2017).

In past research, dmts dance movement therapists (dmts) often described their work referring to concepts originally stemming from psychology, psychotherapy and psychiatry. Indubitably, DMT has developed as a field in relationship to psychotherapy. Pioneers in their own ways framed their practices within psychological theories (Bernstein, 1984). Within the growing DMT community the application of DMT practices broadened to a manifold of settings. The actual content of DMT interventions were adjusted to the given setting and population although still referring to the original DMT techniques such as Chace approach, mirroring or Laban movement qualities (Bräuninger, 2014a).

More recently, the DMT literature has begun to embrace theoretical frameworks that take specific movement or body-related features into account such as embodiment (Meekums, 2006; Panhofer & Payne, 2011; Samaritter & Payne, 2013; Fuchs & Koch, 2014) and phenomenology (Berrol, 2000; Mills & Daniluk, 2002). It is well known that the structure of psychotherapeutic sessions plays a crucial role not only for its replicability but also for its coherence and effectiveness (Hilliard, 1993; Kazdin, 2008). The uniqueness and complexity of creative arts therapies is that they have a dynamic and fluent, often intuitive, structure (Hervey, 2000; Meekums, 2002; Green, 2004). Wengrower (2009, p. 26) discussed the creative-artistic process in DMT as "an exploration of movements, images and metaphors, often in nonlinear paths of thoughts and actions". Therefore, it would be important that therapists' descriptions of their practices provide information about the specific frame of reference and working elements in DMT. Acknowledging the contribution of international research (Bräuninger, 2014a), we especially sought to analyze the dmt's verbal reflections of their clinical practices. Thus, our aim was to systematically inventory how DMT professionals describe their practices and how such contents may contribute to the (mental) health field. By reviewing and categorizing what components these descriptions provide, we aim to collect and describe current theoretical foundations and clinical practices that can be found in DMT articles published between 2000 and 2018.

Such descriptions could serve to elucidate domain-specific DMT practices. A formatted structure may be relevant for the research on effectiveness of DMT interventions. To be replicable over several studies, the structures, contents and activities of DMT interventions need to be well described. As DMT practitioners usually work with relatively small groups, clear description of DMT session structures and applied interventions could support research projects across multiple sites. Moreover, these structures may serve as formats to describe DMT interventions for clinical application and educational objectives in the professional DMT training programs. Also, a clear format on how to describe DMT interventions may facilitate therapists' explication and evaluation of their professional practice.

Based on our clinical and research background in DMT, we expected that (a) many dmts describe mainly the psychological orientation of their sessions (e.g., psychodynamic), and (b) many dmts describe practical applications and structures of their work, such as specific movement activities or DMT techniques. These became the hypotheses of our study.

This chapter will firstly describe the results from a review which inventoried studies that describe specific structures and contents of DMT sessions. Secondly, the chapter will present a conceptual, structural framework for DMT therapeutic models.

METHODOLOGY

The initial literature review was conducted as a scoping review that consisted of four inter-related phases, adapted from Slayton et al. (2010): (1) Identifying the research question, (2) Identifying relevant studies, (3) Study selection and (4) Charting the data.

The scoping review study process started by 'Identification of the research question', i.e., by grouping and discussing themes, theoretical concepts and topics in DMT. This grouping of sources led to a thematic orientation about *how dmts word their professional domain, activities and interventions*. We identified this as the research question for our review. It was important to consider which aspects of the research question are particularly important, and in our case, it was not the particular population or outcome but *how* the intervention was described. Therefore, intervention structures that have been described in manualized DMT treatment protocols (Koch et al., 2014; Pylvänäinen, Muotka, & Lappalainen, 2015) as well as specific evaluation tools (e.g., Bräuninger, 2006) were of particular interest in our study. Like in all research, be it quantitative or qualitative, this phase was informed by our own backgrounds and experiences as dmts originating from different cultures, training programs and work experience.

Based on our research question, we proceeded to the literature search process, i.e., 'identification of relevant studies'. We searched two large databases, the Scopus and Smart-Cat system. To inventory the practices described by dmts, initial searches were conducted with the terms 'intervention' and 'session'. However, the searches with the word 'intervention' provided a large number of hits outside the domain of DMT. Therefore, the final key words were set as: 'dance [and] movement [and] therapy [and] session'. The searches were defined to title, keywords and abstract. Our initial perusal of the 220 hits (99 in Scopus and 121 in SmartCat) indicated that the search strategy had picked up a large number of irrelevant studies, e.g., from other therapy approaches such as music therapy or physiotherapy. It also became obvious that each search engine provided a different amount of hits, i.e., articles. We began 'to funnel' information by extracting from the studies the wordings used to describe DMT as the professional domain, the session contents and activities. Some specific difficulties were faced due to variable terminology used to describe the DMT clinical practices.

It was challenging to be systematic and consistent during 'the selection process', i.e., stage of deciding which articles to include in our study. Our aim was to choose only those studies that provided sufficient description on the applied DMT protocol. Since we had chosen to search for breadth rather than depth, we needed a mechanism to help us eliminate studies that did not address our central research question. We adopted three inclusion criteria to our scoping study to determine the relevance of each 'hit': (1) a DMT professional as the therapist, (2) a therapy setting and (3) a description of activities and interventions with client(s). Exclusion criteria were: (1) Session(s) given by other than a dmt, (2) Session(s) not identified as DMT, (3) Published before year 2000 and (4) Article language other than English. Both reviewers (MC & RS) then applied the inclusion and exclusion criteria to all the abstracts. If the relevance of a study was still unclear from the abstract, then the full article was read. It is important to note that in this review we did not aim to assess quality of evidence and consequently cannot determine whether particular studies provide robust or generalizable findings (Arksey, & O'Malley, 2005).

In the fourth phase, we charted the abstracts to a synthesis table (see e.g., Slayton et al., 2010). It assisted us to exclude the overlapping articles from the two search machines and to make the final choice of abstracts to be included. The content analysis of the reviewed abstracts is described in the Results section.

RESULTS

The scoping review procedure revealed 43 DMT articles (27 tagged in both search machines). The variety between studies was very broad, from single case studies to cohort studies, from personal records to theoretical essays. Thus, although it can be argued that the review was limited by the use of specific search machines, the chosen articles revealed a good range of current DMT literature (See Table 8.1).

Many articles were written as a narrative, without an explicit articulation on how or why the specific techniques, methods or activities were applied. The intention here was to capture the narrative descriptions in a structure that would help to identify the specific contents. The selected articles were initially arranged into two groups based on our initial hypotheses. Group (a) contained studies that described a psychological and theoretical model for the chosen approach, and group (b) contained studies with practical applications. A content analysis of the abstracts within the respective groups led to further specification of the 43 articles. As a result, four thematic groups emerged; one covered information on conceptual references that were described to be relevant for dmts, a second group covered information on the theoretical therapeutic orientation, a third group covered information on specific structures that dmts described for their sessions and a fourth group covered information on specific DMT activities applied during the sessions. Finally, these groups were arranged into a structure consisting of four 'frames', which covered (1) meta-theoretical concepts, (2) therapy theory, (3) structure of the therapy and (4) applied DMT activities.

Face validity between researchers was satisfying for frame 1 and 2, whereas frames 3 and 4 needed some fine-tuning. After this adjustment, the frames were delineated as shown in Table 8.2.

Table 8.1 Table with 43 Studies Included in the Scoping Review

Study Reference	Frame 1	Frame 2	Frame 3	Frame 4
Ho, Fong, and Yip (2018).	1	2	3	4
Young (2017).	1	2		
Ko (2017).		2		4
Wiedenhofer, Hofinger, Wagner, and Koch (2017)	1	2		4
Pylvänäinen and Lappalainen (2017)		2	3	4
Panagiotopoulou (2017)		2	3	
Shim et al. (2017)		2	3	4
Fischman (2017)	1	2		
Ho, Lo, and Luk (2016)	1			4
Seoane (2016)		2	3	4
Houghton and Beebe (2016)	1	2	3	4
Barnet-Lopez, Pérez-Testor, Cabedo-Sanromà, Oviedo, and Guerra-Balic (2016)		2	3	4
Martin, Koch, Hirjak, and Fuchs (2016)			3	
Barnet-Lopez et al. (2016)				4
Doonan and Bräuninger (2015)		2	3	4
Hagensen (2015)		2		4
Koch, Mehl, Sobanski, Sieber, and Fuchs (2015)		2	3	
Pylvänäinen, Muotka, and Lappalainen (2015)		2	3	4
Ho (2015)			3	4
de Tord and Bräuninger (2015)		2		
Dunphy, Elton, and Jordan (2014)		2	3	4
Klasson (2014)	1			
Matherly (2014)		2		
Punkanen, Saarikallio, and Luck (2014)			3	4
Bräuninger (2014a)		2	3	
Anderson, Kennedy, DeWitt, Anderson, and Wamboldt 2014)			3	
Bräuninger (2014b)		2		4
Wadsworth and Hackett (2014)			3	4
Baum (2013)	1	2	3	
Victoria (2012)	1	2		
Bräuninger (2012)		2		
Regev, Kedem, and Guttmann (2012)		2	3	
Crane-Okada et al. (2012)			3	
Blazquez, Guillamó, and Javierre (2010)		2		
Fay, Chaiklin, and Chodorow (2009)	1		3	
Ylönen and Cantell (2009)		2		4
Capello (2007)	1			
Erfer and Ziv (2006)		2	3	4
Bräuninger (2006)			3	4
Grönlund, Renck, and Weibull (2005)			3	4
Nyström and Lauritzen (2005)		2	3	
Sandel et al. (2005)		2	3	4
Dibbell-Hope (2000)	1			4

Table 8.2 Structural Frames From Abstract Content Analysis of Reviewed DMT Literature

I. Frame of meta-theoretical concepts	The structural frame meta-theoretical concepts held information on themes that are found frequently in DMT literature but which do not solely belong to the domain of dance/movement therapy. These are themes that DMT shares with other disciplines, like philosophy, anthropology, psychology, biology, neuroscience.
II. Frame of therapy theory/model	This frame covered information about the characteristics of DMT as a discipline in the creative arts therapies, specific contributions of body- and movement-related work to mental health in general (healing/recovery/well-being) or the use of DMT for specific populations.
III. Frame of therapy structures	This frame was used for the structural components of DMT, such as development of therapy process, as in a manualized intervention, session-structures (open or set structure), leadership styles (improvisational or directive).
IV. Frame of applied DMT activities/working forms	This frame was used for dance-specific methods, techniques or movement activities applied in DMT.

The following section will describe the frames more in detail with some examples from the articles.

FRAME 1 META-THEORETICAL CONCEPTS

Additional examples from the selected studies in **frame 1:** Dance as cultural practice; Dance as healing practice; Creativity/creative process; Body-mind integration; (Movement) expression of inner states; The primacy of movement; Embodiment; Kinaesthetic memory; Metaphors; Aesthetics; Animation; Enactive approach

This frame was indicated when a text presented specific key concepts that are characteristic for DMT but do not solely belong to the domain of DMT. These are concepts that DMT shares with other disciplines, like philosophy, anthropology, psychology, biology, neuroscience. In some cases, such concepts were explicitly discussed or defined, such as the concept of culturally sensitive practice in Ho et al. (2016) or the phenomenological orientation in Wiedenhofer et al. (2017). Professionals in the field of DMT typically contribute from a practice-based and experientially informed epistemology to these conceptualisations, whereas other disciplines contribute typically through theoretical or cognitive models. An example from the selected articles is to be found in Fischman's (2017) conceptualization of transcontextual meta-patterns in group formations in DMT. Some other dmts discussed meta-theoretical concepts directly for their relevance for DMT. An example here would be the discussion of cultural contextualization of movement materials for the use in DMT sessions (Ho, Fong, & Yip, 2018; Ho, Lo, & Luk, 2016).

FRAME 2 THERAPY THEORY

Additional examples from the selected studies in **frame 2:** Models on healing; Models on mental health; Models on well-being; and for the dance informed orientation, models on specific body or movement related aspects, specific working elements; The professional domain was indicated, for example, as Body psychotherapy; Dance Therapy; Dance Movement Therapy

This frame was used when the article delivered characteristics of DMT as a discipline in the creative arts therapies. Decisions for this frame were made from questions such as *'What are specific indications for dance therapy?' 'What does DMT provide that is specifically dance or movement related?' 'What are specific DMT related goals/intentions?'* This frame covered models or explanatory concepts about the way in which DMT may contribute to healing, recovery and well-being. Contributions in this frame were also found to describe the specific contributions of DMT to the treatment of specific symptoms or specific populations. In this frame, authors made the connections between pathological issues and movement-related interventions that would address these issues. Examples: 'grounding' (de Tord & Bräuninger, 2015) and 'the use of touch' (Matherly, 2014).

Closely related to specific therapeutic approaches are choices regarding the therapist's leadership style. Bräuninger (2014b) discusses choices in leadership style explicitly and mentions the interrelatedness of verbal and nonverbal interventions in DMT. Authors mention frequently that leadership style is flexible and dependent on general aims of the DMT and patients' manifest needs as they occur throughout therapy (Dunphy et al., 2014; Sandel et al., 2005; Barnet-Lopez et al., 2016; Shim et al., 2017). Additional examples from the selected studies in Frame 2 in the text box show the broad orientation on theoretical models with psychotherapeutic orientations.

FRAME 3 THERAPY STRUCTURES

Additional examples from the selected studies in **frame 3**: Development of therapeutic process; Session structures; Dyadic and group structures; Autonomous therapy; Adjunctive therapy; Improvisational structures; Directive structures; Choreography

Frame 3 was indicated when the structure of the DMT session was explicitly addressed or when a therapy program was described. Only a few articles explained manualized DMT interventions that give specific descriptions of what happens in the DMT sessions in relation to the individual, interactional, social and environmental factors. Examples for a more detailed description of manualized interventions in our review sample were found in Pylvänäinen et al. (2015), Koch et al. (2015) and Ho (2015). In many cases the information on session contents in terms of the applied interventions was given at a rather general level, such as by listing the phases of the DMT session (from warm-up to closure) or rather general description of session content without specification of the applied technique. Practice-oriented articles in our review did not always provide the theoretical foundation for the choice of a specific session content.

FRAME 4 APPLIED DMT ACTIVITIES

Additional examples from the selected studies in **frame 4**: Chace approach; Authentic movement; Circle dances; Folk dances; Ballroom dances; Improvisation; Relaxation; Breathing exercises

---

This frame was tagged when articles described single interventions or activities in the clinical context, or as examples within a theoretical argument. Typically, this frame would describe the concrete movement activities that dmts apply in their sessions. In some cases, it was difficult to trace the dance-related characteristics of an activity. In these cases, we evaluated the embeddedness of a single intervention in the context of DMT. A physical exercise in the course of a DMT session would not only address the physical engagement of the participants but would be related to the potentially therapeutic effects that stem from the social, aesthetic or cultural dimensions of dance (Samaritter, 2018).

As can be seen from the proportional overview of the 43 studies (see Figure 8.1), most of the studies were categorized into frame 2 suggesting that the scoping review tapped into DMT models and characteristics of DMT as a discipline. Since the least number of studies fell into frame 1, the review suggests that relatively little is written during the last 18 years about metatheory and conceptualization of DMT. Twenty studies fitted into two frames, and 11 studies into three frames. The contents of 17 articles fitted into both frames 2 and 3 revealing that dmts who describe their DMT models also often provide descriptions of therapy structures. Such studies are important for the field in order to build the knowledge base on DMT as a discipline with quantifiable structures. Half of the studies provided descriptions of the actual DMT activities, i.e., frame 4, and 16 of them were combined with frame 3. Only two studies were categorized into all four frames and five studies only with one frame.

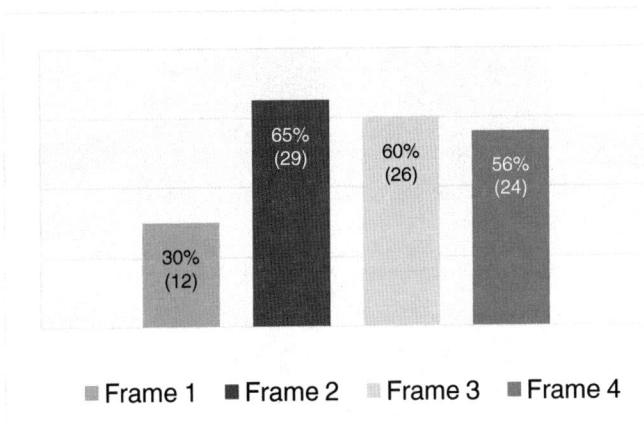

Figure 8.1 Frequencies (n) of the Four Structural Frames

DISCUSSION

The main aim of the scoping study was to review how the dmts describe the contents of their practice. The review included 43 studies from two academic search machines.

It is possible that the results are limited since the chosen search machines may not include all available DMT-related resources. Furthermore, journal articles often have a specific and focused structure, depending on the journals' scope. Also, the choice for specific search terms may have impacted on the outcome of the review.

Summarizing the results, we found that the current review delivered a broad range of DMT-related studies, which offered a considerable diversity of DMT theories and practices. Notwithstanding the variety of the selected articles, the content analysis showed overarching themes and structures between studies. However, in many of them this information was rather implicit. We found it at times difficult to disentangle the information on DMT-specific elements. Also, many studies lacked the argument on why specific interventions would serve a specific target group, symptom or problem. Being dmts by origin, we experienced in the multitude of studies a level of revisiting the well-known, familiar and generalized descriptions of DMT. Reviewing studies that were less explanatory required effort, reorienting and searching for a way in. The contents and definitions of the four frames continued to evolve all the way to the end of our writing process. We felt we had many roles, not just of an external observer but also as a privileged choreographer who combines and structures old and new, having a role in the collective creation of DMT as a specifiable structure.

It seems a challenge for dmts not only to find the right wordings for the experiential content of their work (Panhofer & Payne, 2011) but to also find the right structures for the multiple layers of decision making that go along with the positioning in a professional field that is characterized by a broad variety of theories and applications. Many studies were tagged for multiple frames in various combinations, suggesting that there are studies combining meta-theory (frame 1) with DMT theory and models (frame 2), even together with therapy structures (frame 3) and applied DMT activities (frame 4) (Ho, 2015; Houghton & Beebe, 2016).

In our selection there were also studies that portrayed DMT at just one level, i.e., at a meta-theoretical level as embedded into philosophical, cultural, anthroposophical and psychological fields (Capello, 2007; Klasson, 2014; Ho et al., 2016) or in contrast on a practical level into specific DMT activities and working forms (Barnet-Lopez et al., 2016).

Only a few studies gave explicit information about the specific orientation of the applied DMT intervention, such as psycho-education, revalidation, well-being, prevention, care or cure. In some cases, it was not clear whether the presented model would in fact address therapeutic goals. These results reflect Rush & Imus's overview on the creative arts therapy continuum (2017, p. 173) distinguishing therapeutic, aesthetic, recreational, educational, rehabilitative and psychotherapeutic approaches. For DMT to be recognized within a multi-disciplinary mental health field, it would be helpful if DMT interventions would be indicated with a clear therapeutic orientation.

The formal structure of DMT sessions, which is composed of successive interventions throughout one session, is due to the arts-related contents and dynamics constantly adjusted to the group needs and interactional shifts between group members. The therapist will have to find responsive interventions to alter movement material throughout therapy while maintaining a clear therapeutic orientation to the population and the application of specific working elements. Situating DMT interventions within the interacting structural frames will inform the movement interventions on the spot 'as the body of knowledge behind our intuitive choices increases, perhaps so too will those moments in which the therapeutic process seems to take over on its own' (Bruno, 1981, p. 133).

Ideally, DMT studies would describe a series of choices made, including meta-theoretical concepts and their relevance for the chosen therapy approach. This would enable describing a suitable design of DMT practices and session structures, and finally, would give a rationale for the selection of specific dance and movement interventions. This kind of explicit process description would position DMT more clearly in the broader mental health field or a multidisciplinary context. The four frames may support the process of decision making during the development of a DMT manual. Table 8.3 describes an example about the layered decision making in DMT, focusing on embodiment with a patient with personality disorder.

We would therefore propose the four structural frames as highly interrelated (see Figure 8.2). When viewed together they form a dynamic structure of interacting layers, with the

Table 8.3 An Example of Using the Four Frames to Construct a DMT Manual Focusing on Embodiment for Patients with Personality Disorders

I. Frame of meta-theoretical concepts	Description of the significance of embodiment for patients with personality disorders (PD) and which DMT approaches would support the development of embodiment in PD.
II. Frame of therapy theory/model	Decision on a series of DMT sessions oriented on developing embodiment in PD.
III. Frame of therapy structures	Description of the composition of the single session to support development and maintenance of embodiment in PD throughout a DMT session.
IV. Frame of applied DMT activities/ working forms	Description of specific activities that will afford embodiment in PD.

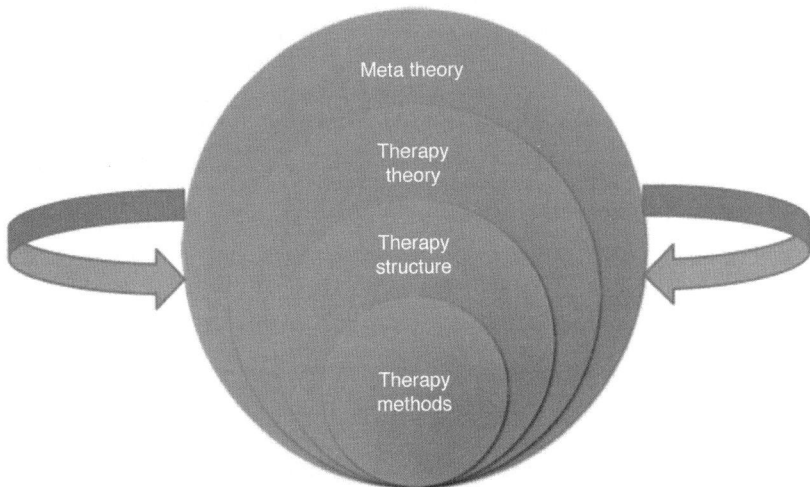

Figure 8.2 The Four Frames as Interacting Structures

meta-theory being the broadest and the dance therapeutic method being the most elementary unit. The description of specific aspects of DMT interventions consisting of all four layers would be useful for dmts. We need to familiarize ourselves not only with different perspectives to acknowledge and take further the existing DMT literature. In order to describe and disentangle the complexity of DMT interventions, we should acknowledge the versatility of studies carried out not only in our own but also in other cultures and traditions. The four proposed frames could serve as a dynamic structure to describe manualized interventions as well as single interventions without losing the complexity of the arts-based nature of DMT.

Choices made throughout the four frames would also have an impact on the leadership style applied during the interventions. In the selected studies, the information on leadership styles was relatively rare. However, some authors have addressed particular variations in DMT leadership styles (Koch, 1984) and their relevance for the effectiveness of DMT interventions (Bräuninger, 2012). Within the structural frames, leadership styles are related to the specific approach or orientation of the intervention, the therapy theoretical choices. For further conceptualization, leadership style could serve as a sub-category of frame 2.

Feasibility of the Four Frames

Parts of our four frames can be considered rather common and thus are also present in other studies that have described specific DMT interventions (Bräuninger, 2014a, 2014b; Bruno, 1990) or specific working factors present in DMT (Wiedenhofer et al., 2017; Koch, 2017). Dmts described a broad variety of techniques, some of them being clearly rooted in dance, such as Chace circle, movement expression and symbolization, folk dances, others with an origin in body- or movement-oriented approaches, such as visualizations, relaxation techniques, grounding techniques. In addition, dance-based procedures such as composition, choreography (Fischman, 2017) and symbolic expression of inner states (Victoria, 2012) are regularly reported but often not clearly placed as part of a specific therapeutic model. It is crucial that dmts strive to provide detailed description of their session contents and specific dance-informed procedures in their therapeutic function. Indeed, this would disclose the specific contribution of DMT to the broader field of mental health.

The challenge is to describe DMT interventions for use in research and/or guidelines without losing the complex nature of DMT. However, evidence-based research is important in order to ensure that DMT is an effective intervention for health-related psychological problems. The demonstration of its effectiveness is essential for promoting DMT to health care and/or education providers, and in a bigger sense, to the survival of the profession (Koch, Kunz, Lykou, & Cruz, 2014). A structural framework as presented here may support dmts in this task.

Future Perspectives

The scoping review responded to the call made to determine more systematically what the contents of specific DMT interventions are, because so little is known about therapists' choices and which specific DMT interventions and their related methods and activities are applied during sessions (Bräuninger, 2014b). The structural frames may help to describe, write and teach the complexity of DMT interventions and develop the notion that a single intervention (even a single movement) may carry information about therapeutic structures, therapy theory models or meta-theoretical models.

The proposed conceptual framework, stemming from the investigation of theoretical as well as practice-based descriptions of DMT interventions, may be helpful for adding much-needed depth to the body of knowledge about the use of DMT and other embodied therapies. We realize the unique position of embodied, arts-based therapies. They provide a distinctive, experiential quality, which may be considered as their specific contribution to the field of (mental) health but which also provides an extra challenge when wanting to formulate coherent interventions for the dynamically changing professional field. Machteld Huber et al. (2011) conceptualized positive (mental) health as the ability to adapt and self-manage in the face of social, physical and emotional challenges. If this is the 21st century concept of health, it invites the dmts to join the development of health care and prevention models— and by doing so, *we are also responsible for being explicit about our theoretical foundations and procedures.*

REFERENCES (*INCLUDED INTO THE SCOPING REVIEW)

*Anderson, A. N., Kennedy, H., DeWitt, P., Anderson, E., & Wamboldt, M. Z. (2014). Dance/movement therapy impacts mood states of adolescents in a psychiatric hospital. *The Arts in Psychotherapy, 41*(3), 257–262.

Arksey, H., & O'Malley, L. (2005). Scoping studies: Towards a methodological framework. *International Journal of Social Research Methodology, 8*(1), 19–32.

Baars, E., Busschbach, J., Emck, C., Hakvoort, L., van Hooren, S., Notermans, H., . . . Spreen, M. (2017). *Strategische Onderzoeksagenda voor de Vaktherapeutische Beroepen.* Utrecht, NL: FVB.

*Barnet-Lopez, S., Pérez-Testor, S., Cabedo-Sanromà, J., Oviedo, G. R., & Guerra-Balic, M. (2016). Dance/movement therapy and emotional well-being for adults with intellectual disabilities. *The Arts in Psychotherapy, 51*, 10–16.

*Baum, R. (2013). In the arms of grief: Working with developmentally delayed children and their caregivers. *American Journal of Dance Therapy, 35*(2), 169–182.

Bernstein, P. (Ed.). (1984). *Eight theoretical approaches in dance-movement therapy.* Dubuque, IA: Kendall/Hunt Publishing Company.

Berrol, C. F. (2000). The spectrum of research options in dance/movement therapy. *American Journal of Dance Therapy, 22*(1), 29–46.

*Blazquez, A., Guillamó, E., & Javierre, C. (2010). Preliminary experience with dance movement therapy in patients with chronic fatigue syndrome. *The Arts in Psychotherapy, 37*(4), 285–292.

Bradt, J., Goodill, S. W., & Dileo, C. (2011). Dance/movement therapy for improving psychological and physical outcomes in cancer patients. *Cochrane Database of Systematic Reviews* (10). Art. No.: CD007103. doi:10.1002/14651858.CD007103.pub2

*Bräuninger, I. (2006). Treatment modalities and self-expectancy of therapists: Modes, self-efficacy and imagination of clients in dance movement therapy. *Body, Movement and Dance in Psychotherapy, 1*(2), 95–114.

*Bräuninger, I. (2012). Dance movement therapy group intervention in stress treatment: A randomized controlled trial (RCT). *The Arts in Psychotherapy, 39*(5), 443–450.

*Bräuninger, I. (2014a). Dance movement therapy with the elderly: An international internet-based survey undertaken with practitioners. *Body, Movement and Dance in Psychotherapy, 9*(3), 138–153.

*Bräuninger, I. (2014b). Specific dance movement therapy interventions: Which are successful? An intervention and correlation study. *The Arts in Psychotherapy, 41*(5), 445–457.

Bruno, C. (1981). Applications and implications of "structural analysis of movement sessions" for dance therapy. *The Arts in Psychotherapy, 8*(2), 127–133.

Bruno, C. (1990). Maintaining a concept of the dance in dance/movement therapy. *American Journal of Dance Therapy, 12*(2), 101–113. doi:10.1007/bf00843885

*Capello, P. P. (2007). Dance as our source in dance/movement therapy education and practice. *American Journal of Dance Therapy, 29*(1), 37–50.

*Crane-Okada, R., Kiger, H., Sugerman, F., Uman, G. C., Shapiro, S. L., Wyman-McGinty, W., & Anderson, N. L. (2012). Mindful movement program for older breast cancer survivors: A pilot study. *Cancer Nursing, 35*(4), E1–E13.

*de Tord, P., & Bräuninger, I. (2015). Grounding: Theoretical application and practice in dance movement therapy. *The Arts in Psychotherapy, 43*, 16–22.

*Dibbell-Hope, S. (2000). From DTR to PhD: The personal story of my dissertation, moving toward health. *American Journal of Dance Therapy, 22*(1), 61–77.

*Doonan, F., & Bräuninger, I. (2015). Making space for the both of us: How dance movement therapy enhances mother–infant attachment and experience. *Body, Movement and Dance in Psychotherapy, 10*(4), 227–242.

*Dunphy, K., Elton, M., & Jordan, A. (2014). Exploring dance/movement therapy in post-conflict Timor-Leste. *American Journal of Dance Therapy, 36*(2), 189–208.

*Erfer, T., & Ziv, A. (2006). Moving toward cohesion: Group dance/movement therapy with children in psychiatry. *The Arts in Psychotherapy*, *33*(3), 238–246.

*Fay, C. G., Chaiklin, S., & Chodorow, J. (2009). At the threshold: A journey to the sacred through the integration of Jungian psychology and the expressive arts. *American Journal of Dance Therapy*, *31*(1), 3–19.

*Fischman, D. I. (2017). Understanding group shaping: Transcontextual metapatterns in dance movement psychotherapy. *Body, Movement and Dance in Psychotherapy*, *12*(2), 83–97.

Fuchs, T., & Koch, S. C. (2014). Embodied affectivity: On moving and being moved. *Frontiers in Psychology*, 5.

Green, J. (2004). Postpositivist inquiry: Multiple perspectives and paradigms. In R. F. Cruz & C. F. Berrol (Eds.), *Dance/movement therapists in action: A working guide to research options* (pp. 109–124). Springfield, IL: Charles C Thomas Publisher Ltd.

*Grönlund, E., Renck, B., & Weibull, J. (2005). Dance/movement therapy as an alternative treatment for young boys diagnosed as ADHD: A pilot study. *American Journal of Dance Therapy*, *27*(2), 63–85.

*Hagensen, K. P. (2015). Using a dance/movement therapy-based wellness curriculum: An adolescent case study. *American Journal of Dance Therapy*, *37*(2), 150–175.

Hervey, L. W. (2000). *Artistic inquiry in dance/movement therapy: Creative research alternatives*. Springfield, IL: Charles C Thomas Publisher Ltd.

Hilliard, R. B. (1993). Single-case methodology in psychotherapy process and outcome research. *Journal of Consulting and Clinical Psychology*, *61*(3), 373–380.

*Ho, R. T. H. (2015). A place and space to survive: A dance/movement therapy program for childhood sexual abuse survivors. *The Arts in Psychotherapy*, *46*, 9–16.

*Ho, R. T. H., Fong, T. C., & Yip, P. S. (2018). Perceived stress moderates the effects of a randomized trial of dance movement therapy on diurnal cortisol slopes in breast cancer patients. *Psychoneuroendocrinology*, *87*, 119–126.

*Ho, R. T. H., Lo, P. H., & Luk, M. Y. (2016). A good time to dance? A mixed-methods approach of the effects of dance movement therapy for breast cancer patients during and after radiotherapy. *Cancer Nursing*, *39*(1), 32–41.

*Houghton, R., & Beebe, B. (2016). Dance/movement therapy: Learning to look through video microanalysis. *American Journal of Dance Therapy*, *38*(2), 334–357.

Huber, M., Knottnerus, J. A., Green, L., van der Horst, H., Jadad, A. R., Kromhout, D., . . . Schnabel, P. (2011). How should we define health? *BMJ: British Medical Journal* (Online), *343*.

Karkou, V., & Meekums, B. (2014). Dance movement therapy for dementia. *The Cochrane Library* (3). Art. No.: CD011022. doi:10.1002/14651858.CD011022.3

Kazdin, A. E. (2008). Evidence-based treatment and practice: New opportunities to bridge clinical research and practice, enhance the knowledge base, and improve patient care. *American Psychologist*, *63*, 146–159.

*Klasson, R. D. (2014). Dance/movement therapists using motivational interviewing: A qualitative study. *American Journal of Dance Therapy*, *36*(2), 176–188.

*Ko, K. S. (2017). A broken heart from a wounded land: The use of Korean scarf dance as a dance/movement therapy intervention for a Korean woman with haan. *The Arts in Psychotherapy*, *55*, 64–72.

Koch, N. S. (1984). Content analysis of leadership variables in dance therapy. *American Journal of Dance Therapy*, *7*(1), 58–75. doi:10.1007/bf02579631

Koch, S. C. (2017). Arts and health: Active factors and a theory framework of embodied aesthetics. *Arts in Psychotherapy*, *54*, 85–91. doi:10.1016/j.aip.2017.02.002

Koch, S. C., Kunz, T., Lykou, S., & Cruz, R. (2014). Effects of dance movement therapy and dance on health-related psychological outcomes: A meta-analysis. *The Arts in Psychotherapy*, *41*(1), 46–64. http://dx.doi.org/10.1016/j.aip.2013.10.004

*Koch, S. C., Mehl, L., Sobanski, E., Sieber, M., & Fuchs, T. (2015). Fixing the mirrors: A feasibility study of the effects of dance movement therapy on young adults with autism spectrum disorder. *Autism*, *19*(3), 338–350.

Mala, A., Karkou, V., & Meekums, B. (2012). Dance/Movement Therapy (D/MT) for depression: A scoping review. *The Arts in Psychotherapy*, *39*(4), 287–295.

*Martin, L. A., Koch, S. C., Hirjak, D., & Fuchs, T. (2016). Overcoming disembodiment: The effect of movement therapy on negative symptoms in schizophrenia: A multicenter randomized controlled trial. *Frontiers in Psychology*, *7*, 483.

*Matherly, N. (2014). Navigating the dance of touch: An exploration into the use of touch in dance/movement therapy. *American Journal of Dance Therapy*, *36*(1), 77–91.

Meekums, B. (2002). *Dance Movement Therapy: A creative psychotherapeutic approach*. London: Sage Publications.

Meekums, B. (2006). Embodiment in dance movement therapy training and practice. In H. Payne (Ed.), *Dance Movement Therapy: Theory, research and practice* (2nd ed., pp. 167–183). London: Routledge.

Mills, L. J., & Daniluk, J. C. (2002). Her body speaks: The experience of dance therapy for women survivors of child sexual abuse. *Journal of Counseling & Development*, *80*(1), 77–85. https://doi.org/10.1002/j.1556-6678.2002.tb00169.x

*Nyström, K., & Lauritzen, S. O. (2005). Expressive bodies: Demented persons' communication in a dance therapy context. *Health*, *9*(3), 297–317.

*Panagiotopoulou, E. (2017). Dance therapy and the public school: The development of social and emotional skills of high school students in Greece. *The Arts in Psychotherapy*, *59*, 25–33.

Panhofer, H., & Payne, H. (2011). Languaging the embodied experience. *Body, Movement and Dance in Psychotherapy*, *6*(3), 215–232. doi:10.1080/17432979.2011.572625

*Punkanen, M., Saarikallio, S., & Luck, G. (2014). Emotions in motion: Short-term group form dance/movement therapy in the treatment of depression: A pilot study. *The Arts in Psychotherapy*, *41*(5), 493–497.

*Pylvänäinen, P. M., & Lappalainen, R. (2017). Change in body image among depressed adult outpatients after a dance movement therapy group treatment. *The Arts in Psychotherapy*, *59*, 34-45.

*Pylvänäinen, P. M., Muotka, J. S., & Lappalainen, R. (2015). A dance movement therapy group for depressed adult patients in a psychiatric outpatient clinic: Effects of the treatment. *Frontiers in Psychology*, *6*.

*Regev, D., Kedem, D., & Guttmann, J. (2012). The effects of mothers' participation in movement therapy on the emotional functioning of their school-age children in Israel. *The Arts in Psychotherapy*, *39*(5), 479–488.

Ritter, M., & Low, K. G. (1996). Effects of dance/movement therapy: A meta-analysis. *The Arts in Psychotherapy*, *23*, 249–260.

Rush, D., & Imus, S. (2017). The same new kid in yet another hood-deep game design as creative arts therapy? In D. Rush (Ed.), *Making deep games: Designing games with meaning and purpose*. Boca Raton, FL: CRC Press and Taylor & Francis Group.

Samaritter, R. (2018). The aesthetic turn in mental health: Reflections on an explorative study into practices in the arts therapies. *Behavioral Sciences*, *8*(4), 41.

Samaritter, R., & Payne, H. (2013). Kinaesthetic intersubjectivity: A dance informed contribution to self-other relatedness and shared experience in non-verbal psychotherapy with an example from autism. *The Arts in Psychotherapy*, *40*(1), 143–150.

*Sandel, S. L., Judge, J. O., Landry, N., Faria, L., Ouellette, R., & Majczak, M. (2005). Dance and movement program improves quality-of-life measures in breast cancer survivors. *Cancer Nursing*, *28*(4), 301–309.

*Seoane, K. J. (2016). Parenting the self with self-applied touch: A dance/movement therapy approach to self-regulation. *American Journal of Dance Therapy*, *38*(1), 21–40.

*Shim, M., Johnson, R. B., Gasson, S., Goodill, S., Jermyn, R., & Bradt, J. (2017). A model of dance/movement therapy for resilience-building in people living with chronic pain. *European Journal of Integrative Medicine*, *9*, 27–40.

Slayton, S. C., D'Archer, J., & Kaplan, F. (2010). Outcome studies on the efficacy of art therapy: A review of findings. *Art Therapy: Journal of the American Art Therapy Association*, *27*(3), 108–118.

Strassel, J. K., Cherkin, D. C., Steuten, L., Sherman, K. J., & Vrijhoef, H. J. (2011). A systematic review of the evidence for the effectiveness of dance therapy. *Alternative Therapies in Health and Medicine*, *17*(3), 50–59.

*Victoria, H. K. (2012). Creating dances to transform inner states: A choreographic model in dance/movement therapy. *Body, Movement and Dance in Psychotherapy*, *7*(3), 167–183.

*Wadsworth, J., & Hackett, S. (2014). Dance movement psychotherapy with an adult with autistic spectrum disorder: An observational single-case study. *Body, Movement and Dance in Psychotherapy*, *9*(2), 59–73.

Wengrower, H. (2009). The creative-artistic process in dance/movement therapy. In S. Chaiklin, & H. Wengrower (Eds.), *The art and science of dance/movement therapy* (pp. 13–32). New York, NY: Routledge.

*Wiedenhofer, S., Hofinger, S., Wagner, K., & Koch, S. C. (2017). Active factors in dance/movement therapy: Health effects of non-goal-orientation in movement. *American Journal of Dance Therapy*, *39*(1), 113–125.

*Ylönen, M. E., & Cantell, M. H. (2009). Kinaesthetic narratives: Interpretations for children's dance movement therapy process. *Body, Movement and Dance in Psychotherapy*, *4*(3), 215–230.

*Young, J. (2017). The therapeutic movement relationship in dance/movement therapy: A phenomenological study. *American Journal of Dance Therapy*, *39*(1), 93–112.

CHAPTER 9

CREATING BREEDS CREATING

Susan Dee Imus

Research has demonstrated that the arts have an impact on our health and can be necessary to our well-being; "the arts can really help people stay healthy or recover when illness strikes" (Crawford, 2018, para. 3). Dance/movement therapists are educated in using their dance/movement expertise and creative process for improving health and fostering wellness. How do dance/movement therapists do this and what language do they use to describe their practice? As a DMT educator in the 21st century, it has become more challenging to consistently describe what dmts do today and how DMT works. The language often varies from one educator, researcher or practitioner to another as well as one educational institution to another. Cultural consciousness is also motivating the discipline to update its taxonomy with a more discerning lens. This chapter attempts to clarify terms such as approaches/methods/theories and accompanying beliefs, assumptions, core concepts and philosophies. The chapter also helps to differentiate a theoretical framework from laws/principles and mechanisms, and it attempts to highlight the power of an intervention as a creative process.

Individual approaches/methods/theories are the description and communication of one's personal practice, while beliefs are assumptions, values, core concepts and philosophies. Individual approaches/methods/theories combined with beliefs/values/core concepts/philosophies are parts of the individual clinician's theoretical framework for the practice of dance/movement therapy. Most of the literature in the DMT field describes theoretical frameworks. Laws/principles define natural phenomena in a discipline. Mechanisms explain how the laws/principles work. It has only been in the past few years that the profession has deepened into an explanation of laws/principles and mechanisms (Caldwell, 2018; Imus, 2012, 2017; Koch, 2018).

The chapter begins with a very brief introduction to laws/principles followed by an introduction to nine fundamental mechanisms. Dance/movement therapy beliefs are briefly introduced followed by an examination of methods and of the term intervention. A teaching methodology called A-FECT, adapted from Imus and Hervey (2004), is introduced at the conclusion of the chapter as a means of bringing the concepts together.

LAWS

A principle is a law, according to author Stephen R. Covey (2004). Laws in science pertain to matter, while laws in psychology pertain to information (Bechtel, 2008). In DMT, we are influenced by both laws of matter and information. Matter exists in form through the body and its movement, while information exists in feelings, thoughts, images and behaviors—the psychological content or story. It is important to note that separation of the laws of science and psychology is only conceptual, as the matter and information cannot be separated in human experience. Some examples of laws/principles applicable to dance/movement therapy can be located in Christine Caldwell's recent book (2018). Caldwell articulated eight principles from anatomy, physiology, neurobiology, physics and information processing that are applicable to DMT. They include—oscillation, balance, feedback loops, energy conservation, discipline, contrast through novelty, change, associations and emotions. Caldwell correlated each principle with symbolic values and combines form and content. A few laws that have also influenced my work derive from psychology and aesthetics—proxemics, symmetry operations, rhythmic synchrony, adaptation, perspective, experience and compensation. These principles are the foundation or scaffolding for the mechanisms. I originally began this chapter with a more in-depth look at the laws and their specific correlations to the mechanisms, but it became impossible to pursue this in-depth line of inquiry within the word limitations of the chapter. Further work is in progress.

MECHANISMS

Mechanisms explain how laws/principles work. Let's take the principle or law of proximity and deconstruct its mechanism within DMT. The law of proximity states that elements that are close together tend to be more related than elements that are farther apart (Moore, 2009). The mechanism for the law of proximity, as in all laws, includes the identification of its component parts. In the case of DMT, one example of component parts in proximity may include the formal descriptors of movement elements through one's orientation to space, weight, time and flow—Efforts. These movement elements can be formed, embodied or concretized through the creation of movement phrases that are closer (proximal) or farther apart (distal or polarity) in their shared or differentiated effort characteristics. The mechanism is the embodiment of the relationship of effort elements into a movement phrase or dance. These movement elements may become co-constructed by the DMT practitioner and their client into movement phrases to assist with feeling identification and mood regulation. Identifying mechanisms has become widespread in the creative arts therapies over the past four to five years (Caldwell, 2018; Imus et al., 2018; Koch, 2017). I identified nine fundamental mechanisms in DMT (Imus, Young, Downey, & Allen, 2018), though they are presented here in an evolved form, as they have continued to develop.

Nine Fundamental Mechanisms of DMT

The nine fundamental mechanisms were identified through an analysis of four sessions from my 40 years of evolving practice, education and research as a creative arts dance/movement therapist. Three were group sessions and one was an individual session; two of the three group sessions were with international participants. One of the international sessions had an interpreter, and one did not. During my analysis, I pursued the question of what is essential in my session and how did 'it' work for my clients' transformation to occur from the beginning to the end of the session? Further development in each category is ongoing as I seek to more specifically articulate the component parts (see Figure 9.1).

Fundamental Mechanism 1: Safety and Risk

Safety and risk include creating an environment within which risk and reward are balanced through the management of biobehavioral stimuli. A receptive nervous system is the goal, allowing the client to receive stimuli and respond without sympathetic overstimulation. Safety includes a shift from a defensive reaction of fight, flight or freeze into social engagement (Porges, 2011). It is, therefore, necessary for dance/movement therapists to prepare

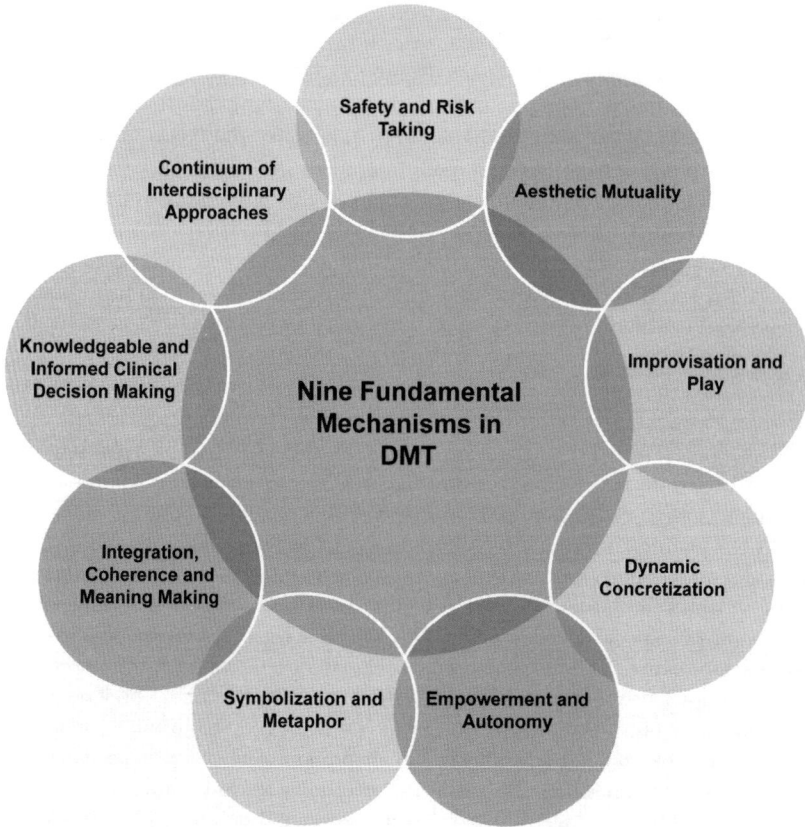

Figure 9.1 Nine Fundamental Mechanisms in DMT

the therapeutic environment to sound, look and mentally and physically be safe. This means that stimuli must be limited at the onset of treatment and throughout the session to prevent emotional dysregulation by the client, or lack of participation, to name just a few defensive responses.

Risk is related to the courage to try something new, seek novelty and shift patterns. May (1974) called it the courage to create, stating "courage is what is necessary to make being and becoming possible" (p. 13). May identified numerous types of courage, including physical, social, moral and creative. He identified creative courage as the most important because it "is the discovering of new forms, new symbols, new patterns on which a new society can be built" (p. 21). Courage is necessary for the client's commitment to treatment. Courage is fostered through the creative inspiration of the therapist at a pace that is commensurate with the client's pace. It includes the therapist's fostering the client's creating. Creative courage is therefore necessitated from the therapist as well as the client. This means that the dmt is willing to take creative risks in co-creating with their client. The therapist learns to embrace their personal fears in facilitation and leadership. I always tell my students that the client will only go as deeply as they are willing to go. Therapists' fears are influenced by their personal history and illustrate the need for their own psychotherapy, particularly to assist with countertransference.

Fundamental Mechanism 2: Aesthetic Mutuality

Aesthetic mutuality is the interactive movement behavior and reciprocal engagement in creating, the purest actualization of one of my personal DMT beliefs that creating breeds creating. Aesthetic mutuality is the therapeutic movement relationship for dance/movement therapy in the same way that the therapeutic relationship functions in verbal psychotherapy. Aesthetic mutuality is accomplished through the discriminating appreciation and participation in making specific qualities reflected in form. It is a relational feedback loop between the client and the therapist that develops bonds within a therapeutic relationship. It includes an additional stimuli and response from and to the creative manifestation—differentiating the creative arts therapies from verbal psychotherapy. Through this process, patterns of attraction manifest through aesthetic sensitivities, aesthetic preferences and aesthetic values. This is a feedback loop like those identified by Caldwell (2018) and Koch (2018).

AESTHETIC SENSIBILITIES

Aesthetic sensibilities are rhythmically coordinated, patterned signals/calls and their responses that are unmediated by thought. This includes temporally organized rhythms of vocal, facial and kinesthetic expressions of affiliation that are unconsciously adaptive within the therapeutic relationship (adapted from Dissanayake, 2009; Porges, 2011; Stern, 2010). Examples of this may be a sing-song vocalization filled with intonation that greets clients or scatting along with someone's movement rhythms, to name just a few examples. This stage of the mechanism relates to sensory information processing and remains more unconscious. The sensibilities will tend to more easily resemble and include developmental and familial patterns.

AESTHETIC PREFERENCES

Aesthetic preferences entail "more complex aesthetic responsiveness [that] requires one to employ and develop a predominately cognitive ability to appreciate (and participate in) the ways in which stimuli are combined with each other and with other humanly features" (Dissanayake, 1982, p. 152). Aesthetic preferences include conscious awareness of favored sensory information processing—iconic, haptic, echoic, gustatory—and their respective arrangement in perceptual forms, which provide the discriminating understanding of and embellishment for our attractions (or things we are drawn to). Aesthetic preferences require the therapist to understand their knowledge about, and bias in, their personal movement predilections. This is called body knowledge/body prejudice (Moore & Yamamoto, 2012) and is influenced through extensive practice of dance technique. It facilitates the dance/movement therapist's quick responsiveness from a solid background in the study of dance and movement. It is, "I know from my body. I have practiced this movement many times throughout my ballet and character dance training, from tap and musical theatre and through this familiarity I can more accurately respond." In addition, culturally informed personal preferences in pedestrian patterns of movement, or the movement signature, have been formed through the repetitive use of movement to meet our needs. This familiarity may perpetuate prejudice in not only how we observe and assess knowledge of movement but in its influence on countertransference with our clients.

AESTHETIC VALUES

Aesthetic values are the set of consciously discriminated and culturally determined beliefs and rules that underlie the dmt's discriminating actions via the call and response. Aesthetic values form patterns of attraction and discriminating appreciation of specific qualities reflected in form. The creation of forms and the representational perception of the forms are "one method of promoting effective interpersonal communication and satisfying relationships" (Hinz, 2009, p. 10). "Representational diversity" is a term that art therapists use to describe differing points of view (Hinz, 2009, p. 10). Aesthetic values previously identified by dance/movement therapists include: the general in the specific, freedom, symmetry (Hervey, 2000), flow (Imus, 2012), beauty, authentic expression and touch (Koch, 2017), though many others may exist. This pattern of attraction includes cultural bias, which may link to the therapist's countertransference.

Fundamental Mechanism 3: Dynamic Concretization

Dynamic concretization is the action-oriented process of making art, dance, music, drama and poetry through an energetic exchange of feelings, thoughts, sensations and memories into an explicit form. This includes "bringing concrete form and containment to sensations, images, feelings, and thoughts, (SIFT) to gain objectivity in viewing one's own creation and forming a new perspective" (Siegel & Bryson, 2011). The forming of objects within the experience is intentional but may have unconscious motivation. In DMT, dynamic concretization may also be referred to as embodiment. Embodiment means a concrete expression of some idea or quality. The concretized form is perceptually understood through formal aesthetic art elements such as space, line, kinesphere, efforts, shape, intonation and so on. Aesthetic mutuality and dynamic concretization together create what Dissanayake (1992, 2009) and Koch (2017) refer to as the aesthetic experience.

Fundamental Mechanism 4: Improvisation and Play

Improvisation and play are the spontaneous expression of imagination, typically without planning. This mechanism does not require concrete form and may not come from guidance from the dmt. Improvisation and play do not need reciprocity or the relational feedback loop. It may be random, exploratory and often nonlinear. This mechanism involves the search for replication through modeling as in play, as well as the search for novelty as in improvisation. These qualities of improvisation and play allow for freedom and are often more unconscious, expansive and may activate divergent thinking.

Fundamental Mechanism 5: Symbolization and Metaphor-Making

Symbolization and metaphor-making are the linkage between matter and the story. It assists one in identifying similarities and differences in patterns. Symbols are simple to complex representations of experiences or implied experiences from past events to new events (Wright, 1979). Symbolization is the action of making symbols and is therefore a creative process. A metaphor is an implied comparison in contrast to an explicit comparison in a simile. Comparing and contrasting creative responses expands possibilities, leading to greater understanding and choices. It is equally as important to identify how a creative call and its response is like something else (simile) or is something else (metaphor) as it is to identify the difference between the creative call and its response. The difference or contrast becomes the springboard for creating something new.

Fundamental Mechanism 6: Coherence, Integration and Meaning Making

Integrate means combining one thing with another so that they become a whole. Dan Siegel (1999) defines it as "the linkage of differentiated elements of a system" (p. 64) and states that it "illuminate(s) a direct pathway toward health" (p. 64). The American Dance Therapy Association's (ADTA, 2016) definition of DMT highlights integration: "DMT is the psycho-therapeutic use of dance and movement for the integration of the physical, mental, social, spiritual, and cultural health of an individual" (para 1). Coherence is systematic, logical or consistency. Siegel (1999) believes that coherence is an outcome of integration and describes it; "as creating balance in the system between sameness and rigidity on one hand, and novelty and chaos on the other" (p. 330). Meaning-making is accomplished when our body/movement logically links together with our information/story. If they do not fit or are incoherent, this creates a tension or call/signal worth examining. Understanding is when the matter of information and the matter of biology fit. As Bechtel previously stated, the transformation in biology is of material. Transformation in psychology is of information (2008). To reiterate—DMT's definition is to transform the whole person (its material body and movement) and its story, thoughts, feelings and beliefs (information). The transformation of the story and meaning-making will be strongly influenced by the psychotherapeutic approach of the therapist. I lean toward a humanistic approach.

Fundamental Mechanism 7: Empowerment and Autonomy

The very nature of making something is a creative process and provides the freedom to make individual choices. Dissanayake (2009) described making art, dance, music, theatre and poetry as competence-building actions. Making art allows the client to feel an internalized locus of control: the client makes it, controls it and can choose to change the specific qualities reflected in any form. Art-making diminishes dependence on the therapist and empowers the client. Empowerment and autonomy promote self-efficacy, which, in turn, promotes empowerment and autonomy. "Self-efficacy and perceived control are the potential for enhancement of mood and of health in general" (Evans, 2007, p 93).

Fundamental Mechanism 8: Informed Clinical Decision Making

Informed clinical decision making is both a systematic classification and a rationale. The mechanism requires the dance/movement therapist to appraise, formulate/develop,

Table 9.1 Integration of Matter and Information

Transformation of Matter (form)	Transformation of Information (content-story)
Biological (bio)	**Psychological** (psycho)
Physical	Thoughts & Feelings
Body & Movement	**Social-Cultural** (social)
(kinesthetic-sensory-perceptual components)	(affective-symbolic-cognitive components)

intervene and evaluate. Decisions on interventions must be informed through assessment of the identified form through movement components and their accompanying content in the form of the story and vice versa. Appraisal tools within dance/movement therapy are required as per the Standards of Education for Approved Master's Programs in DMT. Movement observation and assessment tools that are suggested come from movement observation systems like Laban Movement Analysis, Kestenberg Movement Profile and Bartenieff Fundamentals. The assessment tools provide the difference in making decisions that are intuition driven and decisions that are appraisal driven. The challenge here is in the quickness required to assess and make a decision during practice. According to information processing theory, our sensory memory is no more than three seconds. This is when we pick up or select which movement to develop. How can we rationally go through our entire taxonomy when choosing to intervene when we have only a matter of seconds? A background in dance and movement as previously mentioned is essential to enter the discipline and practice of DMT. It facilitates the therapist's responsiveness from the personal body experience.

Appraisal may also include the psychological paradigm that influences your choice of approach. If you are psycho-dynamic in your approach, the client's developmental history, transference and countertransference will be components that must be examined. They are a part of the story that influences the concretization of movement and the therapist's choice of intervention.

Fundamental Mechanism 9: The Continuum of Interdisciplinary Approaches

The continuum of interdisciplinary approaches is the delivery of DMT interventions along a continuum, including the aesthetic, therapeutic, recreational, educational, rehabilitative and psychotherapeutic (Rusch & Imus, 2016; see Figure 9.2). This mechanism has similarities to

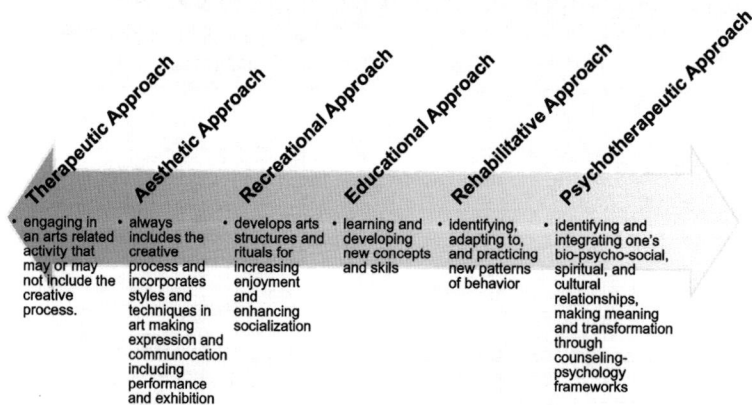

Therapeutic Approach	Aesthetic Approach	Recreational Approach	Educational Approach	Rehabilitative Approach	Psychotherapeutic Approach
• engaging in an arts related activity that may or may not include the creative process.	• always includes the creative process and incorporates styles and techniques in art making expression and communocation including performance and exhibition	• develops arts structures and rituals for increasing enjoyment and enhancing socialization	• learning and developing new concepts and skils	• identifying, adapting to, and practicing new patterns of behavior	• identifying and integrating one's bio-psycho-social, spiritual, and cultural relationships, making meaning and transformation through counseling-psychology frameworks

The seamless flow of intentional and integrated approaches is a part of the therapist's creative process.
An R-DMT and BC-DMT draw from all of their experience in dance and movement.
The DMT's creativity fosters patient's creativity.

Figure 9.2 Continuum of Interdisciplinary Approaches

informed clinical decision making because it is closely affected by the client's diagnosis and the environment where the treatment is taking place.

The continuum is not static. It invites the therapist to be flexible and make creative choices within a session along the continuum. The therapist may ask the client to concretize/embody their feelings into a dance (aesthetic) and then have the client practice it to strengthen muscles and to improve motor functioning (rehabilitative). The client may be asked to perform the dance at home to assist in relaxation and refocusing (therapeutic). The therapist may teach the client (educational) patterns of body connectivity to understand proxemics, physical stability and support. The therapist may then examine the psychological story about relational stability and support from the humanistic perspective of positive mutual regard or examine the psychodynamic perspective of transference and countertransference for further assessment and intervention (psychotherapeutic). The combination of options along the continuum engages the therapist in responding creatively with the most effective intervention from the interdisciplinary approach to the needs of clients within the healing environment. This mechanism provides options for the information processing system that will best work to assist the client in learning. For example, the rehabilitative approach emphasizes the value of repetition and practice essential to working memory. The aesthetic approach focuses on sensory memory. The educational approach highlights the organization of information chiefly through chronology. The psychotherapeutic approach emphasizes meaning-making and its selection into long-term memory.

BELIEFS, METHOD/APPROACHES, INTERVENTIONS

Beliefs/Values/Assumptions/Core Concepts/Philosophies (Beliefs)

Mechanisms explain how DMT works. What explains why dance/movement therapy works? Author Stephen R. Covey (2004) states that beliefs, values, core concepts and assumptions explain why something works within a discipline. I am referring to the vast array of words— beliefs, values, assumptions, core concepts and philosophies as beliefs for this publication. Table 9.2 is a list of dance/movement therapy beliefs that I have accumulated over numerous years but that should not be considered by any means a complete list. The construction of a more complete list would be beneficial for the DMT discipline.

Theories, Approaches and Methods

Theories, approaches and methods are influenced by the therapist's individual beliefs, assumptions, core concepts and philosophies. They differ from principles and laws because they are not phenomena that are considered proven by a discipline. Theories/approaches/methods describe one's individual way of working and ways in which one's practice is described to others (Burnham, 1999). Marian Chace's theories/approaches/methods of DMT included four core concepts—symbolism, therapeutic movement relationship, rhythmic group activity and body action (Chaiklin & Schmais, 1993). Her core belief was that dance is communication. Much has been written about methods and individual beliefs (theoretical frameworks) as exemplified by the founding figures in the discipline. Theoretical frameworks are essential in academic training and have laid the groundwork for the

Table 9.2 Shared Beliefs, Assumptions, Core-Concepts, Philosophies

DMT Core-Concepts, Shared Beliefs, Assumptions & Values Within an Embodied Therapeutic Relationship

– Dance/movement is a physical release of kinetic energy in DMT.
– Body and mind are inseparable. Hence you can move the body to move the mind and vice versa; bidirectional.
– Neuropathways are triggered, altered and created through dance/movement therapy, fostering new behaviors and affective states.
– Dance/movement therapy is developmental, functional, expressive and communicative.
– Creativity is fostered and enhanced through dance/movement therapy; creating breeds creating.
– Dance/movement is contagious and increases one's motivation for action within a DMT session.
– Dance/movement reflects one's personality, culture, gender, race, ability and age within DMT.
– Dance/movement therapy allows for a ritualization of experience.
– Movement is the mediator between our internal perception and external environment within DMT.
– Dance/movement is relational within a DMT session.
– Dance/movement is stabilizing and mobilizing within a DMT session.
– Internal and external consciousness are both elicited through dance/movement therapy.
– Dance/movement is an extension system and helps define one's culture within DMT.
– Dance/movement is both the means of assessment and intervention tool in a dynamic reciprocal relationship in DMT practice.
– Dance/movement may enhance one's sense of autonomy, self-control, mastery and self-esteem within a session.
– Dance/movement fosters beauty and truth as well as their expression within a DMT session.
– Meaning-making occurs through DMT.
– Dance/movement alters one's moods through the creation of biochemical and neuropathways within a session.
– Dance/movement comes from inside out and from outside in within a DMT session.
– Dance/movement therapists trust the wisdom of the body.
– Dance/movement within a DMT session can be receptive, re-creative and creative.
– Dance/movement is embodied culture within a session.
– Dance/movement is adaptive within a session.
– Rhythmic movement increases interpersonal cohesion within a session.
– Rhythmic movement assists in identifying and organizing speech, thoughts, feelings, images, sensations and behavior within a session.
– Dance/movement may be symbolic within a DMT session.

profession. Defining laws/principles and their mechanisms as previously mentioned is necessary for the discipline to grow.

Interventions

A dmt's theoretical framework informs their intervention choices. The DMTCB (n.d.) requires candidates to define their "Movement Interventions and Rationales":

> Demonstrate perception of movement cues and reflection back to client(s) dynamically developing movement to lead to fuller expression. Explain logically and clearly what is observed, what is responded to and why in client(s) movement. Explain what movement intervention is made and why. Describe thematic material and how it reflects intrapsychic issues.
>
> (p. 4)

What is observed, what is responded to, and why, leads us to interventions. Interventions, which are numerous throughout a DMT session, generate action within the mechanisms to bridge the dynamic tension from the current movement presentation/form and its accompanying story/content toward the desired outcome. Interventions are the heart of the therapist's creative process in DMT. The therapist takes what is observed, what is existing and available, and formulates/develops the movement in predictable and unpredictable ways with the client (Rusch & Imus, 2016). An example of an intervention may be to ask your client to create a dance that represents a thunderstorm. A follow-up intervention may be to ask your client to relate the thunderstorm dance to their expression of anger. Formulation and development (from fundamental mechanism 8-clinical decision making) emerge from the therapist's creative process. The less structured and more adaptive the therapist is to the client's call, the more creative the response by the therapist. It is the therapist's *creating that breeds the client's creating.*

Creativity theorist Robert Fritz (1991) stated that structural tension is essential to creativity. Applied to DMT, the tension-seeking resolution is from the current health situation as observed and appraised through the client's movement form and story, the reality, into the form and content of the desired health outcome. The interventions are the experiences or creative opportunities the therapist presents for the client to use to seek resolution. Interventions take the form of both verbal and nonverbal tasks, prompts, cues and instructions. Minor directives may be defined as prompts or cues. I prefer the term transitional task (Wright, 1979) when entering into a specific movement phase in my practice. The term transition assists in explaining the function of the prompt. A prompt during improvisation and play (mechanism 3) may simply be: "Let the music move you." During dynamic concretization (mechanism 4), there is a more complex transitional task: "Create a thunderstorm dance through your movement that has a beginning, middle and end." This task is transitional because it links or attempts to integrate (fundamental mechanism 5-symbolization and metaphor) the content and form to a specific theme. In dynamic concretization, or embodiment, the therapist is taking the story from the client. In this case, the story may be the inability to identify and express anger. The therapist is taking the client's story and transitioning it into a concretized form through a dance that has three phases or phrases.

These two examples presuppose that prompts and transitional tasks are more often verbal. In DMT, the prompts may also take the form of movement development and are called cues. Development of movement through a cue is the nonverbal equivalent of the verbal transitional task. All are transitional, taking what is present and available to the client and changing it in predictable and unpredictable ways (Arieti, 1976; Rusch & Imus, 2016). The client's words may be developed, as well as the client's movement. Interventions are bidirectional—moving the body to move the mind or moving the mind to move the body. Neuroscientists (Caldwell, 2018; Siegel, 1999) call this the bottom-up or top-down approach.

Movement Substances

How do we identify or categorize what we observe, what is present? What is available? What we are trying to seek resolution of or to? Caldwell (2013) called for us to identify what we seek to transform. Bechtel (2008) stated that the way to understand the mechanisms is to identify the various substances within the component parts that are produced or transformed. Bechtel also stated that it is "discovering the various substances that are produced or transformed in operations [that] provides a powerful heuristic for characterizing the operations themselves" (p. 987). This is what I tried to do when I originally analyzed the four

DMT sessions to determine how transformation occurred. The teaching approach called, A-FECT attempts to articulate the movement components and their substances.

What movement is available or is the call and response within aesthetic mutuality (fundamental mechanism 2) and dynamic concretization (fundamental mechanism 3)? What are our substances and formal structures in DMT? Is the DMTCB (n.d.) referring to these substances when they request the certificate applicant identify "movement processes" (p. 4)? Queyquep White referred to the "substances of movement" (Queyquep White, 2009, p. 219) through effort/shape and reported that she and Claire Schmais introduced Rudolf Laban's movement system of effort/shape into the educational content at Hunter College when they created the first degree program in DMT.

The profession of DMT has implicitly agreed upon using the language introduced by Queyquep White and Schmais from Laban, Lamb, Bartenieff, and Kestenberg to identify the substances and components of movement. Although these specific systems are suggested and not required by the current ADTA' s Educational Standards for Approved Master of Arts Programs in DMT (2017), a system for observing and analyzing movement is required in DMT training. Recently, Laban's system has been challenged (Caldwell, 2013) for its Eurocentric bias. As language and synthesis, Laban's taxonomies are invaluable. As a form of analysis, well-trained dance/movement therapists know that they must validate their assumptions and aesthetic preferences with their clients, as in the formation of all good analysis. Interpretation is not usually made in isolation by the observing dmts but is co-created with the client.

In 1999, when preparing for a conference presentation, I designated movement within a DMT session into three categories: functional/developmental, expressive and communicative. These categories are also included within the current Educational Standards for Approved Degree Programs (ADTA, 2017) and are labeled developmental, multicultural, expressive and communicative aspects of verbal and nonverbal behavior.

A-FECT MOVEMENT PHASES AS A TEACHING METHOD/ APPROACH

Today, I define these movement phases as aesthetic, functional, expressive, communicative and transformative (A-FECT), as adapted from my work in 1999 and with Lenore Hervey (Imus & Hervey, 2004) when designing a pedagogical approach to teaching DMT theory to students enrolled in a DMT master's program.

The phases are not completely exclusive or discrete, as they may overlap and occur simultaneously. They are roughly progressive. Each phase is not only related to the kinds of movement but appeals to particular client characteristics, fundamental mechanisms and modes of information processing such as kinesthetic, sensory, affective, perception, cognition and symbolic. Particular pathologies may influence how a client presents in relation to these movement phases, but the movement phases are not in and of themselves indicative of any pathology. Through an identification of movement phases, dance/movement therapists can better create interventions that will be most appropriate at a given time in the therapy, with a specific population and whether working with a group or individual. All populations may benefit from A-FECT because of the adaptive nature of the therapist's creative process within the development of the intervention.

In A-FECT, transformation occurs through both the psychological content (the story) and from the transformation of form (matter) through the body and its movements. It is

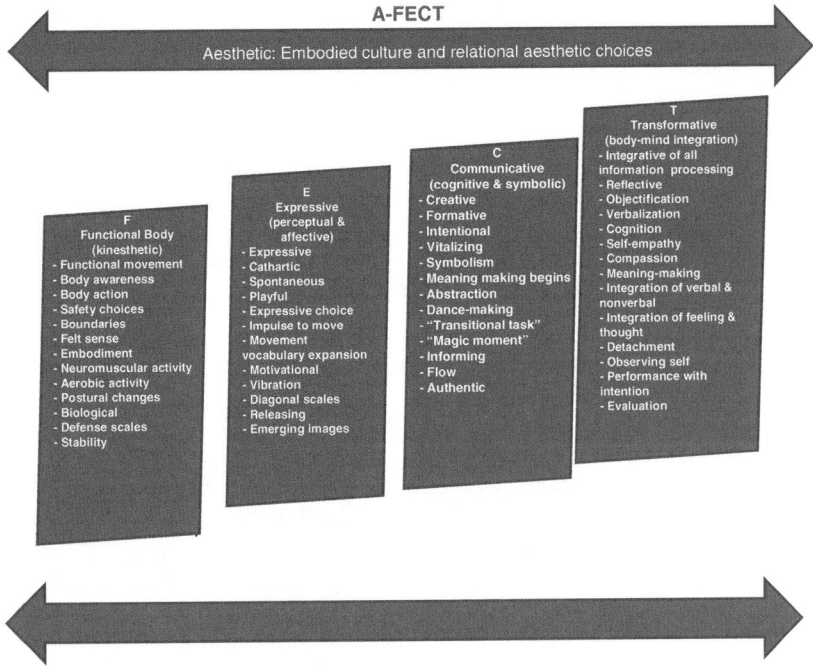

Figure 9.3 A-FECT

important to once again remember that the separation of matter from form and content is conceptual. The movement becomes objectified and is described through formalized aesthetic descriptions in order to be considered the media or substances which become formed. This teaching methodology provides an example for understanding the taxonomy in DMT as presented in this chapter. The A-FECT method includes a brief reference to the laws/ principles, mechanisms and interventions (see Figure 9.3). The laws/principles need further articulation as they relate to the mechanisms, but to do so is beyond the depth of the introductory nature of this chapter. I invite the reader to deconstruct their personal methodologies/approaches in the manner presented here to facilitate an understanding of how DMT works (mechanisms) and can best be communicated (approaches/methods) to others.

Aesthetic Movement

The "A" in A-FECT is set aside in writing because it is not a specific phase of movement. Rather, it defines aesthetic mutuality (fundamental mechanism 2) and dynamic concretization (fundamental mechanism 4); the aesthetic experience (combination of 2 & 4) and acts as the platform for the entire DMT session. All the movement phases are influenced by the embodied culture and our relational aesthetic choices. The aesthetic choices of what the therapist "picks up" (Chaiklin & Wengrower, 2009; Sandel, Chaiklin, & Lohn, 1993) determine the movement relationship, aesthetic mutuality and an understanding of the formalized movement language (e.g., Laban's Body, Effort, Shape, and Space; KMP rhythms; Bartenieff's connectivities) that describes the movement and its formation, dynamic concretization. Dance/movement therapists pick up the components or substances of movement that they are drawn to, through their aesthetic sensibilities, aesthetic preferences and aesthetic values (see aesthetic mutuality-fundamental mechanism 2). Dance/movement therapists make transitional tasks both from their personal aesthetics and from what they pick up and respond to from the client through the therapeutic movement relationship. Creating breeds creating, so there is reciprocity—co-creation. The entire session becomes a work of art (fundamental mechanism 2-aesthetic value of flow), which is why I prompt the client(s) to name the session at its conclusion (fundamental mechanism 5-symbolization and metaphor). The influential beliefs here are: culture is embodied, dance/movement within the therapeutic movement relationship is adaptive, dance/movement is contagious and increases one's motivation for interaction, dance/movement is relational and creating breeds creating.

Functional/Developmental Movement

The "F" in A-FECT stands for functional/developmental movement and is the practical operations of the body to perform movement tasks to meet the needs of the individual. Dance/movement therapists often respond to the quality or dynamics of the movement performed by the individual through effort/shape and/or developmental movement patterns. This includes encouraging in the patient the observation of not only kinesthetic action but body sensation: interoception, exteroception, proprioception and visceroception.

This phase is a very common place for the therapy to begin. The client may be completely new to DMT, may feel uncomfortable or embarrassed about moving and may be restricted in movement vocabulary. The primary goal is getting the client moving and identifying accompanying felt senses, or kinesthetic awareness. Interventions are often educational (mechanism 9-continuum of approaches) and are focused on functional movement, sensory and body awareness or attention to basic physiological functions like breath, perspiration or heartbeat. Movement may be simply action-oriented, consisting of warm-up suggestions to release physical tension, making safe choices (mechanisms 1-safety and risk) in the movement or establishing appropriate physical intrapersonal and interpersonal boundaries (mechanism 1-safety and risk).

The movement may be aerobic or strength building (mechanism 9-continuum of approaches) rehabilitative and/or focused on postural changes and total body connectivities to improve basic body functioning. Dance/movement therapists intervene with the quality of the movement as it relates to the specified therapeutic outcome. If symbolization is used (mechanism 5-symbolization and metaphor), they will tend to be assigned concrete meaning: "This movement is like chopping wood." In terms of the relationship, the goal of this phase is the establishment of physical safety and control, stability and trust, on a body level (mechanisms 1-safety and risk and mechanism; 7-empowerment and autonomy). An example of a belief here is that functional and expressive contents of movement are interrelated to activate the physical body and motivate its expression (Bartenieff & Lewis, 2002).

Expressive Movement

The "E" in A-FECT represents expressive movement and relates to the physical channeling of emotional energy and tension discharge. This may be improvisational and playful (mechanism 3-improvisation and play) and may not require a transitional task, nor reciprocity with the therapist. Movement may come more from the unconscious and need for motoric release as related to unconscious motivation and affectual impulses, not functional.

Expressive movement is also a place where many people begin therapy. These clients may be more comfortable with their bodies and may be able to enter spirited, playful, exploratory or spontaneous movement without much concern for appearances (mechanism 4-improvisation and play). The movement may be associated with feelings, and it may have a cathartic or releasing effect. Interventions are focused on the impulse to move and expansion of movement repertoire; clients make expressive choices based on feelings. Images and metaphors may emerge spontaneously with the movement (mechanism 5-symbolism and metaphor), but the meaning may remain unclear. Much of the work is autonomous (mechanism 7-empowerment and autonomy). A transitional task may not be necessary from the therapist. Although safety remains important, there is an emphasis on risk taking in working with expressive movement phase (mechanism 1-safety and risk).

The assumptions and beliefs of this phase include but are not limited to: creativity is fostered and enhanced through moving, dance/movement reflects the personality, the unconscious may surface as mobility shifts, dance/movement alters one's moods and the dance/movement comes from the inside out—not the outside in like in the functional phase.

Communicative Movement

The "C" in A-FECT stands for communicative movement which becomes more symbolic and metaphoric (mechanism 5-symbolization and metaphor) as it intentionally seeks to be understood and communicated. Communicative movement is defined as movement that must be witnessed and requires a sender, receiver and the creative manifestation. This is when patients have responded to a transitional task that is thematic based, as per the call of the therapist. The movement responses take on a new form through dynamic concretization (mechanism 3-dynamic concretization), are more symbolic and metaphoric (mechanism 5-symbolization and metaphor) and work to achieve coherence and meaning (mechanism 6-integration, coherence and meaning making). The dance/movement therapist's interventions are more individualized in this stage because they aim to more coherently bridge the structural tension within the current reality to the desired health outcome.

Communicative movement is rarely where people begin DMT, and working with this phase takes work to achieve. There is a distinct shift from the two earlier preparatory phases, Functional/Developmental and Expressive, into this movement phase, which is more intentional in its transitional task of deliberate formation of content into form and form into content. Material that arose in earlier phases in images or spontaneous movement is now intentionally embodied into phrases of movement or into narratives. The therapist intervenes by designing specific transitional tasks that help the client shift into making purposeful movement phrases or dances. The role of witness and mover is essential here. The call and response feedback loop are crucial to this communication movement phase, highlighting the power of aesthetic mutuality (mechanism 2-aesthetic mutuality). Symbolism and/or metaphor development tend to be more abstracted in the movement, evidenced by associated images or words (mechanism 5-symbolization and metaphor).

In this phase, the goal is communication. The client makes aesthetic choices in order to communicate affect and/or inform the dance more effectively with newly realized meaning. Formalized descriptors of the movement are often intentionally selected and developed by both the client and the therapist to foster coherence (fundamental mechanism 6-integration, coherence and meaning-making). The results of the movement phase are often in subtle but profound shifts into intentional meaning and vitalization. The fundamental mechanisms in this movement phase are dynamic concretization; symbolization and metaphors; integration, coherence and meaning-making; empowerment and autonomy; continuum of interdisciplinary approaches and clinical decision making. Clinical decision making, which is pervasive throughout a session, is more selective here. This is where the role of evaluation is crucial. The therapist may have to encourage the client to re-form their concretized forms if there is not progress toward session goals or if the dynamic tension between current reality and intended reality is not coherent and/or progressing. The DMT beliefs at this phase are: dance is communication, dance reflects the personality and dance/movement is both the means of assessing and intervening—to name just a few.

Transformative Movement

The "T" stands for transformative with a core task in this movement phase of conscious reflection and integration (mechanism 6-integration, coherence, and meaning-making) of form and content brought forth from the previous phases. It may involve the repetition of created movement phrases or performance of complete dances (mechanism 9-aesthetic choices on the continuum of approaches). In either case, the function is to reflect back upon, or objectify, the creation with the intention of greater conscious understanding, self-empathy and rational evaluation through the development of an observing self (mechanism 6-integration, coherence, and meaning-making). Making meaningful links to life outside of the therapy session is central to this phase. The work at this level may eventually lead to greater compassion with self and others, as well as detachment from previously self-identified material (mechanism 9-psychotherapeutic on the continuum of approaches).

Interventions may include encouraging the client to write or talk about the created dance with the goal of integrating tacit and explicit knowing, feeling and cognition, body and mind or somatic awareness. This phase is the culmination of coherent communication between the self, the concretized creative material and the dance/movement therapist (mechanism 6-integration, coherence, and meaning-making). The results are transformational.

The values, beliefs and assumptions from Figure 9.2 influencing this phase include: the development of congruency between verbal and nonverbal communication, dance/movement is the mediator between internal perceptions and one's external environment, and dance/movement integrates the body-mind.

CONCLUSION

Working to clarify a common set of beliefs and assumptions takes time, but it is essential to transform a practice and make it successful (Covey, 2004). The time has come in the discipline of DMT to clarify our common, not individual, set of beliefs, principles/laws and mechanisms. How do we do what we do and why do we do what we do are the guiding questions. Early DMT theorists set the stage by describing what they did (methods) and why (beliefs, assumptions, core concepts, philosophies and values) by developing *individual* theoretical frameworks. How DMT works—or mechanisms—is still the discipline's growing edge. With such a multitude of choices toward transformation, what movement phases (A-FECT) do I accentuate to assist my client in meeting their health goals? What interdisciplinary approach (continuum of interdisciplinary approaches) do I take to assist the client with understanding? How do I develop a therapeutic movement relationship (aesthetic mutuality)? What content and movement form do I develop (dynamic concretization)? How (symbolism and metaphors, empowerment and autonomy) do I formulate transitional tasks (creative interventions) to assist clients in resolving the structural tension between where they are and what their desired outcome may be? I have outlined how my personal beliefs inform my choices. My strongest assumption is that creating breeds creating. It is a belief that all of the therapist's intervention choices lead to co-creation with their client of new forms, followed by their integration into meaning. More needs to be written to reach agreement on the discipline's laws and mechanisms, not just the approaches and methods from the founding few. This is particularly true as the discipline has advanced and become more culturally diverse. The founding few, however, have created a platform upon which we can further create. Their creating has brilliantly bred ours.

REFERENCES

American Dance Therapy Association. (2016). *What is dance/movement therapy?* Retrieved from https://adta.org/faqs/

American Dance Therapy Association. (2017). *Standards for education and clinical training.* Retrieved from https://adta.org/wp-content/uploads/2015/12/ADTA-Standards-for-Education-and-Clinical-Practice-effective-January-1-2023.pdf

Arieti, S. (1976). *Creativity: The magic synthesis.* New York, NY: Basic Books.

Bartenieff, I., & Lewis, D. (2002). *Body movement: Coping with the environment.* New York, NY: Taylor & Francis Group.

Bechtel, W. (2008, December). Mechanisms in cognitive psychology: What are the operations? *Philosophy of Science, 75,* 983–994. https://doi.org/10.1086/594540

Burnham, J. (1999). Approach, method, technique: Making distinctions and creating connections. *Human Systems: The Journal of Systemic Consultation and Management, 3*(1), 3–26. Leeds: Leeds Family Therapy & Research Centre & Kensington Consultation Centre.

Caldwell, C. (2013). Diversity issue in movement observation and assessment. *American Journal of Dance Therapy, 35,* 183–200.

Caldwell, C. (2018). *Bodyfulness: Somatic practices for presence, empowerment, and waking up in life.* Boulder, CO: Shambhala Publications.

Chaiklin, S., & Schmais, C. (1993). The Chace approach to dance therapy. In S. Sandel, S. Chaiklin, & A. Lohn (Eds.), *Foundations of dance/movement therapy: The life and work of Marian Chace* (pp. 75–93). Columbia, MD: American Dance Therapy Association.

Chaiklin, S., & Wengrower, H. (2009). *The art and science of dance/movement therapy: Life is dance.* New York, NY: Routledge.

Covey, S. (2004). *The 7 habits of highly successful people.* New York, NY: Simon & Schuster Publishers.

Crawford, P. (2018). *The arts are a shadow health service: Here's why.* Retrieved from https://theconversation.com/the-arts-are-a-shadow-health-service-heres-why-105610

Dance/Movement Therapy Certification Board. (n.d.). *Application for board certified-dance/movement therapist.* Retrieved from https://adta.org/wp-content/uploads/2017/08/BC-DMT-application-new-2.pdf

Dissanayake, E. (1982). Aesthetic experience and human evolution. *Journal of Aesthetics and Art Criticism, 41*(2), 145–155.

Dissanayake, E. (1992). *Homo aestheticus: Where art comes from and why.* New York, NY: The Free Press.

Dissanayake, E. (2009). The artification hypothesis and its relevance to cognitive science, evolutionary aesthetics, and neuroaesthetics. *Cognitive Semiotics, 5,* 148–173.

Evans, J. (2007). The science of creativity and health. In I. Serlin, J. Sonke-Henderson, & J. Graham-Pole (Eds.), *Whole person healthcare* (Vol. 3, pp. 87–103). Westport, CT: Praeger Publishers.

Fritz, R. (1991). *Creating.* New York, NY: Fawcett Columbine.

Hervey, L. (2000). *Artistic inquiry in dance/movement therapy: Creative alternatives for research.* Springfield, IL: Charles C Thomas Publisher Ltd.

Hinz, L. (2009). *Expressive therapies continuum: A framework for using art in therapy.* New York, NY: Routledge and Taylor & Francis Group.

Imus, S. (2012, October). *Soaring to new heights.* Paper presented at the 47th Annual American Dance Therapy Association Conference, Albuquerque, NM.

Imus, S., Downey, L., Young, J., & Allen, L. (2018, October). *Fundamental mechanisms in DMT deconstructing and reconstructing our use of relationship.* Paper presented at the 53rd Annual Dance/Movement Therapy Conference, Salt Lake City, UT.

Imus, S., & Hervey, L. (2004, December). *Unpublished self-study for the American Dance Therapy Association's committee on approval.* Symposium conducted at the meeting of the American Dance Therapy Association's Committee on Approval, Columbia, MD.

Koch, S. (2017). Arts and health: Active factors and a theory of embodied aesthetics. *Arts in psychotherapy, 54,* 85–91.

Koch, S. (2018, October). *Why DMT works: State-of-the-art research design to investigate therapeutic factors of dance therapy.* Presentation at the annual American Dance Therapy Association's 53rd Conference, Salt Lake City, Utah.

Moore, C. (2009). *The harmonic structure of movement, music, and dance according to Rudolf Laban: An examination of his unpublished writings and drawings.* Lewiston, NY: The Edwin Mellen Press.

Moore, C., & Yamamoto, K. (2012). *Beyond words: Movement observation and analysis* (2nd ed.). New York, NY: Routledge.

Porges, S. (2011). *The polyvagal theory: Neurophysiological foundations of emotions, attachment, communication, and self-regulation.* New York, NY: W.W. Norton & Company Ltd.

Queyquep White, E. (2009). Laban's movement theories: A dance/movement therapist's perspective. In S. Chaiklin & H. Wengrower (Eds.), *The art and science of dance/movement therapy: Life is dance* (pp. 217–236). New York, NY: Routledge.

Rusch, D. C., & Imus, S. (2016). The same new kid in another hood: Deep game design as creative arts therapy? In D. C. Rusch (Ed.), *Making deep games: Designing games with meaning and purpose* (pp. 167–191). Boca Raton, FL: Taylor & Francis Group.

Sandel, S, Chaiklin, S, Lohn, A, editors. *Foundations of dance movement therapy: The life and work of Marian Chace.* Columbia: Marian Chace Memorial Fund of the American Dance Therapy Association.

Siegel, D. (1999). *The developing mind.* New York, NY: Guilford Press.

Siegel, D., & Bryson, T. P. (2011). *The whole-brain child: 12 revolutionary strategies to nurture your child's developing mind.* New York, NY: Bantam Books.

Stern, D. (2010). *Forms of vitality: Exploring dynamic experience in psychology, the arts, psychotherapy, and development.* New York, NY: Oxford University Press.

Wright, J. (1979). Concept of a symbol. Lecture in *Introduction to Creative Arts Therapy course,* Drake University, Des Moines, Iowa.

CHAPTER 10

CREATING THE DANCE OF SELF
A Stage Theory of the Creative Process in
Dance/Movement Therapy

Kristine Purcell

INTRODUCTION

Dance/Movement Therapy, as one of the creative arts therapies, utilizes a creative movement process to facilitate change (Goodill, 2010). The foundation of DMT is the intrinsically creative and healing power of dance, discovered as a result of the modern dance movement (Bernstein, 1979; Levy, 2005). In exploration of the art form, teachers, dancers, and choreographers discovered expression more deeply meaningful than technique and aesthetic. Pioneers of DMT began focusing less on the dance product, such as a performance or technical perfection, and more on the process of expressing the internal, emotional content of movement (Levy, 2005). The body–mind connection sets the stage for the creative process in dance due to movement's ability to access preverbal states and unconscious material (Bernstein, 1981; Blatt, 1991; Koch & Fischman, 2011; Rodriguez-Cigaran, 2000; Sheets-Johnstone, 2009; Wengrower, 2016). The relationship between the two is reciprocal, meaning that a change in the body's movement/ posture effects a change in the mind both in patterning and insight, and vice versa (Bernstein, 1979, 1981; Halprin, 2003; Koch & Fischman, 2011; Levy, 2005; Wengrower, 2016). Creative exploration of movement leads to developing new patterns, repertoire, and insights, which are then integrated through the embodiment process (Levy, 2005). Koch and Fischman (2011) discuss theories of embodiment and enactment as applied to DMT. In enaction, the client simultaneously engages in formation and discovery of his or her world: movement creates this world which is then expanded upon by the contributions of the therapist and other members of the group. Dance expresses one's inner world as thoughts and feelings take physical form; reciprocally, movement triggers thoughts, feelings, and memory. These founding principles mentioned earlier—creative potential and healing power of dance, emotive quality of expressive movement, access to unconscious and preverbal material, reciprocity of body–mind connection, and embodiment/enactment—build part of the DMT creative process that will be defined in stages and components and explored through the remainder of this chapter.

COMPONENTS AND STAGES

Creativity is a complex concept involving a number of stages and components, unconscious and conscious material—all encompassed within the art of dance and subsequent theory of DMT. This chapter describes the creative process of the client in DMT, delineating how its stages and select components lead to therapeutic change.

In the research phase of the theory explained in this chapter, a concept analysis was completed on the topics of creativity, therapeutic change, and DMT to define and clarify the former two as they are manifested within the latter. Through literature review, the author extracted stage theories proposed in each concept and elements necessary to each. Components and stages were compared across all three categories (creativity, change, DMT) through the tables pictured here (see Tables 10.1 and 10.2). Similar processes in each stage

Table 10.1 Theorist/Author and Stages in Models of Creative Process (1–3), Therapeutic Change (4–6), and Dance/Movement Therapy (7–12)

1. May	Encounter	Engagement	Brewing	Sudden insight		
2. Evans, J. (2007)	Inspiration	Preparation	Incubation	Insight	Execution	Evaluation
3. Nachmanovitch (1990)	Invocation		Work		Thanks	
4. Prochaska, DiClemente, & Norcross	Pre-contemplation	Contemplation	Preparation	Action	Maintenance	
5. C. Hill (3-stage helping model)	Exploration		Insight		Action	
6. Gladis (2008)	Figure/Energetic Formation	Wants/Needs	Contact/Receiving	Satiation Signal	Integration	Completion/Closure	Opening to new experience
7. Chace	Warm up		Theme Development		Closure	
8. Kleinman	Explore	Discover	Acknowledge	Connect	Integrate	
9. Fletcher	Subjective Experiencing	Identifying & Reflecting on Content	Identifying the Actions and/or Mechanism	Linking		
10. Meekums	Preparation	Recognize	Incubation	Illumination	Evaluation	
11. Shreeves	Experience		Deepen	Communicate		
12. Goren-Bar	Contact	Organization	Improvisation	Central Theme	Elaboration	Preservation

(Adapted and expanded from table designed by Ellen Schelly-Hill, 2007)

Table 10.2 Components Delineated Within Integrated Stage Model

Stages Combined →	Experience	Exploration	Development	Insight/Action	Resolution
Components					
Present Moment	x	x	x	x	x
Unconscious		x	x	x	
Conscious	x	x		x	x
Cognitive Processes	x	x		x	x
Affective Processes	x	x	x	x	x
Interaction/Solitude	x	x			x
Receptivity	x	x		x	
Improvisation	x	x	x		
Play	x	x	x		
Self-actualization				x	x

were identified, the stage progressions were explored through movement by the author, and titles were selected that encompassed the work of each stage.

The completion of analyzing and comparing the theoretical tenets of DMT with creativity and therapeutic change revealed how the components common to creativity and therapeutic change were manifested in the movement principles of DMT. The findings of this research explained in this chapter includes a description of the stages and the components as they occur, which then lead to progression through the stages. Tools and concepts in dance education and composition will provide examples of how each component and/or stage manifests through the unique healing, moving art.

Ten components falling in various combinations under five stages emerged from analyzing the concepts and theories of creativity, therapeutic change, and DMT. The stages are as follows: Experience, Exploration, Development, Insight/Action, and Resolution. The following ten elements appear in unique combinations within each stage, present in some, absent in others, facilitating a complex creative change evolution: present moment awareness; interplay of conscious and unconscious processes; cognitive processes; affective processes; interaction vs. solitude; receptivity; improvisation; play; and self-actualization (Bernstein, 1979; May, 1975; Purcell, 2012; Zinker, 1977).

In order to fully understand the interrelationship between the constituents and the stages during which they actively contribute to the creative process, a brief definition of each is necessary:

- Present moment: simply put, this is awareness of the here-and-now; movement and the body are the vehicle through which the present moment is immediately experienced (Sheets-Johnstone, 2009).
- Unconscious processes: movement accesses unconscious material (Bernstein, 1979; Levy, 2005; Wengrower, 2016); improvisation mirrors primary process thought and often provides the inroad to this material: "internal states are made conscious through external expression" (Schmais, 1985, p. 20).
- Conscious processes: act of defining and exploring movement metaphor or creating representational movement or motifs, as well as assignment of meaning to movement expressions (Meekums, 2002).
- Cognitive processes: Kleinman's (2016, p. 154) cognitive markers most succinctly summarize cognitive processes within DMT. The Exploration marker describes a

process of divergent thinking often facilitated through improvisation as the individual explores possibilities of movement and expression; Discovery and Acknowledgement mirror problem finding (Runco, 2007) in which a theme is selected; Connecting relates to analogous thinking (Runco, 2007) or application of a self-discovery; and Integration correlates to transformative abilities in which the individual incorporates a new insight and changes his or her behavior because of it.

- Affective processes: movement is a direct expression of emotion, providing the vehicle through which emotion can be expressed (Bernstein, 1979; Sheets-Johnstone, 2009).

- Interaction versus solitude: relationship with therapist and group members; this can occur through therapist mirroring the client's movement, bringing awareness to affect, attitudes, patterns (Chaiklin & Schmais, 1993; Levy, 2005); additionally the unique movement of the therapist and group members contributes to the repertoire of the individual (Koch & Fischman, 2011). Solitude will relate to those moments of focusing internally; of personal movement expression versus group movement expression; of personal relation/interpretation of movement metaphor.

- Receptivity: openness, awareness, often facilitated through mirroring or reflection of movement or inviting exploration.

- Improvisation: spontaneous experimentation with movement; unplanned movement. In dance technique, improvisation can be a tool for discovering movement potential or capacity, to become more aware of the moving self, become more empowered and integrated through free explorations of movement with others (Lavender & Predock-Linnell, 2005). Utilized similarly in DMT to access the unconscious, discover new ways of moving, explore a theme, shift between levels of consciousness, and free oneself from a pattern (Bernstein, 1979; Meekums, 2002; Rodriguez-Cigaran, 2000; Wengrower, 2016)

- Play: a way to transform, structure, and work through unconscious material in a non-threatening way (Russ & Fiorelli, 2010); used in DMT to explore new behaviors and to work with metaphors.

- Self-actualization: realizing one's potential, becoming whole. In DMT, this may manifest in expanding one's repertoire (Blatt, 1991); integration of the mind, body, spirit that occurs through expressive movement (American Dance Therapy Association, 2010, *What is dance movement therapy?*; Bernstein, 1979).

Stages in the Creative Process in DMT

Each of the five stages will now be presented, with a discussion of how each component defined earlier contributes to the facilitation and progression of the stage.

Experience

The first stage in the creative process requires an encounter with a source of inspiration. In DMT attention is brought to the body in the present moment through the warm-up. The warm-up begins to facilitate the conscious body–mind connection through physical sensations inherent in activating the muscles. Divergent thinking, a cognitive process of brainstorming several ideas around a concept, is achieved through movement play and improvisation, when the client explores a variety of movement in order to open the self to the possibility of development and expression. The therapist may encourage the client to explore variations in size, speed, location of a movement in the body or the dynamic and qualitative aspects of movement as set forth by such movement analysts as Laban[1] or Kestenberg (Levy, 2005). By introducing a variety of movements, the client may begin to unlock unconscious material held at the nonverbal body level. Rogers (1954) discusses openness as a necessary component of the first stage in the creative process, welcoming all stimuli into awareness. Other such stimuli are affective processes, due to the interrelationship between body movement, sensation, and emotion; feelings begin to arise as the client connects to his or her body in the present moment and as unconscious material begins to surface. The client will not yet have full awareness of the connection, as this kind of development occurs further on in the creative process, but may simply feel the significance of the associated emotion. Acolin (2016) outlines how movement expresses inner states, is a mode of communication, and reveals personality, and how one can interpret emotion from observable movement qualities. Simple examples might include buoyant movement evoking joy, or use of space correlating with level of confidence. Interaction fuels the first stage of Experience, through the cooperative and reciprocal navigation of the warm-up between therapist and client(s). Chaiklin and Schmais (1993) describe the acute observations and receptivity of Marian Chace as she guided her clients in warm-up: she did not enter the room with a plan or prescription for movement but picked up on affective and interactive cues from her clients to determine how to start, always beginning with the clients themselves. She mirrored the emotional states and communications of her group members to understand, offer acceptance, and begin a process of cohesion with the rest of the group. With the awareness and inspiration engendered through the warm-up, and the sense of safety and community, the group or session can progress to the second stage in the creative process.

Exploration

This second stage engages all components except self-actualization, as no new insights have been made to integrate into oneself. The Experience of the body and movement expression during the warm-up sets the stage for further and more conscious present-moment exploration of a theme. Again, the therapist enters the equation as an interactive component through movement reflection, labeling of movement, verbal prompts, or provision of structure encouraging this exploration. Conscious and unconscious processes overlap during the second stage; movement draws up unconscious material from its connection to preverbal experiences while the client and therapist work on bringing awareness to movement expressions and patterns and shaping them into representational movement (Sheets-Johnstone, 2009). This may take shape in the therapist attuning to a select movement and encouraging repetition or clarification of this movement. Play and improvisation are tools for the exploration of the second stage (Bernstein, 1979; Halprin, 2003; Levy, 2005; Rodriguez-Cigaran, 2000; Wengrower, 2016). Improvisation accesses primary process thinking, in which spontaneous movements flow from one to the next. Like the cognitive process of divergent thinking, movement improvisation provides a multitude of variations on a theme. Play gives form and structure to the unconscious material and inherent emotions accessed through improvisation (Greenacre, 1959) and an opportunity to experiment with these new behaviors in a safe way; through the imagery and symbolism of play, difficult situations and emotions can be confronted, yet the individual is protected in the fantasy of the play, the separation provided through metaphor. Additionally, through embodied play, the client can feel more assertive and confident in the experimentation with newness. Both components elicit feelings of freedom, permission, spontaneity, enjoyment, fluidity, and openness or receptivity (Hayes, 2006), all of which serve the creative process through encounter and experimentation with a variety of coping options and solutions. As can be gathered from this identification of feelings, affective processes simultaneously contribute to and arise from the Exploration stage. Firstly, feelings of safety are necessary to freely explore unconscious and symbolic movement material and must be present to engage in improvisation and play. Secondly, movement is the direct and external expression of internal feeling states (Bernstein, 1979; Sheets-Johnstone, 2009; Young, 2017). As mentioned in the chapter's introduction, the emotional content of dance expression may constitute part of the healing processes inherent in dance (Levy, 2005). Exploring movements related to an initial source of inspiration—a movement or sensation that arose in the warm-up—provides the opportunity for the individual to connect with and communicate a personal feeling. Choreographic tools, such as changes in size, tempo, quality, embellishment, or instrumentation—performing the movement with a different part of the body (Blom & Chaplin, 1982)—may be ways the therapist utilizes her dance background to assist in variation or exploration of the movement that aids the progression of the creative process and further exploration of emotions. Concretely in the session, this stage may manifest as synchronous or reciprocal movement between client and therapist. The client may make a movement, which is then mirrored by the therapist, perhaps with a chosen quality, such as strength, accentuated to emphasize this affective content of the original movement. The client may then repeat this movement and both may go on in call-and-response manner, echoing this movement to one another, continually playing and improvising with variations, honing in on the relevant thematic and affective content.

Development

The continued movement exploration of a feeling or theme through the use of tools for movement variation leads to a period of incubation during the third stage in the process. Shifting focus from exploring a variety of movements, the movement expression begins to narrow onto a central theme (Goren-Bar, 1997). This is likely one of the most familiar stages of any creative process, as the individual becomes submerged in the process of creation. Unconscious processes dominate, as "spontaneous movements become more obviously expressive of the intrapsychic material" (Meekums, 2002, p. 17). The dance contains more affect as spontaneous movements flow into one another, each coming from and leading to an emotive place, succumbing to the primary process. Enactment (Koch & Fischman, 2011), as mentioned in the introduction, summarizes this process: the client moves, giving form to the unconscious through symbolism and imagery and thus creating an imaginary environment to be explored and discovered; simultaneously, the client experiences and makes discoveries in this environment through the felt experience of movement. The process occurs in the present moment, as the movement cannot be planned but must be discovered. At this point in the session, the therapist becomes less active as a "choreographer" of variation, as she may have done in the second stage, and drops into holding the space to provide containment for the deepened exploration. This occurs through the therapist's presence—not simply physical but emotional presence, sense of grounding, and kinesthetic empathy (Young, 2017). The acceptance of the client is communicated both verbally and through the reflection of the client's movements, allowing the client to deepen their movement expression. True reflection of the client's movement can only occur through the therapist's thorough knowledge of his or her own body and an understanding of the symbols and metaphors inherent in movement. By dropping into this deeper felt sense in his or her own body, the therapist likely sets the stage for the client to sink into this stage of incubation. During this stage, imagery likely arises, its content potentially rich in emotion, metaphor, and symbolism; the deep meaning of these arising images, however, still lies beneath the surface of consciousness, not yet in the conscious awareness of the mover. The "world" of the client, as referenced in enactment (Koch & Fischman, 2011), is created and discovered through this imagery, and the therapist's presence, her ability to be with and support this imagery of the client's, can contribute to the deepening of the creative process (Young, 2017).

Insight/Action

It is during the fourth stage that connections form between the movement exploration/ improvisation and personal meaning for the individual (Fletcher, 1979; Hill, 2004; Kleinman, 2016; Meekums, 2002; Shreeves, 2006). Meanings may suddenly become clear as a memory is triggered through the movement, and metaphor may arise from the imagery of the third stage. Unconscious processes allow for new associations to be made between seemingly unrelated movements or expressions, a characteristic aspect of creativity as something new comes into existence (May, 1975). This stage again requires receptivity, in the openness required to allow for such new connections.

Of note, this is also a prime opportunity to briefly address the concept of everyday creativity, a potential of all humans—as opposed to eminent creativity, a more advanced cognitive function, in which an artistic masterpiece results (Kaufman & Sternberg, 2007; Rogers, 1954; Wengrower, 2016). Everyday creativity simply results in something new evolving from already existing parts, put together in a unique combination to result in a novel solution to a problem. Such could be said about the therapy process with individuals whose cognitive, emotional, and social selves suffer from some impairment or disintegration. Artistic genius, or a resulting product, is not the goal or intention of therapy; instead, personal therapy calls for increasing self-awareness and self-integration. Thus the therapist and client work together to uncover strengths already existing in the client, and with the added creativity of the therapist and/or group members to devise a new solution to the client's present state of discomfort.

Returning to the fourth stage in the creative DMT process, consciousness comes into play through meaning-making. The creative dance weaves together the experience of the body's expression, exploration of this expressive potential, and development of the movement theme. Metaphors arise and are explored. The metaphor is an important piece of DMT, as it can hold meaning on several levels, revealing the client's deeper thoughts, feelings, and behaviors that were previously unconscious (Bernstein, 1979; Blatt, 1991; Halprin, 2003; Meekums, 2002; Rodriguez-Cigaran, 2000; Sheets-Johnstone, 2009; Shreeves, 2006; Wengrower, 2016). Transformation, a cognitive process of making a new combination of information (Russ & Fiorelli, 2010; Standler, 1998), may appear through further movement exploration of the metaphor, consciously and intentionally, thus putting the Insight into Action. A movement motif or performance of a movement experience may be used but is not necessary. In Kleinman's (2016) description of cognitive markers, Connect relates one's movement and emotional expressions to one's present life, and Integrate provides a summary and learning opportunity for how to handle a similar experience in the future.

By applying or embodying the insight discovered, finally the individual reaches the component of self-actualization. The new discovery or new awareness is moved, felt, acted upon by the dancing individual, incorporating the change into one's self and adding to realization of one's potential. Personal expansion occurs through the broadening of one's movement repertoire, and the individual changes as a result of embodying these new qualities or actions. An example of this stage may be to try on and practice a new movement through play to experiment with the new movement or gain assertion and mastery over the action (Hayes, 2006). The movement, the action, powered by affective processes inherent in the connection between movement and emotion, is "essential to embodied learning and change" (Halprin, 2003, p. 230). Again, the link between dance movement and emotions deserves emphasis. The power of the modern dance movement existed in the authentic expression of human experience and emotion (Levy, 2005). Observers could relate to the realness of the dance, the truth of the feeling in the movement. Without this connection, dance was merely a spectacle, as ballet had begun to fade into pure technical feats. Similarly in therapy, true personal change is much more likely to occur when tied with a strong emotion (Fink, 2010). DMT pioneer Trudi Schoop's idea of "full feeling expression" (Bernstein, 1979, p. 42) supports the movement toward self-actualization in this fourth stage, facilitating acceptance and ownership over all parts of oneself by embodying one's emotions fully, thus leading to greater integration of the self.

Resolution

This fifth and final stage is a process of closure and containment. While verbalizations likely occur throughout the process to bring awareness to the self or to encourage and develop exploration of a theme, verbal processing of the session typically classifies it as dance/movement therapy and not simply therapeutic dance. However, as noted in Acolin (2016), "movement need not enter consciousness to be meaningful and cause change" (p. 324). Changes made on the body level have been seen to effect change on a mental level and do not always necessitate conscious awareness or analysis. The limitation to the evidence supporting this statement, however, is that it was drawn from a short-term study and could not predict lasting change. When appropriate and necessary, a conscious process of verbalization facilitates insight into events in the client's life from the dance expression, leading to greater self-awareness and understanding. Catharsis of emotion may occur through the expressive movement of dance, but is not sufficient for therapeutic change. Transformation, whether large or small, is the goal of therapy, and this is done through conscious integration of the movement experience and the discoveries made—through identification of symbols and their meaning in reality. Kleinman's (2016) cognitive markers, Connecting and Integrating, involve relating the movement experience to an issue in the client's life and reorganizing oneself around this new discovery, respectively. Interaction contributes to these connections, as therapist and/or fellow group members make their own observations, thus adding to the individual's interpretation and insight. Affective processes persist now and run the gamut of emotion; the movement expression may have given form and awareness into, for example, deep, viscerally felt grief from a loss, or strong assertion in finally (literally) standing up to a "foe" in movement play. In the stage of Resolution, however, it is this writer's belief that an overall encompassing feeling should be of completion or resolve; just as Chace worked to wrap up her clients' movement expressions to provide closure and prepare them for life outside the therapy room (Chaiklin & Schmais, 1993). Often, this finalization begins through a movement cool-down or closing ritual such as a series of deep breaths or stretches, and completed through the verbal processing, the latter grounding the experience in conscious awareness.

Finally, self-actualization enters once again. According to May (1975), creativity expresses the self as a manifestation of one's unique thoughts and feelings. The self, and one's potential, is more fully realized through its creative expression and all the more deeply through the physicality of that expression. A selection of the author's master's thesis summarizes this point:

> Movement is the most fundamental expression of one's being because it is pure self expression. All parts of the self reside in the body: the physical, emotional, and psychological. The body and its movement *are* one's being, and communication through symbolic use of the body creates a profound connection to and formation of the self. In this way, movement can create deep, self-actualizing change.
>
> (Purcell, 2012, pp. 95–96)

We Do Not Dance a Straight Line

While the stages of the creative process in DMT have been described in a sequential manner, it is necessary to discuss the true non-linear pathway the dance takes. This is best described through the metaphor of a spiral, an image that arose through analysis of literature and themes during the author's thesis process (Purcell, 2012). Therapeutic change and creative products are not the result of completing one stage, ticking off a list of requirements, and moving onto the next stage. Both involve beginning, exploring, deepening, narrowing, resurfacing to incorporate new information, broadening, deepening again, and so on and so forth as one would follow a spiral into and out of its coil. Stages may be revisited or repeated, as is inevitable in the process of personal change (Prochaska, DiClemente, & Norcross, 1992). Similarly, a choreographer does not simply set a series of dance steps and leave it unchanged, unmodified. The DMT client may continuously discover and develop new ways of expressing an emotion to deepen his or her self-understanding and improve upon themself. These processes do not have an end point but do have endless potential. New insights fuel further processes of self-exploration, and self-exploration opens the individual to new sources of inspiration, thus igniting another creative process.

An additional similarity between the spiral and the creative process is that it cannot be fully represented concretely; the infiniteness of a spiral cannot be drawn in finite form. The creative process of DMT can be described but to be fully understood and integrated, it must be experienced. This may be a difficulty, yet it is also a unique strength of the field: a difficulty in the limitations of words to describe the embodied, expressive, experienced process of DMT, yet a strength because of its uniqueness. There is nothing like dance—to integrate and express the fullness of the self in body, mind, and spirit.

THE ROLE OF THE THERAPIST

Through the author's years of clinical experience, the integral role of the therapist has become all the more apparent in the progression of the creative DMT process. DMT itself cannot in fact, occur without a therapist. As a master of dance and movement expression, the dmt holds an array of tools necessary to make interventions appropriate to the stage of the creative process and functioning level of the client or group. These tools spring from both psychotherapy and dance as they necessitate knowledge of group processes, psychodynamics, movement observation/assessment, choreography, and perhaps most importantly, the therapist's own self-awareness. The therapist's experience as a dancer is central to his or her role as dmt. Marian Chace utilized her own feelings in response to the kinesthetic empathy when reflecting her clients' movements (Chaiklin & Schmais, 1993). The technique of mirroring allows the therapist to become attuned with the client by "feeling with" in movement expression (Levy, 2005; Young, 2017). The safety and acceptance that is communicated through this attunement allows for each participant to influence one another. Recent writing on the therapeutic movement relationship more explicitly defines the unique aspects of this relationship and addresses the concept of mutual creativity. Young (2017) found through phenomenological research that several dmts experienced reciprocal creativity as they became attuned with their clients in the movement relationship. Additionally, as creativity occurs between therapist and client, the relationship between the two is deepened. A conclusion can thus be drawn that the therapeutic movement relationship and the creative process can continuously and reciprocally build on one another.

It is this writer's proposition that in the cases of psychiatric populations with multiple or severe deficits in cognitive, emotional, or social functioning, the therapist promotes or embodies the components necessary to facilitate a creative process; for example, the therapist can suggest variations of movement shapes and qualities to promote divergent thinking or become playful in interaction with the client in order to promote play. Simultaneously, as the creative arts therapies draw on the strengths of the individual, the dmt will have the awareness and observation skills to recognize the already present attributes of the client, utilize these to facilitate creativity, and add only where necessary with appropriate interventions. With the therapeutic relationship in place, the therapist can aid in increasing the client's self awareness through embodiment, mirroring, and labeling of the client's movements; reflect latent emotional content; and communicate acceptance and therefore provide safety for exploration through mirroring and structuring of movement material. The therapist can model components such as improvisation and play, and suggest meaning through movement metaphors and identification of patterns in the client's expressions. All of these interventions contribute to the creative process, reflecting necessary components delineated in the stage and component section of this chapter.

ADDRESSING CLINICAL POPULATIONS

It is one thing to consolidate a concept analysis into a theory, as has been done in this chapter; it is quite another to be aware of and facilitate this with a clinical population, given the complexity of the process. However, it is the goal of this section to simplify these concepts and describe the role of the therapist as a model or catalyst for components of the process. A narrative of how the creative process presents in a session will further concretize the process for readers.

Reach Out, See Me

A group of four individuals gathered in a bright, stuffy dayroom on an inpatient psychiatric unit one warm June day. The group consisted of a man (J.), a woman (E.), a transmale (C.), and a transfemale (F.); all commonly struggled with chronic depression, several attempting or considering suicide. The therapist entered and provided a brief and simple introduction to DMT: it was about connecting with oneself and one another through movement; expressing feelings for which words were not sufficient; understanding oneself in a new and different way. The four participants presented with flattened, restricted affect, even flow, narrowness, and concave torsos—classic indicators of depression. This group was in a place to start with slow and small movement, perhaps simply shape-flow (role of therapist in sensing and responding to existing repertoire). Members were invited to begin connecting their feet with the floor, then to notice their breath (Experience—present moment, conscious awareness, receptivity). The therapist noticed subtle movement and encouraged connection of this movement with the breath; the group was invited to allow movement to grow from the breath. The focus of each participant was on themself: eyes closed, shifting, breathing, rolling, tensing in a dance of shape-flow (initial solitude). One movement led to another as flexions extended, fingers gently tapped from pinky to thumb (perhaps beginning stages of improvisation), torsos subtly grew and shrank with the breath. This internal process was interrupted, though not apparently to the upset of the original members, as two additional female patients (T. and M.) entered the room; their entrances mirrored the already even and quiet atmosphere of the room. Gazes shifted to the door and micro-smiles crossed the faces of the movers. To address the changing dynamic and facilitate the component of interaction, the new members were explicitly welcomed. At this moment, for the therapist at least, a symbolic movement emerged of "opening our eyes." As members continued to explore movement impulses connected with their breath (Exploration), they were invited to open their eyes, to begin not only welcoming their new fellow members into the room but also to the movement, and into acceptance through seeing one another. Were there similarities between any pairs of movers? In shape, body part, rhythm? Synchronous movements rippled through the group. The previous quiet of the room was punctuated by expressions of amazement—exclamations and moments of laughter (affective processes).

A sense of commonality was felt through the room. Then a pause; perhaps the resonance of this connection (Development, present moment, unconscious, affective process). As the therapist looked around the room, each participant was observed to have become more internally focused and in some form of self-touch, just after this connection with one another (interaction versus solitude). A question was posed to bring attention to the self-directed tender, caring gestures: Do each of you notice how one part of you is holding another? As this was labeled, the theme of self-touch and care restarted the movement process and members caressed and cradled their own hands, arms, and torsos (Development). As each person's arms enclosed around his or her own body, E. commented "It's like a hug." Then almost immediately, M. responded quietly, "No one hugs." Sadness crossed her face and swept like a soft, yet chilly shadow over the group. The group sat there, holding themselves—the gesture was both a symbol of the self-care needed in the group and a stark sense of aloneness. It was such a far stretch to move from this place of enclosure and simultaneous isolation to openness, connection, and vulnerability with each other—it would feel rushed and unnatural (therapist's sense of own body and understanding of organic movement transitions). The earlier theme of "opening our eyes" was reiterated and the group was asked how they might reach out with gaze, then possibly gesture, and finally reflection of a peer's movement (proceeding into Insight/Action through bringing movement to conscious awareness; cognitive process of transformation by intentionally exploring metaphor). Eyes glanced across the circle. Hands stroked down their own arms and hands encircled one another. Implicit in the light, careful, slow and deliberate self-touch was profound care and tenderness (affective processes, body–mind connection). Slowly, each pair of hands, at first one curled around the other, began to open, expand, extend out; fingers like the delicate petals of a flower blossoming in the warmth of the group. The movement ended with a cohesive gesture of arms partially extended, cupped hands directed into the middle of the circle. And breath. Although not all participants actively moved the symbolic expression or joined in the synchrony—F. moved between sitting back in her chair and leaning forward, supported by resting her elbows on her knees—all did end in an advancing posture, hands forward, if not yet reaching. The group ended up mirroring F.'s posture, whether consciously or unconsciously, effectively communicating acceptance and solidarity to this lone member who did not intentionally, though likely did unconsciously, join in the group movement.

After a brief pause for resonance and Resolution of the movement, the group began sharing. They discussed connection and acceptance felt in seeing their peers imitate the movement. E. expressed wonder in the immediate and organic mirroring between her and her peers, unplanned and without conscious intention, even noting the connection as "magic." J. said he felt understood. The room grew quiet again with these revelations; a sense of resolve gently settled in the same way as the sadness had fallen before, yet this time calmly and reassuringly (affective processes). It even took the form of the slight drowsiness that accompanies relaxation. C. stated he needed a nap; when this feeling of tiredness was reflected he said, "I won some battles today." He went on to share how members of his family had accepted his gender transition—he finally felt SEEN and shed tears as he acknowledged the weight of this acceptance, his own self-acceptance and that from his family (application of symbolism accessed through movement, conscious processes, self-actualization). After affirmations were shared with C., the group turned their attention to F., still in a sunken posture, with sad, hopeless affect. Likely she felt some resonance with C. in their similar transgender journeys—yet F. had not yet felt the acceptance from her family. "I don't feel like trying," she said, so softly it was barely audible. She barely had a voice and with little voice, with little sense of self, she had a limited ability to access her creativity, to dive into that process with her peers. Yet her peers were there to fill in the missing pieces (interaction). J. labeled depression as "quicksand": the more one struggles, the faster one sinks. He related to F., reaching the point of wanting to give up and give in to the quicksand, feeling that struggling and fighting got him nowhere. A final question was posed: what is something from this metaphor we can use? What is the way we escape the quicksand? (Application of symbolism, Insight). And C., without speaking, reached her hand up and out (Action).

CONCLUSION

In support of DMT's foundation in the creative art of dance, this chapter set out to explain the creative process of dance/movement therapy. As described earlier, dmts and their clients move through stages of Experience, Exploration, Development, Insight/Action, and Resolution to create therapeutic change. Orientation to the body's sensations and impulses awakens the client to an inner experience in need of exploration and discovery. The creative influence of the dmt contributes to broadening the client's repertoire and possibilities for exploration, providing the client with the opportunity to access relevant unconscious material stored in the body and in movement. Movement symbolism provides a vehicle through which the client can play with psychic material on a more concrete level through the use of imagery. In playing with these symbols, the client may discover a particular insight in how the movement expression holds meaning in his or her life. Once this meaning is discovered, the client may deliberately act on it, integrating the new feeling or action. Finally, the movement process reaches a point of resolution. With conscious awareness, the client processes the multifaceted meaning of the movement that arose from the unconscious to facilitate new self-understanding and access to the resources to integrate it.

Recognizing some of the cognitive and emotional limitations of the clinical populations with which many dmts work, the author's hope is that further understanding of this theory will contribute to more informed practice. The increased insight into the creative change process as delineated in this chapter will allow the therapist to utilize each intervention and component at the appropriate stages in the process in order to address the presenting problem and create an opportunity for change.

Finally, the author hopes that the ideas put forth in this chapter reconnect dmts with the founding theory of the field: the power and wisdom of dance.

NOTE

1. There are currently differing opinions surrounding the continued use of the Laban Movement Analysis system, due to recent news about his role in Nazi Germany. Historically, Laban's system has been used widely in dance/movement therapy observation and assessment.

REFERENCES

Acolin, J. (2016). The mind-body connection in dance/movement therapy: Theory and empirical support. *American Journal of Dance Therapy, 38*(2), 311–333.
American Dance Therapy Association. (2010). *What is dance/movement therapy?* Retrieved from www.adta.org/Default.aspx?pageId=378213
Bernstein, P. L. (Ed.). (1979). *Eight theoretical approaches in dance-movement therapy.* Dubuque: Kendall/Hunt Publishing Company.
Bernstein, P. L. (1981). *Theory and methods in dance-movement therapy* (3rd ed.). Dubuque: Kendall/Hunt Publishing Company.
Blatt, J. (1991). Dance/movement therapy: Inherent value of the creative process in psychotherapy. In G. Wilson (Ed.), *Psychology and performing arts* (pp. 283–288). Amsterdam: Swets & Zeitlinger.
Blom, L., & Chaplin, L. (1982). *The intimate act of choreography.* Pittsburgh: University of Pittsburgh Press.
Chaiklin, S., & Schmais, C. (1993). The Chace approach to dance therapy. In S. Sandel, S. Chailkin, & A. Lohn (Eds.), *Foundations of dance/movement therapy: The life and work of Marian Chace* (pp. 75–97). Columbia, MD: The Marian Chace Memorial Fund of the American Dance Therapy Association.
Evans, J. (2007). The science of creativity and health. In J. Sonke-Henderson, R. Brandman, I. Serlin, & J. Graham-Pole (Eds.), *Whole person healthcare: The arts and health* (Vol. 3, pp. 87–105). Westport, CT: Praeger Publishers.
Fink, B. (2010). Against understanding: Why understanding should not be viewed as an essential aim of psychoanalytic treatment. *Journal of the American Psychoanalytic Association, 58,* 259–285.
Fletcher, D. (1979). Body experience within the therapeutic process: A psychodynamic orientation. In P. L. Bernstein (Ed.), *Eight theoretical approaches in dance movement therapy* (pp. 131–154). Dubuque: Kendall/Hunt Publishing Company.
Gladis, M. F. (2008). *Tales of a wounded healer.* Malvern: Wind Whispers Press.
Goodill, S. (2010). The creative arts therapies: Making healthcare whole. *Minnesota Medicine, 93*(7), 46.
Goren-Bar, A. (1997). The "creation axis" in expressive therapies. *The Arts in Psychotherapy, 24*(5), 411–418.
Greenacre, P. (1959). Play in relation to creative imagination. *Psychoanalytic Study of the Child, 14,* 61–80.
Halprin, D. (2003). *The expressive body in life, art and therapy.* London: Jessica Kingsley Publishers.
Hayes, J. (2006). Dance/movement therapy with undergraduate dance students: Special ingredients in the development of playfulness, self-confidence, and relationship. In H. Payne (Ed.), *Dance Movement Therapy: Theory, research and practice.* East Sussex: Routledge.
Hill, C. (2004). Theoretical foundation of the three-stage model of helping. In *Helping skills: Facilitating exploration, insight, and action* (pp. 25–37). Washington, DC: American Psychological Association.
Kaufman, J., & Sternberg, R. (2007, July/August). Creativity. *Change,* 55–58.
Kleinman, S. (2016). Becoming whole again: Dance/movement therapy for individuals with eating disorders. In S. Chaiklin & H. Wengrower (Eds.), *The art and science of Dance Movement Therapy: Life is dance* (pp. 139–158). New York: Routledge.
Koch, S. C., & Fischman, D. (2011). Embodied enactive dance/movement therapy. *American Journal of Dance Therapy, 33*(1), 57–72.
Lavender, L., & Predock-Linnell, J. (2005). From improvisation to choreography: The critical bridge. In J. Chazin-Bennahum (Ed.), *Teaching dance studies.* New York: Routledge.
Levy, F. (2005). *Dance Movement Therapy: A healing art* (Revised ed.). Reston: National Dance Association.
May, R. (1975). *The courage to create.* New York: W.W. Norton & Company Ltd.
Meekums, B. (2002). *Dance movement therapy: A creative psychotherapeutic approach.* London: Sage Publishers.
Nachmanovitch, S. (1990). *Free play: The power of improvisation in life and the arts.* New York: G. P. Putnam's Sons.

Prochaska, J. C., DiClemente, C. C., & Norcross, J. C. (1992). In search of how people change: Applications to addictive behaviors. *American Psychologist, 47*(9), 1102–1114.

Purcell, K. (2012). *Creating the movement of self-change: A concept analysis on the creative process and nature of change in dance/movement therapy* (Unpublished master's thesis). Drexel University, Philadelphia.

Rodriguez-Cigaran, S. (2000). *Becoming more of who you are: A literature review on the creative process in dance/movement therapy* (Unpublished master's thesis). Drexel University, Philadelphia.

Rogers, Carl R. (1954). Towards a theory of creativity. *ETC: A Review of General Semantics, 11*, 249–260.

Runco, M. A. (2007). *Creativity: Theories and themes: Research, development, and practice.* Burlington, MA: Elsevier Academic Press.

Russ, S., & Fiorelli, J. (2010). Developmental approaches to creativity. In J. Kaufman & R. Sternberg (Eds.), *The Cambridge handbook of creativity* (pp. 233–249). New York: Cambridge University Press.

Schelly-Hill, E. (2007). Components and phases of dance/movement therapy. In E. Schelly-Hill (Comp.), *ARTS 552: Therapy Relationship Skills I.* Philadelphia, PA: Drexel University.

Schmais, C. (1985). Healing processes in group dance therapy. *American Journal of Dance Therapy, 8*, 17–36.

Sheets-Johnstone, M. (2009). Why is movement therapeutic? *American Journal of Dance Therapy, 32*, 2–15.

Shreeves, R. (2006). Full circle. In H. Payne (Ed.), *Dance Movement Therapy: Theory, research and practice* (pp. 232–245). East Sussex: Routledge.

Standler, R. (1998). Sternberg's theory of creativity. *Creativity in Science and Engineering.* Retrieved from www.rbs0.com/create.htm#anchor1000010

Wengrower, H. (2016). The creative-artistic process in dance/movement therapy. In S. Chaiklin & H. Wengrower (Eds.), *The art and science of dance/movement therapy: Life is dance* (pp. 13–32). New York: Routledge.

Young, J. (2017). The therapeutic movement relationship in dance/movement therapy: A phenomenological study. *American Journal of Dance Therapy, 39*(1), 93–112.

Zinker, J. (1977). *Creative process in Gestalt therapy.* New York: Brunner/Mazel.

Part III

PRACTICE

CHAPTER 11

DANCING ACTIVISM

Choreographing the Material with/in Dementia

Beatrice Allegranti

INTRODUCTION

This chapter introduces feminist interdisciplinary dance movement psychotherapy (DMP)[1] and choreographic research, practice[2] and activism with people living with the rare diagnosis of young onset dementia (YOD), their families and the artistic team—Beatrice Allegranti Dance Theatre.[3] The international project builds on previous practice and research investigating the role of artistic processes in DMP (Allegranti, 2011, 2019), with a specific focus on challenging dominant discourses of relating in dementia.

Dementia is a worldwide concern, with an estimated 135 million people living with the diagnosis by 2050. As an umbrella term, the 'dementias' include several variations that are characterized not only (and in some instances not even) by loss of memory, as is public perception, but also significant impairment of language and communication and relating in the world.

There has been little impetus to provide specialist services for YOD in the UK, where services for older people can have a detrimental effect on a younger person (Burton-Jones, 2015). The body politics of age reverberate when people are mid-life and mid-career, often with families and living actively at the time of diagnosis. The medicalization of dementia framed as a pathological condition, while intended to reduce stigma and taboo, has often resulted in more stigmatization. A biomedical bias emphasizes cognitive deterioration and does not take into account personal and social experiences where it is understood that affective resonance endures (Allegranti, 2019). Within this complex milieu, the lives of partners, children, parents and friends are impacted, and a new way of relating must be found for all. This account of my work—to creatively reimagine dementia in the arts, health and justice together with notions of what constitutes 'self' and 'bodies'—speaks to these pressing sociopolitical needs in somatic, relational and aesthetic ways. To paraphrase Rosie Braidotti (2013), I seek to put the dancing body back into activism.

The urgency of this dancing activism speaks to dominant discourses across the Western world where dementia is depicted as a devastating 'loss of self' or even loss of humanity. A hypercognitive model of dementia equates the notion of 'self' with mind and mental function and language residing within bodies as 'containers' (Post, 2000). The limits of this 20th-century Anthropocentric humanism predicated on separation and binaries such as body/mind, nature/culture, subjective/objective, maintain the long-held view of the bodies as discrete entities.

Comprehensive critique of this Cartesian view of self/body has been in the area of posthumanism and feminist new materialisms (Harraway, 2016; Braidotti, 2013; Manning, 2013; Barad, 2007) or 'PhEmaterialism' as coined by Ringrose, Katie, and Zarabadi (2019), where *PhEm* refers to the blend of posthumanism and feminisms, materialism from the new materialist movement, and the capital 'E' highlighting education. I have adapted this term to include a capital 'M': PheMaterialism, thus foregrounding the material multiplicity across conceptual and political discourses that work towards counterhegemonic (anthropo-centric) understandings of bodies, affect and relating. In doing so, this writing considers what happens when insights from DMP, choreography and dementia are read through one another—with the aim of opening pathways for alternative narratives of human-environment relations to ethically flourish.

PHEMATERIALISM IN MOTION

Drawing on Erin Manning's (2013) use of the verb *bodying*, the PheMaterial Möbius (Figure 11.1), is a specially commissioned illustration offering a starting point for discussing the process of human-environmental relations. Inspired by Karen Barad's "agental realism: a shift away from representationalism—reflecting on the world from outside—to a way of understanding the world from within and *of being of the world in its dynamic specificity*" (Barad, 2007, p. 377, author's emphasis), this möbius moves beyond representation or metaphor for the body. Imagining this strip in motion, where inside and outside are continuous, leans towards a posthuman bodying of permeable, dynamic, dispersed, spatially and temporally specific (contingent) relating.

Bodies, therefore, do not only 'exist' in a network of human (bio-psycho-social) forces but are in Barad's (2007) terms '*intra*-acting', denoting the mutually constitutive process of

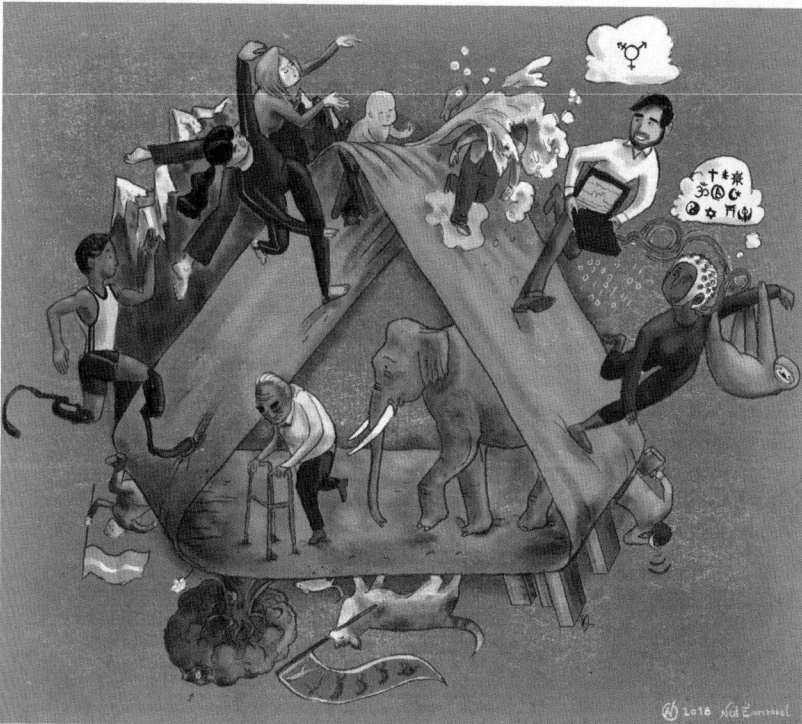

Figure 11.1 PheMaterial Möbius

Artist: Neil Max Emmanuel.

being *within* and *part of* the world rather than the interaction of separate entities. Bodying, *infolds* (Manning, 2016) where the line between body and environment is smudged and 'life' can be seen as an 'entangled' (Barad, 2007) system of relating. The entanglement includes human and non/more-than human bodies *intra*-acting with/in a network of language, biology, affect, cognition, ecologies, technology, embodied practices and power structures. As Barad states, "[E]xistence is not an individual affair" (2007, p. 3), and all these human and non-human things matter; they are all given equal value in this co-constitutive process.

Consequently, *bodying* can be described as a material-discursive process. This way, language does not need to be understood in simply discursive terms—but materially, too. Therefore, within DMP and dance practices, language can be considered as a product of material flows where the emphasis is not on what is said in terms of linguistic or speech acts but on "that which constraints and enables what can be said" (Barad, 2007, p. 146).

Working towards understanding the politics of discourse with/in dance and movement-based practices is a crucial counterhegemonic endeavor. A clear example of bodying as a necessarily material-discursive process is the intersectional body politics of age, gender, sex, sexuality, class, race, ethnicity and dis/ability. These material-discursive processes are ever present, subtle, in/visible, intersecting and changing throughout our lifespan. The implicit and explicit power differentials are often taken for granted, inside and outside the therapy room and/or artistic process. Much is at stake, and an ethical imperative involves generating our attention to intersectional body politics as they manifest within therapeutic and/or artistic practices and research. PheMaterialism, then, implies a progressive politics for the ethics of health and well-being with an enlarged sense of community (Braidotti, 2013).

Equally, materiality constitutes the assembling of human and non/more than human bodies such as, objects, entities and forces that together produce agentic power. By not reducing agency to what humans do and say, or to fix meaning based on one's articulation of 'experience', humans can be viewed as part of the wider vital materiality of the world. Given this tangle, I work towards what Alaimo and Heckman (2008) call *trans*-corporeal understandings: the inseparability of self and environment. In practice, I attend to distributed networks of agency across heterogenous elements and on different spatial and temporal scales, such as choreographic or clinical material (which is always movement material anyway), therapy room, dance studio, a song, objects, gendered bodies, family histories—all these are part of what can be described as an 'agentic assemblage' (Barad, 2007; Jackson & Mazzei, 2016). This writing aims to articulate agential relations between the connections of the assemblage (Ringrose et al., 2019) and in doing so, to illustrate how dementia is an ecological process distributed in the environment.

MATERIAL FOR LIFE

Resisting the singular agentic anthropocentric I/eye in research who authoritatively interprets and presents research findings (Taguchi, 2013), my intent is to present a multiplicity of realities and subjectivities in collaboration with the artistic team and families living with YOD.

Instead of the research 'data' and 'findings', I conceptualize the combined research and practice as '*spacetime* events' (Allegranti, 2019). The series of events act as both method and content and do not unfold chronologically, but 'infold' (Manning, 2016) across temporal and spatial scales. Past, present and future life stories of people living with YOD, their family carers and the artistic team are archived with/in moving-relating bodies, objects and texts. As such, the content of these events is always already in us as words, experiences, stories, movements, sounds and more-than-human environments (Allegranti, 2019; Jackson & Mazzei, 2016). Hence, of relevance is not only *who* but *what* participates in knowledge production. In PheMaterial terms, *knowing* comes from a direct material engagement with the world. My intent, therefore, is to describe how the profoundly relational nature of 'knowing' and 'being' are both inseparable and an ethical imperative in this project.

In what follows, I speak to this imbrication of *spacetime* events that pave the way for constantly evolving material-discursive (affective, bodily and political) changes. In this sense, the events enact micro and macro bodying activism for human others and for the dancer-choreographer-therapist-participant who is relating with the (movement and environmental) material.

Listening with Movement

The first *spacetime* event is interview-conversations in family homes, the hub of intimate relating. The (audio-recorded and transcribed) interviews[4] are a material-discursive process: I *listen with movement* and in doing so hear the 'vibrant' material moments (Jackson & Mazzei, 2016) in our exchanges, for example, expressions such as prosody of speech, vocal tension, volume of voice but also the more-than-human processes such as wider social and environmental structures. Also, by modifying my conversational approach to suit the person that I am speaking with (in the same way I might with someone who does not speak the same language as me) my intent is to collaborate in producing knowledges.

With this gesture of listening, I heard the body politics of family life: people living with YOD finding it increasingly difficult to navigate the geography of their own home, couples in their mid-life, single mothers with an adult child caring for them all making sense of their lives with dementia and how this affects their intimate relationships and everyday material engagements. As I listen, I am moved to recognize that the very process of engaging in all these activities are small acts of resistance, an everyday activism.

Making (the) Material

A constant in my creative process is my shift between authoethnographic (Allegranti, 2014, 2019) writing, movement improvisation and choreographic co-composition as part of choreographic or therapeutic relating. I employed this process when creating bespoke choreographic and accompanying sonic material in the studio with the four professional company dancers and musician. During this studio practice, the impetus for movement exploration and composition is the transcribed interview-conversations and my autoethnographic writing together with movement responses following the family interview-conversations.

Making (the) material was not only a space where choreography was undertaken. It was, in the Winnicottian sense (1971), also a 'holding' space. With the dancers, I facilitated movement improvisational tasks and verbal reflections[5] where the visceral and felt sense impact of lost, incomplete words, family relationships in turmoil, changing identities, fading memories, relationships with environments (natural, medical), symbolic and literal references was explored by the dancers, see Figure 11.2. As a team of artists working together, we articulated the impact of working with *this* dementia material on our own bodies, and in doing so, the bespoke material became a performance of selves (Allegranti, 2011), layered from the families' autobiographical, often intimate stories, whilst also combining the artistic teams'

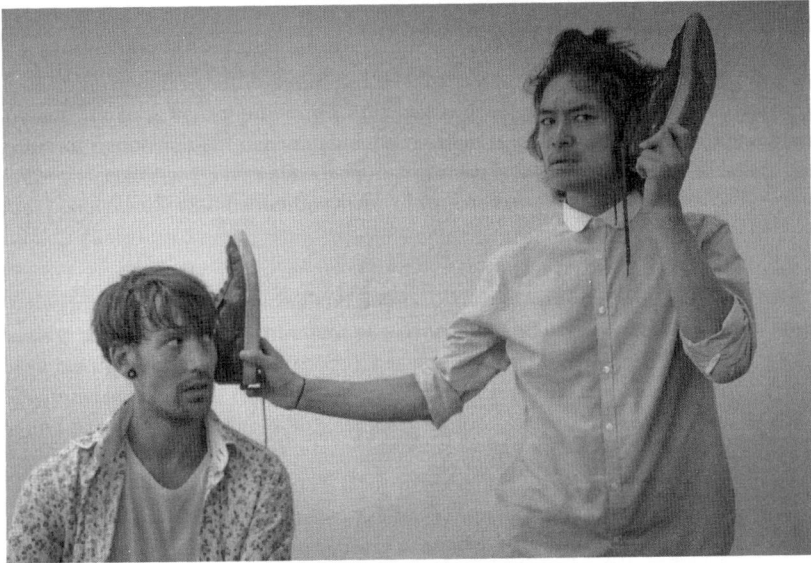

Figure 11.2 Luke and Takeshi, Public Performance at Crouch End Festival

Photo: Julia Testa.

verbal and movement responses to that material. Sabrina speaks to this tangling of stories, affects and memories after one of the studio practices:

> We're not pretending to have dementia; we put ourselves, as well, in it. I felt like in [the] rehearsals I was receiving something in return about my life that I can carry. It's something that really shifted my life.

The artistic import during this process allows for a disruption of participants' stories and working against representation (Ringrose et al., 2019). In doing so, we began to inhabit the other—as well as reinhabiting ourselves—the resultant bespoke choreography became a process of 'storying' life material. The dancers were not 'pretending to have dementia' as accessed through forms of role play or 'verbatim' performance. Instead, I facilitated the dancers through a process of *kin*-aesthetic prompts. I have adapted the word *kin*-aesthetic to include three aspects: the sense of movement, including interoceptive and proprioceptive awareness; the vital aesthetic process in forming movement (in artistic and therapeutic contexts) and the emergent material kinship during the process of witnessing and engaging in movement. This intersecting trinity of *kin*-aesthetic co-composition provides an epistemological gateway towards an intuitive understanding of the dynamic inseparability of selves and environments and allows the dancers to engage with the ubiquitous and tangled material layers of loss and life with dementia and thus extend their own understanding and capacities of relating in this context. The process highlights several ubiquitous factors crucial for artistic and therapeutic practice: how (the) material holds affective and intimate parallels as well as vastly different experiences from our own and, how the evolving choreographic process became a movement form of consciousness. It also highlights that the process of storying is not flat and fixed but open-ended; offering somatic, movement-based and political layers of dementia and everyday life.

Participatory Ecologies

The third *spacetime* event troubles embodied intersubjective relating (Allegranti, 2011, 2014) and is more akin to Manning's (2013) proposition of *participatory ecologies* inasmuch as an ecology touches on the everyday while moving beyond the individual and beyond the event. These one-and-a-half-hour events include an average of three to six families each session. The events comprise bespoke performances witnessed by families, followed by an invitation for families to join us in a collective movement improvisation response, see Figures 11.3 and 11.4. An option for verbal and written reflections is offered at the end. These events take place in a variety of spaces such as art galleries and studios, libraries and hospital wards. Shifting between artistic and therapeutic facilitation (Allegranti, 2011), I pay attention to the ethics of engagement

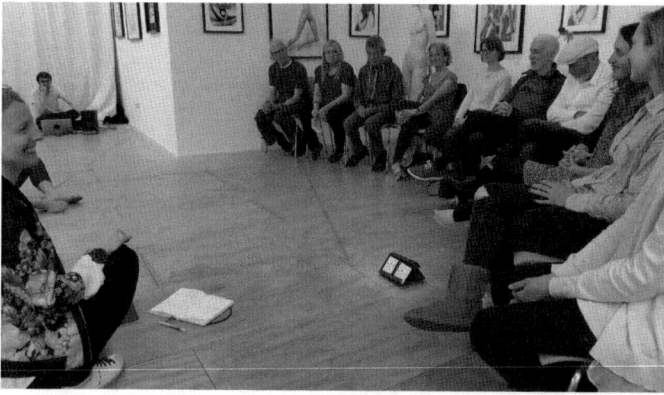

Figure 11.3 Participatory Ecology

Photo: Julia Testa.

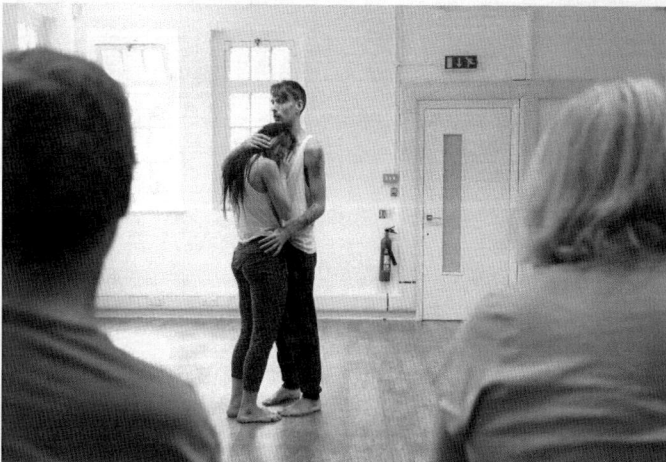

Figure 11.4 Bespoke Performance for Family

Photo: Aidan Orange.

such as trust, consent, safety, level of participation, and choice, and I maintain a strong witness position, assisting me to hold group process and enfolding material.

Performing bespoke choreographic and sonic material is the first step where the witnessing families, who have been interviewed, are already invested in the material and are perhaps 'reminded' of people in their personal life stories, their singular and collective identities, and their value as a collective. This collective remembering is a crucial aspect of relating, particularly for people living with dementia where control, independence and voice are personally and publicly challenged.

The act of witnessing and being witnessed during the bespoke performances holds neuro-affective impact both for dancers and families. Takeshi speaks to the unmediated nature of what is getting 'done' in this moment of performing and being witnessed by the families, by describing the process as "very special, because it allows us to be very attentive and very careful with what we do [it] feels like we are creating an umbilical cord between the performance and participants". Takeshi's visceral observation is also echoed by Luke, who speaks of the impact of being witnessed, "face-to-face, flesh-to-flesh, that is a bit more loaded or charged; allowing emotion to come". This neuro-affective recognition in witnessing and being witnessed (Calvo-Merino, Grèzes, Glaser, Passingham, & Haggard, 2006) during the bespoke performances offers opportunities to recognize and work with the tangle of personal and collective (family) processes. For people living with young onset dementia and their families, this may be crucial since it allows for an immediately *kin*-aesthetic way of facing the changes in their lives with a view to redefining and reimagining, as Jacquie, whose husband lives with Alzheimer's, said, "[T]he dances surfaced a lot for me as a carer and made me realise that I could use some sort of help, counseling or therapy. I've buried a lot".

The second participatory ecology component involves participant-led movement improvisations, including responses to the performance material, see Figure 11.5. The aim is to

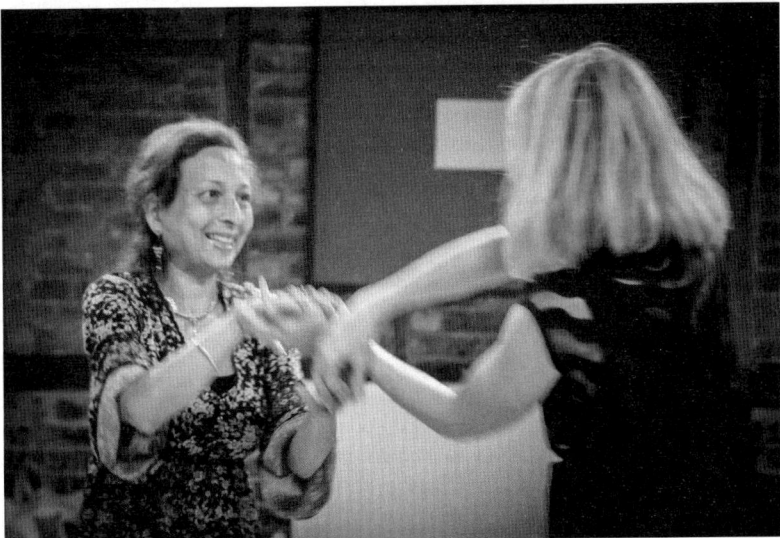

Figure 11.5 Movement Improvisation with Participant

Photo: Julia Testa.

invite participants to playfully make the material their own and in doing so, to creatively and affectively co-compose through gaze, gestures and micro and macro movements and voice. Luke referred to an 'elastic structure' capturing the process of overall safe holding and being prepared to let go of structure when participants take the lead and choose their own level of engagement. Elasticity also refers to the creative incipience of movement and relating (Manning, 2013) and notably, this is a distributed process: between people living with dementia and their family carers. Zaki, the adult son of Forhat, who was diagnosed with young onset dementia at 52, speaks to this distribution:

> We were both able to experience something in our own ways and get something independently out of it. It was incredibly liberating to see mum enjoy and be so engaged in dancing. It was the first time in a while I was able to leave her to herself and her own enjoyment without feeling guilt or responsibility.

Our *participatory ecology* became a *kin*-aesthetic assemblage for shared agency through a recursive loop of performing, witnessing and moving together. During this process, kinship extends beyond immediate family ties to other families, the artistic team and *with* the choreographic material and all the human and more-than-human forces that the material evoked.

Giving-Back

The material emerging from the bespoke dances contributed to the creation of an internationally touring dance theatre work *I've Lost You Only to Discover That I Have Gone Missing*, see Figure 11.6. Troubling the linear causality of 'story', this dance theatre piece opens into a wider ecology during every relationally contingent performance. The work aims to disrupt sociopolitical taboos about loss, intimacy and resistance and acknowledges the tensions of

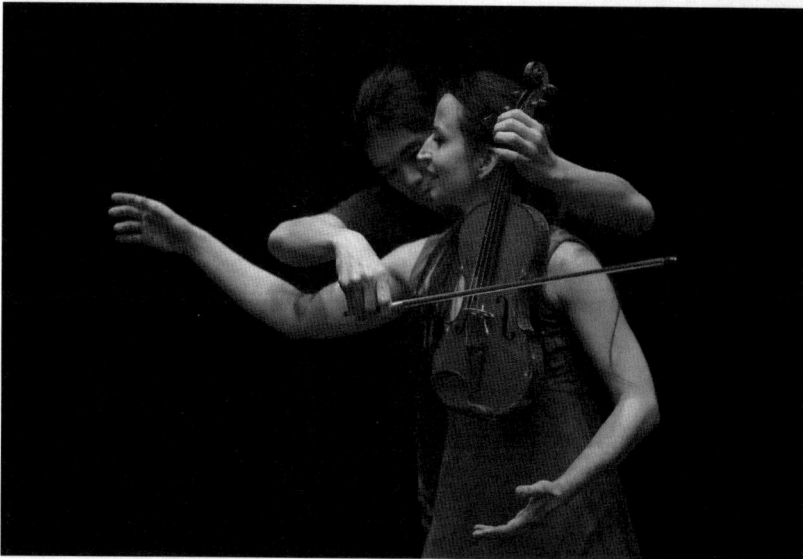

Figure 11.6 Takeshi and Aneta, Public Performance at Utrech Centre

Photo: Martha Kamminga.

our entanglements with others, with our environment and the paradoxical sense of dispossession in loss and grief, and every audience engages with this in different ways. To date, there have been 12 international public performances of the work. Some have been dementia-friendly studio performances and others in more traditional theatre spaces.

Detailed discussion about the choreographic process for performance is presented elsewhere (Allegranti, 2019), but it is worth noting the overall impact of the work in the wider public arena as a continued distribution of the *material*. Following a dementia-friendly studio performance that many of our participants attended an insight from Takeshi about 'giving back' was offered:

> [It] felt like opening some precious gift, like it was giving-back today . . . being witnessed by [the families] was a crystallization of these last few months. And also makes me think about this process of dementia, transforming or becoming different, it's becoming a positive thing. Beautiful.

Performing each iteration allows for new possibilities of consciousness-raising with public audiences in different ways, and journalist Pippa Kelly captured the bigger picture in her review, writing that "what you'll see is about the ties that link and sustain us, verbal or not. It's about what it is to be human, and surely we all have a stake in that".

In the writing that follows, my intent is to produce multiple, colliding, *intra*-acting subjectivities—for people living with dementia, their families, the artistic team and my own as practitioner-researcher. Drawing from choreographic vignettes, photographs, memories, interviews with participants and discussions within the artistic team, I demonstrate how DMP, choreography and dementia 'diffract' (Harraway, 2016; Barad, 2007): how ongoing insights from each can be read through one other. In doing so, I highlight how the work has challenged perceptions and ways of movement relating for everyone taking part, particularly around themes of loss, voice, vulnerability and agency.

Shouting Silently

One of the early interview-conversations in London was with Takeshi, a collaborating professional dancer in the project whose father—Souji—lives with YOD in Japan, see Figure 11.7 for an early family photo taken by Takeshi's mother, Kimika. Takeshi has spent time being his father's carer, and as I listen to him speak about their relationship, I feel warmth and groundedness together with sparks of agitation. It is with these affective layers that I start to imagine into their current relationship. I reach for a deep breath when Takeshi tells me that he does contact work with his aligning father, "back-to-back, and then holding hands and leaning back and forwards. Sometimes turning together". Takeshi, invites his father, Souji, into a way of knowing in the world, and into the present moment through tactile-*kin*-aesthetic conversation. Touch awakens deep-rooted somatic memories and in doing so, as Manning (2013) describes, it animates the politics of an event. This *kin*-aesthetic conversation was not something that father and son engaged with before dementia, and Takeshi notices that taking his father's weight (in all senses) agitates the father-son balance of power:

> Father always wants to be 'father' rather than be taken care of. Also, I think it's my tendency to become like a teacher and I think my dad doesn't like that. I see it with his facial expression . . . and he also says 'no, I don't want to do this!'

A different father-son kinship seems to manifest through confronting the boundaries of touch. It seems that this exchange trembles as Manning has it, "between touch-as-tact and touch as the activity through which new constellations for bodying are created" (2013,

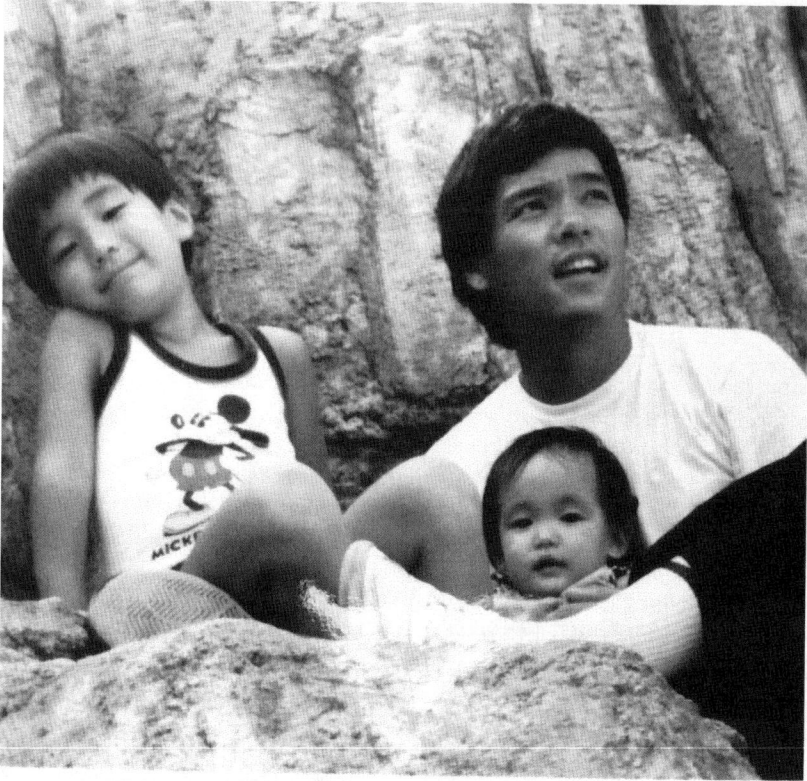

Figure 11.7 Takeshi, Souji and Asami Matsumoto

Photo: Kimika Matsumoto.

p. 125). Souji's clear boundary, his 'no', poignantly resounds with Takeshi's description: his father is a man who was diagnosed with dementia at the age of 56, with a working life, a family and, who in the early stages of diagnosis, developed hallucinations and now, is restless with insomnia, expressing his resistance as he shuffles his way through the family home at night barefoot, speaking quietly into the silence of the night. I sense a man confronted by his own finitude, laying bare some of our most fundamental notions about what it means to be human. Dominant discourses of aging and dementia describe not only a threat to some part of the anatomy, but to a person's mind, their autonomy, their capacity to speak and 'voice' themselves in the world, or even their humanity—thus revealing deeply held, if seldom articulated misconceptions about the nature of selves and bodies, which in turn has consequences for how we assess the very humanity of the elderly. By way of antidote, I am moved when Takeshi considers his father's humanity and potential:

> I've never really looked at him until he gets dementia. So, it's like, 'ok I hear your voice now.' He never complained before. It's hard, because that's dominating at the moment, but at the same time I see him as a whole, and I think it's OK to have these moments, because he's never been like that. I positively try to take dementia as a kind of 'possibility' to do something different to what he never experienced before.

Takeshi challenges the limits of humanism with his inclination towards 'taking dementia positively', allowing for potential to meet the possibility. Preceding PheMaterialism, Japanese anthropological research conceptualizes the self as relational and a process of achieving a social and psychological reciprocity and integration into the wider collective (Traphagan, 2000). From this vantage point, historical Japanese representations of dementia tend to eschew tropes of obliteration and erasure that figure so prominently in Anglo-American narratives and biomedical accounts and are instead attuned to the materiality of memory and its role in making us who we are (Post, 2000). This dwelling in the present allows Souji and many other people living with dementia, for dancers, therapists, to embrace the flux and persistence of somatic habits with/in the dynamic specificity of everyday life (Barad, 2007).

Summer 2017, London-Tokyo

I am working in the studio with four dancers preparing Takeshi and Souji's bespoke performance for other families to witness. I am aware that Souji is both present in this creative process and yet geographically 'absent' as he lives in Japan and is the only participant living with YOD that is not physically present with us in London. This realization becomes paradoxical, it highlights the ontological presence-absence that often characterizes the person living with dementia and, also Derrida's notion of the person 'lost' as inescapably 'in' us (2001).

In an attempt to maintain a response to some of this complex and ambiguous bodily knowing, I support the dancers to work improvisationally with Takeshi's refrain, 'I hear your voice now'. In doing so, I am also aware, from Takeshi's current updates at the time of writing, that his father's capacity to speak words is diminished, leaving him with a permanently open mouth. As I witness Takeshi, I am drawn to the cool, shiny, grey dance linoleum floor as he takes gradual and steady forward steps repeatedly opening his mouth and reaching with both hands, arms extended in front of his body, see Figure 11.8. I sense my own steady

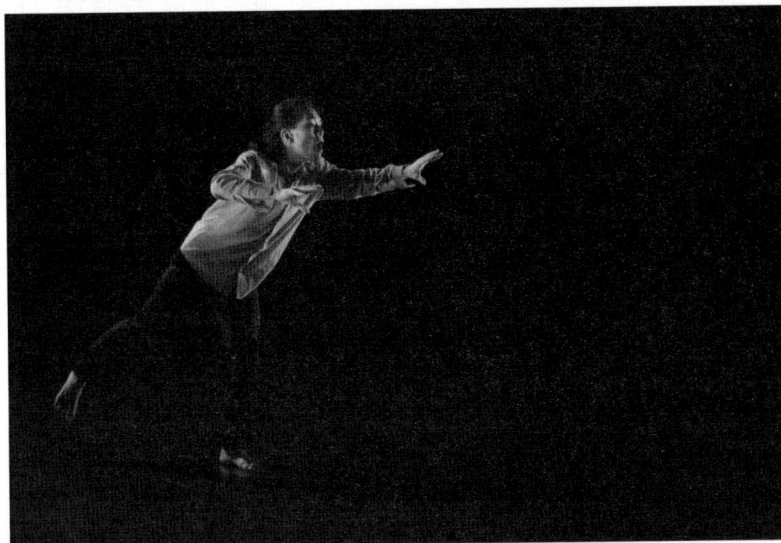

Figure 11.8 Takeshi, Public Performance at Michaelis Theatre

Photo: Thomas Lines.

breathing rhythm and my gut tells me he is not reaching in the singular, his father reaches with him, I am reaching with them both, and the environment reaches. Takeshi, repeatedly opening his mouth as if to shout, remains silent. In this moment, the impact of Souji's voice is kaleidoscopic, across time, space and place, between Tokyo and our London studio. Souji's voice is 'post-verbal' (Quinn & Blandon, 2017, p. 587) extending beyond his individual body and as it does so, the material begins to compose us. For Takeshi, hearing his father's 'voice' in the creative process has articulated the ineffable. Ten months later, Takeshi speaks about this material in his interview:

> I'm shouting towards the void, or loss. Shouting Silently. And someone is assisting me shout. I think more so now, I start to feel anger towards dementia—finally, I just want to shout and express this anger.

We are not defined solely by our intellect. Railing against hypercognitivity and in stark contrast to biomedical prognosis of silence, language impairment and individualism, Takeshi's silent shouts have an acoustic presence that draw attention to the articulacy and agency of this bodying act. Becoming a choreographic refrain, shouting silently is not less than human, it does not render those living with dementia as 'disposable' (Braidotti, 2013, p. 15), shouting silently is a worlding, as Manning (2013) has it, of equity, solidarity between father, son, dementia, bodies and choreographing the political—all at once a reconfigured *kin*-aesthetic assembling of otherness and reciprocity. This fleshy act of resistance summons a constructive politics of illness, silence, anger, loss and of relating with fathers.

Winter 2017, Florence-London

The politics of shouting silently evokes a parallel process that churns in my gut. I too want to shout from a primal, rage-filled place as I remember shifting uncomfortably between sitting and standing in the intensive care unit of Florence's university hospital, the hospital where I was born. I am dimly aware of the bright January sun filtering through the vertically slatted blind. This suggestion of light from the natural world is something I crave but is in stark contrast to witnessing my dying father in a coma, silenced, no longer speaking for himself. And yet, as I pay close protective attention to his micro-movements, his heart rate changes, mechanically captured by the clicking and beeping of the monitor, my dad has become-with-machine (Braidotti, 2013), *it* will do the telling. I carefully breath-with his fluctuating rhythms, the rise and fall of his chest, a chest I have rested my head against all my life, and I do so one more time, again and again, because I know that soon I will no longer be able to do this. Reaching for his body I squeeze his feet, gently hold his head, grip his hand, a conflicting intimacy both treasured and resisted. In his near-death state, I am summoned to speak for my father, I want to release my breath from a deep place and to shout out his suffering and mine. I cannot. As we both confront death's "final silence" (Lorde, 2017, p. 3) this moment wrenches, it viscerally marks my understanding of kinship as an entangled materiality and Barad reminds me that "the *other* is not just in one's skin, but in one's bones, in one's belly, in one's heart, in one's nucleus, in one's past and future" (2007, p. 393). This silent shouting becomes a *trans*corporeal inheritance where affective intensities, vital organs, life support technology, father-daughter bonds, an Italian January assemble for the first and last time.

Destabilizing the linearity of past, present and future (Barad, 2007), I do not yet know how this material will dispossess me. Braidotti (2013) tells me that it will be part of my 'future-present' and I begin to see how it is part of the wider creative process of living. As the

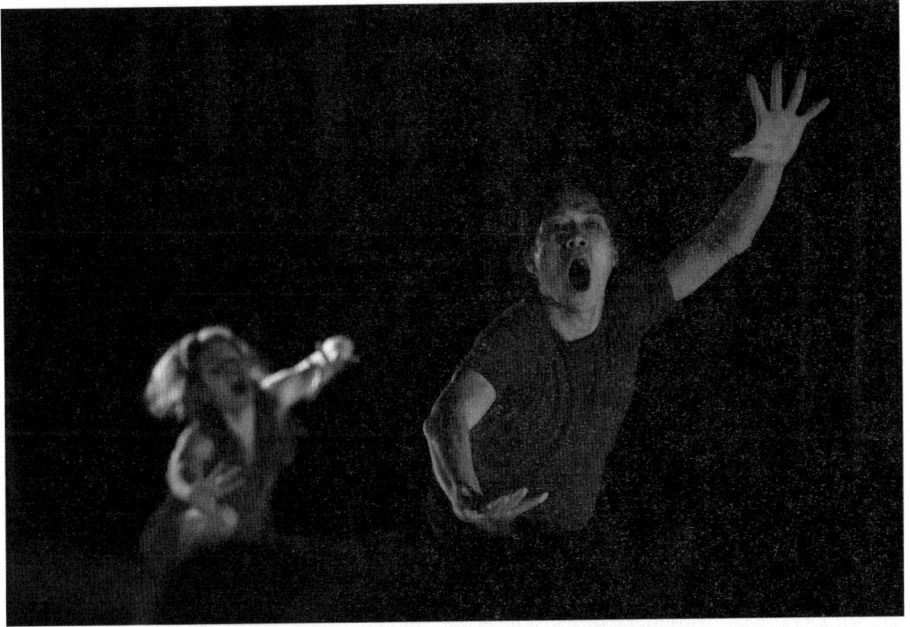

Figure 11.9 Maria, and Takeshi, Public Performance at Michaelis Theatre

Photo: Thomas Lines.

co-compositional process takes hold, I invite Sabrina to stand behind Takeshi and, rooted to the spot she gradually begins to find a deep resonating shout from her belly, see Figure 11.9. I witness the intersecting body politics of this moment and am caught off guard: Sabrina's small-boned, muscular body shape-shifts, she becomes-animal (Braidotti, 2013) emitting a deep howl that seems to propel Takeshi forward. Sabrina *becomes* with Takeshi, Souji and dementia:

> Takeshi starts in front of me very close, we are gathering our breath from the previous scene. I can see his back swaying. Slowly, I start to breathe, my exhalation will be the engine for him to move. As I breathe a force from the ground reaches my lungs and my throat—my voice is out. I can see his back breathing and expanding, I'm talking with his back, my voice now is powerful and through it he can reach further. He wants to scream but he can do so just through me, we are connected. He is me and I'm him, he talks because of me and I walk because of him.

Sabrina's somatic 'force from the ground' summons Braidotti's words on art as "cosmic in its resonance and hence posthuman by structure, as it carries us to . . . the limits of life itself and thus confronts us with the horizon of death" (2013, p. 107). Sabrina's becoming-with is an affirmative endurance of rage, loss, dementia, since it articulates how, as Manning has it, that "movement is not of a body. It cuts across, co-composing with different velocities of moment-moving. It bodies" (2013, p. 14). In a similar vein, Kate Swaffer (2016), diagnosed with dementia at the age of 49, proposes a dementia carer as a 'back up brain', an extension of 'self-other' binary. Sabrina, Takeshi and Souji, voice, breath, dementia—are also prosthetically entwined (Manning, 2007). This *trans*corporeal moment of *shouting silently* offers an extension of a capacity for relating, beyond the imagined stability of individualism, beyond

identity, a posthuman shouting, highlighting material-discursive flows, incompleteness, inde-
terminacy and continual reconstruction.

Winter 2018, London

In a continued web of relating, the un/voiced rolls across the studio and through eleven public and international performances of *I've Lost You Only To Discover That I Have Gone Missing*.
As it does so, the *shouting silently* material sensorially widens in a way that Luke describes as
a "disruption":

> I remember first working with this material from Takeshi and his father . . ., I always work
> with clenched fists, disturbing the space. As I was doing it, it felt really emotional and I felt
> really affected by it . . ., the tension. And then, the more times I've done it [t]he material has
> emptied out in relationship to Takeshi, but in relation to my role with Sabrina, it's loaded up.
> So, yes, just feeling and seeing the different content that comes and goes emotionally with the
> material and knowing when to let go. Every time I perform that piece, it couldn't have been
> about Takeshi's father, otherwise I would have looked at him on stage and burst into tears
> (see Figure 11.10).

The material is *intra*-activated and transformed through Luke's performative acts where
voice is distributed and becomes part of an agentic assemblage. Luke's response somatically
unsettles relating with the material, and his deliberate provocation demonstrates how his
movement has *created* space and time (Manning, 2007). In doing so, *shouting silently* gathers
affective momentum, interfering with hegemonic expressions of anger and voice residing in

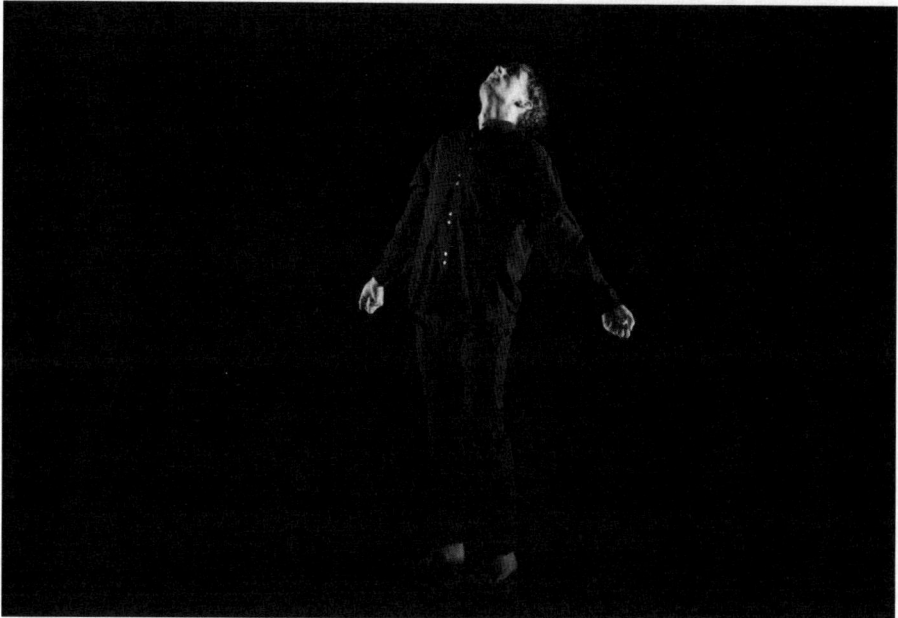

Figure 11.10 Luke, Public Performance at Michaelis Theatre

Photo: Thomas Lines.

individual bodies. Instead, moving affects constitute this event that in turn becomes bodying multiplicity (Manning, 2013).

The bodying multiplicity of *shouting silently* points towards clinical and/or artistic material being self-evidently in flux, and as Luke clearly demonstrates, a distributive process. All these affectively affirmative layers—father, son, daughter, vocal chords, acoustic resonance, geographical locations, movement across oceans and time zones, technology, becoming-animal, studio floor—have assembled and are nonsemantic companions in birthing *kin*-aesthetic clusters of resistance. This is our dancing activism.

WE'RE DOING THIS TOGETHER

The wide open patio doors reveal a long garden dissected by a rose bush trellis. Seated in Jacquie and Tony's kitchen for their interview-conversation, Tony has silently witnessed Jacquie and me talking for some time. He then puts on his Ray-Bans, moves out into the garden and stands under the roses in full bloom. Jacquie explains Tony's previously professional legal life which relied on his outstanding communication skills and that now, at this stage of his dementia, "he knows his limitations and recognises his inability to find the, right words". I feel a pang of guilt as I hear this, being able to summon words at my own volition and witnessing Tony's vulnerability in this conversation, in the safety of his own home, and yet demonstrating his resistance by maintaining contact from a distance. Jacquie hands me a tiny piece of paper and on it are the words that Tony wrote to his future self, ten years pre-diagnosis, "he lapsed back into that contented solitude of an only child going his own way in silence, without reference to anyone at all".

Any life-changing illness causes ruptures in everyday life and can divulge values, ideals and mental habits that would have otherwise remained implicit and unrecognized—perhaps challenging notions of responding in socially prescribed ways. And yet Jacquie quotes her son, "it took dementia to reveal dad", and I hear Takeshi's words chiming with his experience of his own father, far from 'loss of self' another layer of Tony has been revealed, changed, become apparent *because* of dementia. Is this the struggle of that 'all too human' striving for survival to which Braidotti (2013) alludes?

The Dance Studio

When I bring Jacquie and Tony's stories into the studio, I am compelled to set a task that mobilizes the vulnerability I sensed from my visit to the family home. My invitation to 'do your dance of courage' produces a stunning assembly of bodies evoking vulnerability as a form of activism (Butler, 2015, p. 123). Here, in this private dance studio, we open a space for small acts of activism, not yet a 'public' performance (for families or for theatre); instead, an unknown creative process. What emerges is material *for* and *with* life. Luke, like Tony, is an only child, and in response to my suggested task, he begins an internal dialogue where speaks to his five-year-old self, "You'll be OK, you can jump, you're deserving"; he then proceeds to run blindly—t-shirt covering his head—towards the stretchy cloth boundary held by Takeshi and Sabrina. Aneta tells us how, as a child she was "mummy to my younger sister" and begins to ceremoniously pick up every dancer, one by one and carry them from the edges of the room into the centre. I am struck by what I witness as the simultaneous expression of her vulnerability in evoking her younger self and her current physical strength as she lifts Luke and Takeshi, see Figure 11.11. The dancer's guided movement responses become

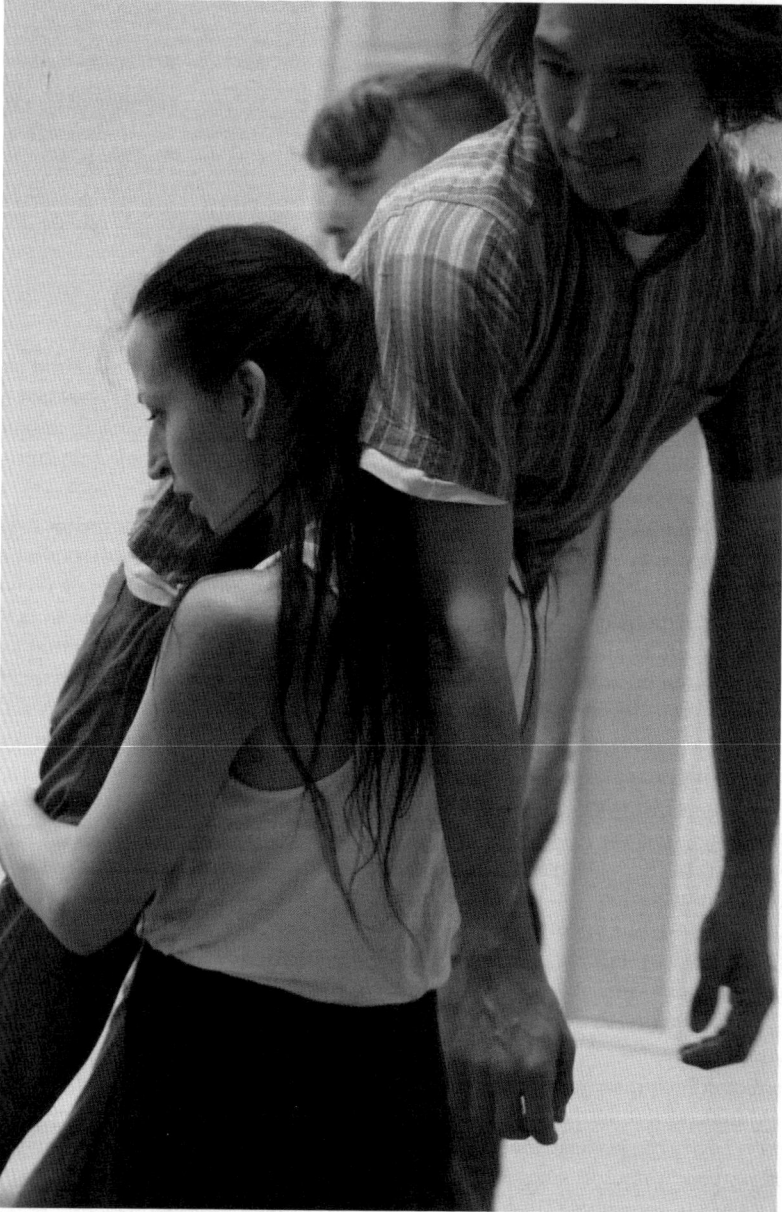

Figure 11.11 Aneta and Takeshi, Making the Material in the Studio

Photo: Julia Testa.

interstitial connections between the family home and the dance studio. In this creative process, mobilizing vulnerability shows how it is not a gendered characteristic. By co-composing this material, it is possible to glimpse how vulnerability and resistance coexist and pave the way for dancing collective recognition.

Ties That Bind

Tony and I are walking side by side, through the South London public library and into the art gallery that we have transformed into our participatory ecology. As we reach the door, Tony stops, a small act of resistance, perhaps. It is as if he anticipates the affective potential inside this room. We are at a threshold, between a public space and a smaller, more intimate one. I look through the door and gesture towards the pianist, Frankie, motioning him to play something welcoming. It seems to work and Tony moves, slowly, through the door, where the dancers await in the gallery room heated by the summer sun.

Within seconds of Tony and Jacquie's bespoke performance starting, Jacquie cries tears of recognition. As the four dancers scatter paper, there is an immediate reminder of the mess tangled with the 'thing power' of this paper (Jackson & Mazzei, 2016, p. 98; Bennett, 2010), see Figure 11.12. With/in this paper is the ethics and decision making that Tony was faced with, signaled by the moment when Jacquie entered Tony's office and witnessed his legal documents in complete disarray covered with nonsensical writing. Later Jacquie comments on the immediacy of witnessing the performance, "It's quite shocking how quickly we felt things".

Minutes later, Sabrina and Takeshi are enacting a tug of war with a cloth-covered stretchy elastic cord. Takeshi has his back to Sabrina and Sabrina is pulling Takeshi backwards, towards her, see Figure 11.13. This moment becomes a trigger: Tony, suddenly stands bold upright from his chair, ready to intervene. Offering a barely audible commentary, it is striking that Tony may be trying to make sense of his losses in the same way we all are in

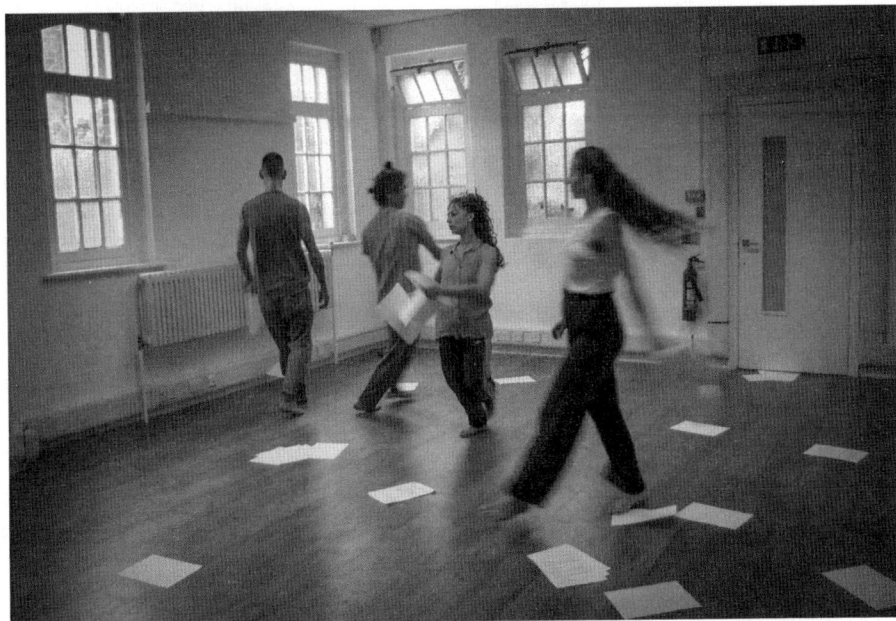

Figure 11.12 Luke, Takeshi, Sabrina, Aneta, Bespoke Performance for Tony and Jacquie

Photo: Julia Testa.

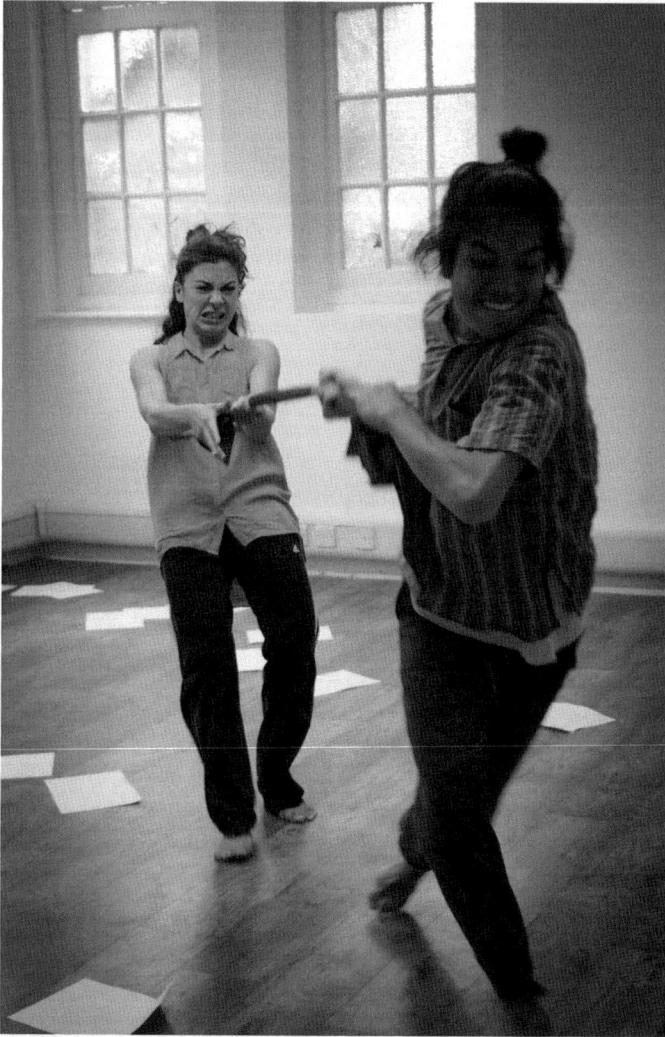

Figure 11.13 Sabrina and Takeshi, Bespoke Performance for Tony and Jacquie

Photo: Julia Testa.

this room today. Jacquie remains sitting, gaze fixed ahead whilst also reaching out for Tony's hand as if to steady him. What are we all facing in this moment? Perhaps we are becoming-with the material in a stretching, grasping, pulling, tussle. This performance becomes more than the sum of its parts, and the 'umbilical' cord has agentic force, and it becomes a means of survival.

During this moment, I strain to hold the tension and am concerned how long everyone can endure. Bodying the ubiquitous ties that bind has taken us all to our edges: those processes that bring up information that is difficult for us to accept. I am faced with the ethics of acknowledging "the ties that bind us to the multiple 'others'" (Braidotti, 2013, p. 100): we are not in charge of these irrepressible flows, affects, movements, and we are tangled. Tears sting my eyes and once again I turn to Frankie, imbuing him as acoustic leveler and ask him to play something soothing. Sabrina tears down the fourth wall, looking directly at Tony, and Tony looks back at her, still standing, gaze scrutinizing as he is 'infolded' into performance (Manning, 2016). Sabrina then looks at Jacquie and later comments on this tangling of human and no-human agents:

> I felt for the first time that I'm carrying this, and I'm showing to him, to her, it must be diffi-
> cult, especially when we were with the elastic-cord. I kind of wanted to protect her. I decided
> to look at her, and kind of like: 'we are with you, don't worry, we're doing this together'. And
> she was aware of this, we exchanged a smile.

In a striking resonance, after the performance, Jacquie recounted, "What surprised me about the dance was how painful and how raw it was to watch"; she is feeling *with* the dance and this process is neuro-affectively unmediated, since when the feeling evokes a response there is a physiological marker on a visceral level (Damasio, 2000). Like the PheMaterial möbius, bodying is an unmediated process. Tony, too, has grasped the affective content of this performance and Jacquie later comments "how he was drawn to intervene". The 'loss' of his cognitive and linguistic function does not endanger the status of his 'self'. Tony's visceral response affirms his presence: he experienced an aspect of himself. It becomes clear that affect and memories, far from being unique and personal, can be reconstructed through dance movement relating.

Later still, when we invite Jacquie and Tony to join the improvisation, Tony allows himself to be with us in another way, see Figure 11.14. In contrast to his solitude, Sabrina comments on how Tony is present, not only in his witnessing, but also by participating:

> It was really powerful when Tony [was] in the middle of the room, stretching. Because I
> thought . . ., he's a solitary man and yet, we were all around him.

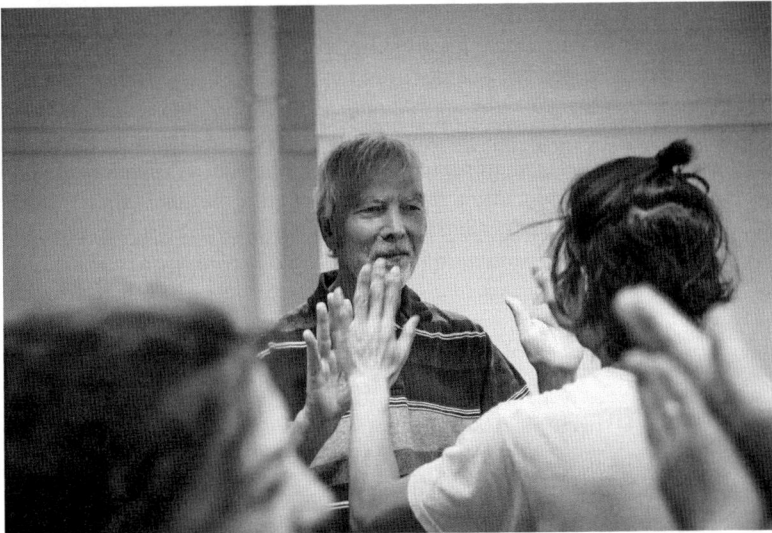

Figure 11.14 Movement Improvisation with Tony

Photo: Julia Testa.

Our dance *with* and *for* Tony and Jacquie becomes political; it is a 'collective assembly' (Butler, 2015) where we open a space for making physically and spatially visceral, otherwise hidden vulnerabilities and social arrangements. The evocative and recursive impact of witnessing, being witnessed and participating in improvised movement responses, expands beyond anthropocentric intersubjective relating (Ammaniti & Gallese, 2014) and towards entanglement: we are all becoming *with* this moment of vulnerability. In this dance, dementia leaks beyond the confines of diagnosis; instead, human relating and agency is distributed across the bodies of dancers, families, through the choreographic material, with objects and into everyday life. We become-with our vulnerabilities and become more-than-dementia.

MOVING WITH THE TROUBLE

In this global time of sociopolitical and environmental crisis, we are faced with multiple forms of social exclusion and economic inequality that challenge core values of equality and respect for human and animal rights. Securing peace and prosperity for future generations in the face of such challenges requires a reinstating a bodying activism, a generative change with innovative solutions that address social inequalities, reconcile conflict and have lasting impact, in short, a more-than-human revolution in relating.

My intent in this chapter has been to demonstrate how the ability to affect and be affected is in constant motion. The affecting process is more than anthropocentrically intersubjective—it is *trans*corporeal and has the potential to *kin*-aesthetically reshape the micro-politics of relating. How we make (the) material and the multiple colliding subjectivities and *intra*-action of these events (in clinical or artistic contexts) will help us to pay attention to how change and transformation occur, in turn changing our relating in micro and macro ways. This work goes some way towards rethinking the relations through which the human is made possible, specifically with and through an assembling of choreography, DMP and dementia. To this end, choreography and performance as potent artistic processes—within or without the therapeutic process—allow for neurodiverse, transversal ways of relating. Choreography is not a luxury but an ethical imperative yielding constantly renewable *kin*-aesthetic insights into ways of relating for people living with YOD, their family carers as well as for broader healthcare and medical practitioners. In this way, dementia (and any other 'diagnosis') becomes an ecological process distributed in the environment rather than a pathological manifestation of a human subject.

When stories of crisis and othering become part of us, as they do ubiquitously in therapy, art and everyday life, we must cultivate the capacity for "response-ability" (Harraway, 2016, p. 2). The dancing activism discussed in this chapter is an artistic contribution to nourishing equitable citizenship and counterhegemonic narratives of aging, agency, illness, vulnerability, living and dying. Dancing activism is, to paraphrase Harraway (2016), a *moving* with the trouble. In a time where a hypercognitive view holds currency in the global North and where neo-liberalist ideals permeate education, health and arts policies and cultivate a culture of anthropocentric individualism, dancing activism is a *kin*-aesthetic antidote, a response to moving with the complexity of the more-than-human in everyday life. Dancing-with human and more-than-human others enacts subtle and incremental changes and makes space for our unimagined hopes.

NOTES

1. The UK name for the profession.
2. The project, is funded by Arts Council England (2016–2021), with commissions from Bergen International Festival and in partnership with Dementia Pathfinders, Merton Arts Space, Dementia Action Alliance UK, Public Health (Merton), University of Bergen, Alexandra Palace.
3. Beatrice Allegranti Dance Theatre comprises artistic director and choreographer Beatrice Allegranti; producer Nancy May Roberts; professional dancers Luke Birch, Sabrina Gargano, Takeshi Matsumoto, Maria Palliani, Aneta Zwierzyńska; composer Jill Halstead, and musicians Robert Howat and Frankie Burrows.
4. At the time of writing, 12 (audio-recorded and transcribed) interview-conversations have taken place with a cumulative total of 30 family members. Ethical clearance is from the University of Roehampton, London.
5. At the time of writing, five studio practice discussions were audio-recorded and a further five individual interviews conducted with the company dancers.

REFERENCES

Alaimo, S., & Heckman, S. (Eds.). (2008). *Material feminisms*. Indiana: Indiana University Press.
Allegranti, B. (2011). *Embodied performances: Sexuality, gender, bodies*. London: Palgrave Macmillan.
Allegranti, B. (2014). Corporeal kinship: Dancing the entanglements of love and loss. In J. Wyatt, & T. E. Adams (Eds.), *On (writing) families: Autoethnographies of presence and absence, love and loss*. Rotterdam: Sense Publications.
Allegranti, B. (2019). Moving Kinship: Between choreography, performance and the more-than-human. In S. Prickett & H. Thomas (Eds.), *The Routledge dance handbook*. London: Routledge.
Ammaniti, M., & Gallese, V. (2014). *The birth of intersubjectivity: Psychodynamics, neurobiology and the self*. London/New York: W.W. Norton & Company Ltd.
Barad, K. (2007). *Meeting the universe halfway: Quantum physics and the entanglement of matter and meaning*. Durham/London: Duke University Press.
Bennett, J. (2010). *Vibrant matter: A political economy of things*. Durham: Duke University Press.
Braidotti, R. (2013). *The posthuman*. Cambridge: Polity Press.
Butler, J. (2015). *Notes toward a performative theory of assembly*. Cambridge, MA: Harvard University Press.
Burton-Jones, J. (2015). *Approaching an unthinkable future: Understanding the support needs of people living with young onset dementia*. Dementia Pathfinders Resource Publication. Retrieved from www.youngdementiauk.org/sites/default/files/approaching_an_unthinkable_future_lr.pdf [accessed 2017 05 20].
Calvo-Merino, B., Grèzes, J., Glaser, D. E., Passingham, R. E., & Haggard, P. (2006). Seeing or doing? Influence of visual and motor familiarity in action observation. *Current Biology, 16*, 1905–1910.
Damasio, A. (2000). *The feeling of what happens: Body and emotion in the making of consciousness*. London: Vintage Books.
Derrida, J. (2001). *The work of mourning* (P.A. Brault & M. Naas, Eds.). London/Chicago: University of Chicago Press.
Harraway, D. (2016). *Staying with the trouble: Making Kin in the Chthulucene*. Durham: Duke University Press.
Jackson, A., & Mazzei, L. (2016). Thinking with an agentic assemblage in posthuman inquiry. In C. A. Taylor & C. Hughes (Eds.), *Posthuman research practices in education*. London: Palgrave Macmillan.
Lorde, A. (2017). *Your silence will not protect you*. London: Silver Press.
Manning, E. (2007). *Politics of touch: Sense, movement, sovereignty*. Minneapolis: University of Minnesota Press.
Manning, E. (2013). *Always more than one: Individuation's dance*. Durham: Duke University Press.
Manning, E. (2016). *The minor gesture*. Durham: Duke University Press.
Post, S. G. (2000). The concept of Alzheimer's disease in a hypercognitive society. In P. J. Whitehouse, K. Maurer, & J. F. Ballenger (Eds.), *Concepts of Alzheimer disease*. Baltimore & London: John Hopkins University Press.
Quinn, J., & Blandon, C. (2017). The potential for lifelong learning in dementia: A post-humanist exploration. *International Journal of Lifelong Education, 36*(5), 578–594.
Ringrose, J., Katie, W., & Zarabadi, S. (2019). *Feminist posthumanisms and new materialisms in education*. London and New York: Routledge.
Swaffer, K. (2016). *What the hell happened to my brain?: Living beyond Dementia*. London: Jessica Kingsley Publishers.
Taguchi, H. L. (2013). Images of thinking in feminist materialisms: Ontological divergences and the production of researcher subjectivities. *International Journal of Qualitative Studies in Education, 26*(6), 706–716.
Traphagan, J. W. (2000). *Taming Oblivion: Aging bodies and the fear of senility in Japan*. Albany: SUNY Press.
Winnicott, D. (1971). *Playing and reality*. London: Tavistock.

CHAPTER 12

SEEING WITH THE HEART

The Aesthetics of Dance/Movement Therapy with
Older Adults and People with Dementia

Donna Newman-Bluestein

INTRODUCTION

After almost 30 years of practice as a dance/movement therapist, as I began working exclusively with older adults and especially those with advanced dementia, I found myself wondering about the role of aesthetics in my practice. Because there was little that looked or felt like dance—only the most minute movements, barely expressive, and lacking much physicality or beauty—I was no longer experiencing aesthetic satisfaction in my work. I wondered where the dance was in this particular dance/movement therapy (DMT) work. Simultaneously, in an online forum for dance/movement therapists working with older adults, we discovered that many of us felt marginalized. Because our work was not in a mental health setting, it was often considered an extension of recreation therapy by other dance/movement therapists. As we shared our strategies within groups and in affecting the environment, I felt validated and began to realize that we actually had much of significance to contribute to the field of gerontology. In yet another online discussion, several of us wrangled with the differences between DMT and other body-oriented psychotherapies, which led to further discussions about the aspects of dance essential for dance/movement therapists to be effective clinicians. It was then that I began to consider how an aesthetic perspective in dance could make my DMT work more effective and fulfilling.

Wondering exactly what my personal aesthetic in dance was, I initially found that reading did little to answer my questions. As a way of grounding this topic experientially in dance, I took a week-long workshop with the Liz Lerman Dance Exchange, seeking to better understand my personal aesthetic. Repeatedly during that week, we were asked both as dancers and as audience members "Where in the piece did you feel drawn in? What was interesting? Exciting? Most memorable? What were you curious about? Which parts had meaning for you? What surprised you?" Those were the questions I learned to ask to discern aesthetic preferences. I have since found this corroborating statement by Alma Hawkins (1991): "The movement event should have the power to evoke an aesthetic response. What is it about a piece of choreography that causes the audience to be drawn into the experience, to respond imaginatively, and to feel aesthetic satisfaction?" (p. 2).

This chapter looks at the specific challenges I faced in my DMT work with people with dementia, elements of my particular aesthetic in dance, and where and how my aesthetic intersects with and supports DMT with people with dementia.

THE CHALLENGES

Looking back at that time when I first began to consider the aesthetic of dance in my DMT work, what stands out in my memory was greeting people as the nursing assistants brought them into one group in particular. This group was my most demanding, as the residents had significant cognitive and physical challenges and were also behaviorally challenging. These older adults were often still wearing their paper bibs from breakfast, with food accumulated on their faces and hands.

As a dance/movement therapist, grooming was not part of my role or training. Yet as I imagined what they might feel like in their skins, practicing kinesthetic empathy as it were and putting myself in their places, I imagined that part of my attention during the group would be on the food stuck on my face, making my face tighter, less expressive. Dirty, sticky fingers would also distract me from what was going on, to say nothing of being a public health hazard. Wondering if this were "part of my job", I concluded that using a warm, wet paper towel and asking their permission, gently cleaning their faces and hands, restoring dignity to the person in front of me was indeed part of my role.

In addition, the participants in this DMT group did not follow directions or mirror movements, mine or group members', and generally appeared unaware of one another. They seemed to need individual attention if they were to participate at all. They barely moved. Where was the beauty, the aesthetics, the dance, in this work?

DISCOVERING MY PERSONAL AESTHETIC

In the workshop with Lerman, I found in choreographing a solo, the most important and pivotal movement was one where I was balanced on my sitting bones, the back of my wrists resting on my knees. I was fascinated that this movement had found its way into my solo. It was a position which recalled one of my early modern dance classes 40 years earlier, and a rare moment in a dance class when I received positive kinesthetic feedback. The teacher of that class had come around to demonstrate that if we had a good abdominal contraction, when she attempted to pick us up from under our arms, our bodies would remain in position. As she spoke, she put her hands under my arms, and lifted; my body remained in position. This abdominal contraction, characteristic of Graham technique, was something I had not practiced for many years. I loved the dramatic element of Martha Graham's choreography, the sharply contrasting shapes, and the sensations deep in my gut. I felt those movements helped me express emotional anguish; that my dance was the silent song of my soul. Dancing in such a way took a strong internal focus and helped me find my centered self.

I have found repeatedly when dancing that when my internal focus is strong, it seems to draw the viewer in, despite my lack of technical prowess. The audience in Lerman's class provided feedback that that movement was compelling for them, and subsequently, the trio I worked in chose that movement to incorporate into our group choreography. Perhaps what makes a strong focus compelling is that it allows the viewer to find his or her own story in the particularity of the movement. Dance/movement therapist Lenore Hervey (2000), referencing Kant, Heidegger, and Schopenhauer, said that "art uniquely reveals the universal in the particular" (p. 13). Apparently, my strong internal connection acted as a magnetic force for the audience.

The fact that this movement emerged spontaneously from unconscious sources spoke to its authenticity. I found that movements that connected to memories or which elicited images brought a sense of meaning and coherence to the dance. According to Donald Blumenfeld-Jones (1997):

> A search for meaning . . . is a search for experiencing connection with others in our world as well as with our physical and social environment. This connectedness carries with it an experience of wholeness (however temporary this experience may be).
>
> (p. 315)

In another dance with Lerman, we were working with partners in a structure she called "One to Ten". Each person was to move into a still pose, to which the other person then responded, creating their own pose. This sequence was repeated ten times. After the exercise, my partner noted my tendency to create movements which contrasted with hers. In these positions, she discovered an increased sensation of energy because of the dynamic tension between our contrasting shapes.

In addition to the dramatic contrasts, balance, strong center, and the dynamic tension of a strong internal focus on my kinesthetic sense even while looking outward toward the audience, I also appreciate the playfulness, spontaneity, and present-centeredness I experience when dancing improvisationally. Because my DMT teacher and mentor, Norma Canner, had studied with Barbara Mettler and encouraged her students to as well, I spent two summers learning from Mettler.

Mettler's first movement structure each time we began was what she called "arrangement of group". Later in this chapter, you will see how this sensibility has permeated my work as a DMT. As she wrote in *Materials of Dance as a Creative Art Activity* (1960):

> Your first creative problem is both an individual and a group problem: go out into the room and find a place for yourself where you can be all alone with plenty of space around you . . . not close to anyone else . . . everyone should have an equal amount of space so that someone looking down from above would see the space equally divided among you in a regular pattern.
>
> (p. 19)

> In this first problem (arrangement of group) the seed of all future creative work is sown by requiring the individual to adapt his own needs for free expression to the needs of the group as a whole.
>
> (p. 18)

I remembered another element of my personal aesthetic in dance as I recalled placing myself directly in front of the drummer at high school dances and letting my entire body simply express the rhythm. I didn't recognize at the time how deeply healing it was to let go of my conscious mind. I also came to understand later that that dance was mostly about the elements of Weight & Flow, that particular combination of Efforts, or qualities of movement, that Rudolf Laban associated with dream state (Dell, 1977, p. 115). The Effort state of Weight and Flow is thought to be related to bodily sensations and emotional feelings (Bloom, Adrian, Casciero, Mizenko, & Porter, 2017), which was certainly borne out by my experience.

The elements of Weight and Flow are typical of West African dance. For many years, I took classes and performed traditional dances from West Africa and the Caribbean in a dance company. In addition to activating my propensity for Weight and Flow as we danced to the poly-rhythmic djembe drum music, the emphasis on the collective appealed to me greatly. Our place within the community of dancers was clear and equal; all of us were responsible for forming a clear line or circle. Fellow dancers in the West African dance classes were much more likely to assist in learning a new step than in the often competitive and hierarchical atmosphere of modern dance classes.

I continued to learn about my dance aesthetic by noticing what I was most drawn to as an audience member. I find that I am captivated by dances which move me emotionally and awaken my kinesthetic sense, the feeling inside my muscles of moving like the dancer. Dances which drive me to think about challenging issues or what I think of as beauty emerging out of suffering are especially salient. In fact, seeing Alvin Ailey's lead dancer Judith

Jamison's seemingly effortless floating across the stage and effortful scrubbing the floor in *Cry* in 1973 inspired me to return to see her perform the following two nights. After the third night, I dreamt that I would teach dance to children. Serendipitously, when I shared my dream with a friend, he asked if I knew of dance therapy, which I did not. He gave me the name of a dance therapist whom I contacted immediately and that was my first step in pursuing a career in DMT.

The Bill T. Jones/Arnie Zane Dance Company is another company which moves me similarly. His works are always provocative, his company inclusive of diverse body types, and the physicality of the dancers inspiring. I also appreciate Twyla Tharp's choreography, which I admire for the quirkiness and element of surprise. Sometimes I appreciate small, local dance companies more than acclaimed professional companies, when the former's performances are defined more by excellence, commitment, and passion and less by a glossy veneer.

Until now, I have been speaking of distinct elements of dance which I find compelling. Importantly, however, the arts touch us only to the extent that the relationship between the parts and the whole is satisfying. It is not the colors or the shapes that create the aesthetic experience of visual art, but how the whole comes together. Elements such as proportion, harmony, balance, symmetry, or asymmetry may appeal to and move us. Similarly, as an art form, it is the dance as a whole that provides us with an experience that inspires. Sondra Fraleigh (1980) suggests:

> Dance is the aesthetic archetype of a process understanding of life. Dance is a constant becoming. Perceptivity in dance is the awareness of changing values in relation to a total gestalt. . . . Because dance unfolds through time in a relentless process of becoming, we do not view the whole as we might see the whole of a picture. . . . As we follow the dance through time, however, the whole is manifest. The completeness of the work is sensed as we perceive its interrelated values . . . as sense awareness of total patterns. If I can see only one gesture of the dance, I am nonetheless aware of this gesture's contingency. It has lost its meaning apart from the whole. I am always perceiving total form because any part of a work relates to and calls forth the unified whole.
>
> (p. 25)

In the ensuing years since my first explorations, aesthetics has remained a vital lens through which I see my work. My understanding has become both simpler and more layered. The primary questions I am curious about are "What am I drawn toward? What do I avoid?" in relation to my aesthetics in dance, and by extension, the lens through which I see DMT with my clients: What are my clients attracted to, and what do they avoid?

If my personal aesthetic in dance involves dramatic contrasts, balance, a dynamic tension between internal and external focus, authenticity, meaningfulness, playfulness, spontaneity, present-centeredness, surprise, and the elements of Weight and Flow as manifestations of bodily sensations and intuition, individuality and the collective, do these elements manifest in my DMT groups with people with dementia, and if so, how?

AESTHETICS IN DANCE/MOVEMENT THERAPY WITH PEOPLE WITH DEMENTIA

I start from a Rogerian perspective (Rogers, 1995); a basic tenet of Rogers is that humans tend toward self-actualization. I believe that just as grass grows, people grow, given a nurturing environment. I find that people with dementia can also continue to grow—perhaps not cognitively, but physically, emotionally, and spiritually. When we tap their internal motivation by inviting them to move through the use of music, props, and relating to them as dance partners, they build strength, endurance, and flexibility, expanding their physical and expressive range of movement, A meaningful aesthetic experience furnishes the nourishing environment people with cognitive limitations need to grow and heal. The value of such an aesthetic experience can be found in this statement by Donald Blumenfeld-Jones of Arizona State University: "Living aesthetically is an active participation in the world through one's senses . . . having a profound effect on one's sense of place and value in the world (1997, p. 315).

Belief in the therapeutic process is the deepest underpinning of my practice. I trust that healing wants to happen, just as I trusted my intuition that DMT was my path. Similarly, I have faith that if I bring my intention to be a vessel for healing, setting ego and personal concerns aside, I strengthen the container for therapy. I have come to understand setting an intention and recognizing the images that emerge as perhaps the most important aspects in my creation of an aesthetic DMT experience for groups of people with dementia.

Intention

In her elucidation of Irmgard Bartenieff's Fundamentals, Peggy Hackney wrote "Intent organizes the neuromuscular system" (Hackney, 2002, p. 262). While Bartenieff and Hackney may have been speaking of an effectively functioning body, I find that to be equally true of our actions in life. Setting a clear intention enables the greatest likelihood of achieving our desired outcome.

My intention in leading groups for people with dementia is to create a safe space for healing relationships through dance, music, props, caring, humor, and joy (Newman-Bluestein, 2005; Newman-Bluestein & Hill, 2010). Through exploration, as we play with various rhythms and colors, I hope to motivate people, stimulating their individual energy and shaping the group energy. My purpose is to transform the space into a dance of interaction where people can be, and know they are seen, heard, and valued. I envision people feeling a greater sense of vitality as they express themselves, leading to genuine, heartfelt exchanges which are intimate, joyful, and uplifting. I aim to provide an aesthetically satisfying experience in which each person feels an essential part of a group, a larger whole, one that is vibrant and alive with possibility and which they can then internalize (see Figure 12.1).

Without a curtain rising and falling, movement rituals establish the beginning and end of the group as a time and space outside the ordinary, where movement will be the primary medium for our relating. This makes it more likely that even participants without the ability to verbally understand will grasp our nonverbal communication. The following paragraph contains the words that accompany the movement ritual with which I begin each session:

> Let's begin by wrapping our arms around ourselves in a big hug. Now let's open our arms and our hearts, making room for a group hug. Our theme is love, because it takes work to grow love. Living in a world where it is much easier to hate than it is to love, we need to work on growing love. Now we bend over and gather up some of the love that is in this room, as much or as little as you want. Let's lift the love, raising our arms over our heads, and let the love shower into our hearts. And now, we give it away. The best way to grow love is to give it away.

From the outset, I am inviting participants to recognize themselves simultaneously as an individual and a member of a group, focusing on their internal, kinesthetic sense, even

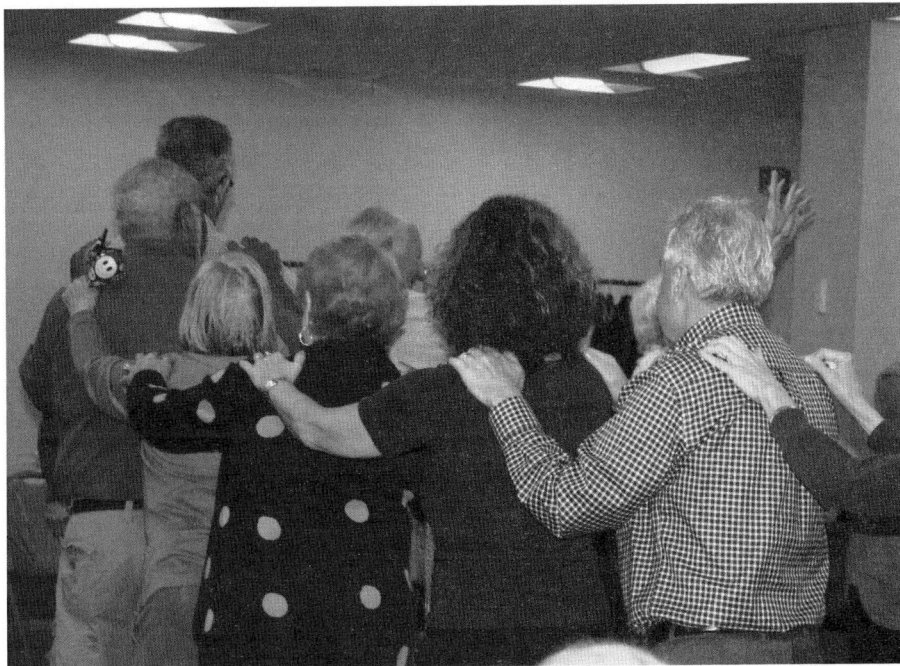

Figure 12.1 This Conga line spontaneously emerged in an environment where each person had a choice

Source: Courtesy of JF&CS of Boston.

while looking beyond themselves. As they open their arms, reaching out to the sides, they often adjust their chairs so as not to make accidental contact with their neighbor. They have begun adapting to both their individual and group needs. As far as the theme goes, I have learned over the years that love is what they appear most interested in. The theme of love also helps create a safe space. In terms of the movement itself, we are changing our shapes as we enclose and spread, gather and scatter, moving in space in the horizontal, vertical, and sagittal planes. We are using different body actions as we lift and flutter and different body parts as we move our arms and our spines, hopefully engaging several of the body connections Irmgard Bartenieff identifies, namely, the arm-scapula, head-tail, and upper-lower connections, as we bend over (Bartenieff & Lewis, 2002; Hackney, 2002).

To ensure safety given their physical challenges, we do most of our moving while seated. For many older adults living in an institution, joint pain and stiffness due to prolonged sitting as well as neurological issues often lead to poor balance. They and the staff around them are fearful of their falling, so they sit more. When they do walk, they tend to be cautious, using considerable tension to hold themselves erect. That tension, while natural, is counterproductive to fluid, grounded, well-balanced movement. While seated, we have the opportunity to safely move off-center. Only when I am confident of their ability to stand will I encourage them to do so, providing support to those who need it. My goals for them individually are to increase spontaneous self-expression, reach into their far kinesphere, move off their center of balance, and most of all to move their spines:

> In doing this and in every way I can conceive, I am attempting to get each person to release as much personal energy, take risks and give as much of themselves to the group as possible. It is not necessarily the size of the movement, but the level of engagement I am looking for. Sometimes, it is the smallest movements which are the most profound. I am looking for movements that demonstrate a sense of connection, to rhythm, to their bodies, to themselves, feelings, memories, and thoughts. I want them to move with some awareness of, and at least momentarily, in relation to another person.
>
> (Newman-Bluestein, 2005, p. 6)

Of course, many of the people I work with don't follow suggestions. While initially, I found that distressing, as is often the case, I learned the most from my most challenging group, the one I mentioned at the beginning of this chapter. About ten minutes into every group, I wondered why I was even trying to get them to be a group. My efforts appeared futile. At that point in each group, it seemed that I surrendered, giving up what were clearly unrealistic goals. As soon as I let go of my expectations, I began to observe what they *were* doing, rather than bemoan what was missing. As I began to see, name, and applaud their very small efforts, to my amazement, I noticed small shifts. Their kinespheres were expanding, as was their range of expressive movement through the use of various props. When I opened up my auditory field, I began to hear some of the sounds in the environment outside our space, to which they were responding. I could appreciate that despite significant dementia, one woman had a strong empathic response to a woman crying in another room. She interpreted the sound as a baby crying—her baby—and she needed to ease her baby's suffering. Understanding this, I could meet her where she was.

Because people in this group were unable to connect with one another, requiring individual attention to engage at all, I turned to my images for guidance.

Image

As in my own dance, the image I hold as therapist is vital and probably the most cohesive element. In general, as the group leader, I see myself first as container, holding not a circle but a sphere which encompasses the multidimensional group experience involving the movement in planes, the emotional, the imaginal, the liminal, and the unconscious as well as the conscious.

As the group unfolds, my images often shift. In groups where participants are unable to connect with anyone other than the group leader, I find a useful image to be that of a wheel, with the leader as the hub and the interactions between the leader and the members as spokes. I hypothesize that the participants are relating to the group leader as though that person were their primary caregiver. As hub of the wheel, I connect with each member of the group individually and repeatedly, in hopes that they will begin to interact with one another (see Figure 12.2):

> With this image emerging quite frequently, I wondered what would happen if I created a physical representation of the wheel out of stretchy fabric. Would I then be able to occupy a seat at the periphery of the circle rather than continually moving through the center? That image led to my creation of the Octaband®. The Octaband® is made of colorful stretchy fabric shaped like an octopus or the sun, with a center circle from which a number of legs emanate. Because there were hems at the end to slip their hands into, it was easy for them to hold

on, and because they could visually, kinesthetically, and tactually see and feel their connection to the others, there began to be a bit of group cohesion. This did, indeed, allow me to be at the periphery with them, and to see myself as one of the members of the circle, receiving as well as giving. The quality of humility is paramount and is symbolized by this image.

(Newman-Bluestein, 2005, p. 5)

Rather than seeing myself bearing sole responsibility for the group, my image needed to expand to see the participants as also responsible. The Octaband® helped me do that. As soon as I experienced the slightest responsiveness on their part as a gift, I experienced meaning and beauty in our exchanges. The relational aspect of my aesthetics was being fed.

Shifting Focus

As the leader, my primary focus is external, paying attention to the group. However, I find my focus shifts very rapidly from external to internal. I find that my intuition kicks in as my attention shifts briefly and swiftly to my internal kinesthetic sense. In those moments, I am often guided by a brief discomfort, as it were. I check within to better discern what I am feeling, based on what I am seeing. It may be that I am observing an evenness to the energy that lasts a bit too long. As my focus returns to the group, I may notice who is moving little and needs individual attention to express themselves more. I arise from my seat and approach

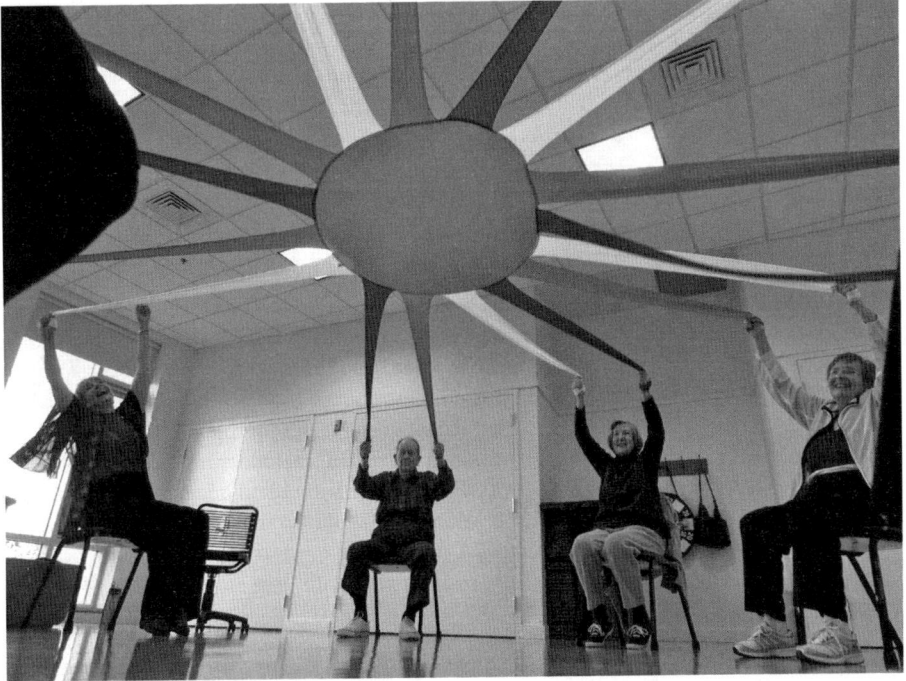

Figure 12.2 The Octaband® affords us the opportunity for mutual play as we each give and receive energy

Source: Charles Daniels Photography.

that person. I may use a gentle touch to get them to open their eyes or I may mirror their movements up close. I crisscross the circle, going from the person who is the least alert to the next least attentive, activating not only the individuals but also the energy at the center of the circle. Again, I find an image helpful. It as though my perspective is a camera lens, shifting rapidly from whole to parts and back to the whole. This shifting between direct and multi-focused aspects of Laban's Space Effort, along with my deep care and concern, is what I believe makes my groups as effective as they are.

Or I may respond to the evenness of the group by changing the pace, introducing suddenness either through what we're doing or by changing the music. When I notice that they or I seem to need a bit of a break, I lower the energy, perhaps bringing our attention to the breath with our hands to our chests, or through sighing, and appreciating a moment of stillness.

Regarding my use of intuition, dance/movement therapist Alma Hawkins wrote:

> When we are functioning at the highly conscious level, we are concerned with the outer world of reality and action. At the deeply unconscious level, our interaction with the outer world is diminished, memory traces are deeply anchored, and there is less interest in action and more concern with self-experience. Between these polarities is believed to be another level of mental activity that has been identified as 'pre-conscious' (Kubie, 1942). This mode of thought makes possible the effortless bringing together of fragments and isolated elements of experience into new constellations. Drawing on affective states and sensory imagery, a spontaneous stream of thought results in clustering around a preconceived goal.
>
> (Hawkins, 1991, p. 7; Kubie, 1942)

In a discussion with a DMT colleague, I once mentioned my use of intuition in leading groups. She advised me not to speak of intuition, that it makes it seem as though DMT has no foundation actually grounded in theory. I am confident that not only is DMT grounded in theory, but intuition is part of that theory. It is also, in part, where our artistry lies.

Optimizing the Environment Through Props

Because difficulty initiating is one of the executive functions often affected by dementia, giving people stimuli to respond to reduces their need to initiate and changes their environment to one that is less stressful and more supportive of ongoing engagement with life (Coaten & Newman-Bluestein, 2013; Newman-Bluestein, 2017). In general, the greater the level of dementia, the more I use props, because they provide a structure, which people with dementia need. Props can help elicit a range of Effort qualities and provide motivation for a person to reach farther into their kinesphere, all of which contributes to a greater aesthetic experience.

In order to focus my attention entirely on them during the group, I create, in advance, a musical playlist beginning with music of their era which I find irresistible, that I think will appeal to them, is culturally sensitive, and that has lyrics they may remember. Using a high-quality sound system, I play music evocative of a range of dance styles. As we warm up our bodies, we begin expanding our physical range of movement.

Ribbon wands are plastic sticks with colorful ribbons attached and are usually the first prop I offer, providing group members with an opportunity to choose colors, to further elicit their rhythmic responses, and to expand the visual component of their movement (Newman-Bluestein, 2017; Newman-Bluestein & Hill, 2010). Regardless of diminishing cognitive abilities, most people have the ability and the desire to make choices, whether of colors or whether or not they want to participate. Honoring their choices reinforces their sense of agency. Observing, mirroring, and naming their movements, i.e., bouncing, swinging, or twirling, side to side, up and down, forward and back, effectively increases their responses (Newman-Bluestein & Hill, 2010).

The ribbon wands tend to boost the individual energy group members expend. As I observe their movement, I am looking to increase their range of movement, both physically and expressively, finding contrasts that make the dance more interesting, for me and for them. Maracas are another frequently used prop, appealing to their auditory engagement. And while balloons may seem to have little to do with dance, there is no other prop I have seen which prompts group members to move to the edges of their kinesphere or to move as spontaneously as the balloon. With the ribbon wands, balloons, and with scarves, I encourage a range of Efforts. All three of these props may be used with lightness. However, flexing the wrist with the ribbon wand with a sudden, whipping type of movement creates a snapping sound that wakes us up and usually generates laughter. Similarly, encouraging group members to hit the balloon with strength, directness, and quickness often results in great hilarity. While we often use scarves to waltz music for lyrical movement, by using a little tango music and changing direction on the count of 4, we begin to create some of the dramatic contrast I long for. With a cognitively higher-functioning population, using derby hats in the manner of choreographer Bob Fosse tends to foster their playfulness and observation of one another as well as to build upon memories they may have of Broadway and movie musicals. Finally, group props such as Octaband®s contribute to an increased level of group awareness and connection.

As Chaiklin (2016) stated, dance allows individuals to relate to their community while simultaneously being able to express their own impulses and needs within the group. The shared energy and strength that comes from being with others enables people to go beyond their personal limitations or concerns. Moving together brings joy, providing validation of our own worth as well as recognition of our personal struggles (p. 5).

Group Leader's Movement Style

In 2010, as part of a grant-funded project, Certified Movement Analyst Jackie Hand analyzed video footage of my movement patterns while leading a DMT group with people with dementia to identify effective elements of my leadership style. Among her findings was considerable attention to Space with both Direct and Indirect focus, a flexible expressive range, and adapting my shape to each participant. She also noted an interesting spatial pathway: in the beginning of the group, I approached each person directly, shaking hands, exchanging names, and making eye contact. I then backed away toward the center of the circle before approaching the person beside them in the circle. I repeated that pattern with every person. I was unaware of that pattern until she reflected it back to me. I realized that my backing away was purposeful so that they would see my leave-taking as deliberate, rather than leaving them to be with someone else. That pattern also seems reminiscent of the Octaband® shape.

Salient Moments

It is in this atmosphere where openness and spontaneity are encouraged that some new movement usually happens, whether in moving with a prop, gesturing as they speak, sharing memories, interacting with others, or entrusting secrets. There is a depth and volume of synergy that emerges from this interdependence which is surprising, energizing all of us. Murmurs of appreciation can always be heard at the end of a group.

Because memories are stored in the body's muscles and tissues, expressive movement often stimulates the release of memories. Within the safe context of a group, people will often share something important. It may be something that they repeat often, such as: "I was the only girl, with five older brothers." It may be something that they say quietly and with great feeling, only to me: "Life is good. There is no slavery in my life since I was released from the concentration camp where my son died." One woman, 100 years old, was in a group where two of us were swinging a jump rope across the circle. She asked for a second rope so that she could swing "double dutch". As she swung the second rope, she said, "I wonder if Jane died. She used to be my partner." Yet another woman with lifelong physical and cognitive challenges cried on remembering an uncle who used to carry her to school. They were tears of sadness and joy. Another Holocaust survivor found herself not wanting to talk about something that was bothering her, yet she continued to speak. She acknowledged, "I didn't tell my children; I tried to protect them. I found out that my daughter knew when I was worried, even though I tried to not let her know. I lost a son." Rather than feeling depressed at these memories, at the end of group she smiled and said, "You're wonderful. You made me feel better." She acknowledged that she felt better because she was accepted for what she was feeling and not pretending. When one woman forcefully threw a balloon to me, I asked her where her strength came from. She answered, "Wisconsin." I asked, "Wisconsin?" She said, "Yes. I grew up on a farm." There are many who cannot verbalize except to say, with great effort at the end of a group, "Thank you" as they look earnestly into my eyes, press my hand with theirs, or blow kisses.

Of course, there are also the stories of those who cannot speak with words. Theirs are the dances of prolonged handshakes prior to group—the physical jokester, who willingly dons a ridiculous hat; the person who doesn't remember how to use a fork but whose spine lengthens elegantly when she hears a waltz; and the man who speaks gibberish but knows to toss the balloon gently to the frail elderly woman and smashes it to me.

Closing Ritual

To mark the end of the group, I close with the following ritual: three times, we slowly take a breath in, bringing our hands up in front of us only as high as our shoulders; we breathe out, bringing our hands down. After the third time, I say with accompanying gestures, "In a gesture that symbolizes what we've been doing, we give a little bit of ourselves to everyone here and we receive a little bit of everyone right back in." We move our hands face up, from the heart, arms extending forward and then out to the sides and back to the heart. I follow that with, "We give with our words, our movements, our voices, our smiles, our presence." Most of the group members, even those who didn't join in the opening greeting ritual, usually do the ending ritual.

SUMMARY

Dance is ephemeral. As an art form based in the kinesthetic sense, it can only be experienced in the here and now. Barbara Mettler's thoughts are relevant to our understanding:

[Improvisation] is our dance here and now, to be created and performed with all the skill at our disposal. . . . Each dance is unique according to the time, the place, and the people. . . .

Our improvisations need not have impressive climaxes and conclusions. They are not interpretations of life, they are authentic life experiences—casual, flowing, irrevocable and
precious—to be begun, continued and ended as simply as any other phase of life.

(1960, p. 401)

Our group dance is a time and space set aside for playing with others, expressing ourselves
through the medium of dance as well as through our voices. It's a time when we are all more
in our bodies, expressing our rhythmic responses through movement, hopefully in synchrony,
but where every person's movement is appreciated for its uniqueness as well. There's a certain satisfaction is seeing people come alive, feel emboldened to express themselves, and
make choices, internally led.

The physical contrasts may not be as striking as would be the case for professional
dancers, but compared to how they are at the beginning of a group, the difference is often
dramatic. Prior to group, people are often sitting inert, passively settled into their chairs, not
relating to other people or their environments. Sometimes I feel like a magician, where, with
a few words and gestures, we move from a still tableau into a dance of interaction. Watching
their focus shift from internal to external in our initial greeting as my presence invites theirs is
itself quite moving. With props and the relationship to motivate their engagement and without an internal censor to inhibit them, people with dementia are generally quite playful and
spontaneous. While some people may still participate in activities because of social propriety,
there are many who will not unless their intrinsic motivation is tapped. It must be meaningful
for them to engage. It is a rare group where I am not surprised by their contributions. The
synergy that happens when every person brings their self as fully as possible, which happens
in most groups, is a remarkably joyous and fulfilling experience—for me, for them, and for
any staff who happen by.

Expressive arts therapy pioneer Shaun McNiff (2004) wrote:

Groups are capable of generating much more energy and power than a person acting alone.
The leader activates the energy of community, setting in motion a dynamic interplay among
the people, the space, the images, and the spirits of expression. This creates the atmosphere
of authenticity and healing only available in a safe and sacred space.

(p. 30)

In my work with these older adults and people with neurocognitive impairments, I am
continually moved by their genuineness, which further feeds my sense of aesthetics. As people age, they seem to become more of who they are, more themselves. I love working with
people in a way which is authentic, unlike the everyday world where there is so much artifice.
These people have to be who they are—it seems as if they have no choice. At a time in their
lives when they need care, surrounded by people they don't know, slowed down, avoiding
risks, rarely moving suddenly or off balance, they and I delight in our dance together.

REFERENCES

Bartenieff, I., & Lewis, D. (2002). *Body movement: Coping with the environment*. London: Routledge.
Bloom, K., Adrian, B., Casciero, T., Mizenko, J., & Porter, C. (2017). *The Laban workbook for actors: A practical
training guide with video*. London, England: Bloomsbury Publishing.
Blumenfeld-Jones, D. (1997). Aesthetic experience, hermeneutics, and curriculum. In *Philosophy of Education
Archive* (pp. 313–321). Tempe, AZ: Arizona State University.
Chaiklin, S., & Wengrower, H. (Eds.). (2016). We dance from the moment our feet touch the earth. In S.
Chaiklin & H. Wengrower (Eds.), *The art and science of dance/movement therapy: Life is dance* (pp. 3–12). New
York: Routledge.

Coaten, R., & Newman-Bluestein, D. (2013). Embodiment and dementia: Dance movement psychotherapists respond. *Dementia, 12*(6), 677–681. doi: 10.1177/1471301213507033

Dell, C. (1977). *A primer for movement description* (2nd ed.). New York: Dance Notation Bureau.

Fraleigh, S. H. (1980). Aesthetic perception in dance. In C. E. Thomas (Ed.), *Aesthetics and dance* (pp. 24–26). Washington, DC: AAHPERD Publications.

Hackney, P. (2002). *Making connections: Total body integration through Bartenieff Fundamentals.* New York: Routledge.

Hawkins, A. M. (1991). Moving from within. In *A new method for dance making.* Chicago, IL: A cappella books.

Hervey, L. W. (2000). *Artistic inquiry in dance/movement therapy: Creative alternatives for research.* Springfield, IL: Charles C Thomas Publisher Ltd.

Kubie, L. S. (1942). *Neurotic distortion of the creative process.* New York, NY: Farrar, Strauss & Giroux.

Mcniff, S. (2004). *Art heals: How creativity cures the soul.* Boulder, CO: Shambhala Publications.

Mettler, B. (1960). *Materials of dance: As a creative art activity* (3rd ed.). Tucson: Mettler Studios.

Newman-Bluestein, D. (2005). *Seeing with the heart: The aesthetics of dance/movement therapy with the elderly.* 40th Annual Conference Proceedings, ADTA, MD.

Newman-Bluestein, D. (2017, June). Improving quality of life for people with dementia through dance/movement therapy. *Creativity & Human Development Online Journal.*

Newman-Bluestein, D., & Hill, H. (2010). Movement as the medium for connection, empathy, playfulness. *Journal of Dementia Care, 18*(5), 24–27.

Rogers, C. R. (1995). *On becoming a person: A therapist's view of psychotherapy.* Boston, MA: Houghton Mifflin Harcourt.

CHAPTER 13

DANCE-RHYTHM-THERAPY FOR PATIENTS WITH PARKINSON'S DISEASE

Emilie Jauffret-Hanifi, Svetlana Panova, France Schott-Billmann

INTRODUCTION

Dance has always been part of the rituals of healing and celebration in traditional cultures. Over time, it has maintained an important role in various civilizations and can serve various functions. It is an art that allows the articulation of movement through rhythm and the added possibility of sculpting time and space through movement.

Rhythm is everywhere and around us all the time. Our first rhythmic experience is that of the heartbeat and breathing. Thus, rhythm is an activity both perceived by a human being and produced by them: the external rhythm is related to our own inner rhythmic experience.

It is this relationship that we have been exploring for six years in our Dance-Rhythm-Therapy workshops with people with Parkinson's disease (PD).[1] The Primitive Expression method that we use in our work in DRT[2] (Dance-Rhythm-Therapy) is based on the use of rhythm, especially "primitive" rhythms: beating and swaying (Schott-Billmann, 2015a). People with PD have significant physiological arrhythmias, resulting in psychological and emotional disorders and withdrawal into themselves.

Many studies on the use of rhythm (McIntosh, Brown, Rice, & Thaut, 1997; Pacchetti et al., 2000; Sacks, 2007; Nombela, Hughes, Owen, & Grahn, 2013) and on dance practice in PD (Hackney, Kantorovitch, Levin, & Earhart, 2007, 2009; Marchant, Sylvester, & Earhart, 2010; Heiberger et al., 2011) have legitimized these mediations[3] as a method of supportive care in the management of PD which is, after Alzheimer's disease, the most common neurodegenerative disease in France (Moisan et al., 2018).

After a presentation of the Primitive Expression method and PD, we will describe the methodology which allowed us to establish a protocol of practice and experimentation in DRT with the patients. By correlating the symptoms, the tools used, and the benefits obtained, we are then better able to identify the medical and psychological benefits of the Primitive Expression as a supportive care for PD.

A DANCE-RHYTHM-THERAPY METHOD: PRIMITIVE EXPRESSION

Today, there are different approaches in dance-therapy; DRT is one of them. It gives a central place to the rhythm as well as to the social and therapeutic function of folk dances, which for centuries were performed in town squares (Schott-Billmann, 2015a). Among all these dances, one of them held our attention: Primitive Expression.

Herns Duplan, a Haitian dancer and disciple of the African-American choreographer Katherine Dunham, created Primitive Expression in the 1970s. It is a simple and powerful Métis dance, rhythmed by the drum with structured, codified, symbolic, and repetitive gestures and vocalized by asemantic phonemes. He valued the word "Primitive", which should be understood as "primordial." Not meant to be a hypothetical primitive society but the first gesture performed with the first rhythms: the heartbeat and breath. The heartbeat converted in the drumbeat that accompanies dance; the breath converted in the rhythm and balanced movements.

African and Afro-American dances present characteristics close to the dances of therapeutic rituals: energetic and strongly rhythmed by a drum beat. Moreover, the gestures are accessible, repetitive, and liberating. Thus, this type of dance seemed to us adaptable to a dance-therapy method.

The Primitive Expression method, developed by France Schott-Billmann, preserves the ritual elements, the tribal climate and the evocation of a "primitive" imaginary world. But it engages in a different type of relationship with the participants. In this case, Primitive Expression is proposed as a third-party mediating dance. It allows a therapeutic process based on symbolization[4] to discover the right distance between the other and oneself, the imagination and reality, desire and the Law (Schott-Billmann, 2018).

For therapeutic use, we use several tools.

The Ritual

The ritual calls for repetition and rhythm. The latter is given by the drum, struck by a percussionist. His cadence connects to the vital rhythm; beat and cadence imitate the heart and the breath, the first rhythmic and musical experience perceived by the fetus in the womb. To this is added the use of the voice without words that refers to preverbal language. The repetition of sound patterns and gestures recalls the repetitive nature of a baby's play.

The group becomes a sort of autonomous entity in which the dancers wrap themselves and merge, finding solid support and heady resonance. In fact, this method is "choral": in the unison of gestures and the chanted or melodic voice, each dancer becomes in relation to the group that swings in cadence, like the child in the arms of the mother who rocks them (Schott-Billmann, 2018).

Rhythmic Games

Primitive Expression reactivates the transitional space through rhythmic games inspired by those shared by mother and child, from lullabies to exchanges of gestures and facial expressions. We can compare the humanizing, socializing, structuring, and empowering work of the mother to her child and that of the therapist to his or her patient (Winnicott, 2002; Dolto, 2013). Anthropology shows us that the activities of traditional societies which are necessary for social and individual balance make use of the structures of children's games with mothers or peers (e.g., repetition games with words) (Schott-Billmann, 2011, 2013, 2015b).

Creation Times

These are choreographic and rhythmic, gestural and verbal times[5] in the sessions. These creation times are always done in small groups for the dynamics of relationship and communication between its members while respecting the rhythmic framework. These creations are based on themes with strong therapeutic potential (e.g., the ugly duckling that becomes a swan), which then solicit the patients' imaginations.

The Therapist's Function

The therapist is the guarantor of the framework. They give injunctions to the dancers who relive with them an archaic and hypnotic parental relationship. Their injunctions are meant to have intrinsic value and effectiveness. They are gestural and verbal; the gestures are accessible, powerful, and figurative, and the words they pronounce are related to their symbolism. Thus, everyone can extract a particular memory, can appropriate archetypal images from the collective unconscious, can give meaning to the emotional experiences they trigger and can build social bonds (Schott-Billmann, 2018).

The Symbolization of Impulses

The injunctions given to the dancers are therefore symbols that appeal to the imagination. Through these symbolic gestures, the dancers play primary emotions, primary actions (e.g., take/give, attract/repel), first gestures coupled in opposites (e.g., appear/disappear) which are at the source of the symbolization mechanism. For Winnicott (2002), therapy is playing. In Primitive Expression, the dancers play and joy reigns. Since the therapist also plays, it is felt not real, so there is no guilt, we pretend—that is, we say without saying—while saying!

The Self-Awareness Process

Primitive Expression enables us to be more aware of ourselves, of our body. But it is in the unconscious that the true transformation takes place. The gestures emitted by the dance-rhythm-therapist are a symbolic statement; the participants capture them; the gestures are repeated, they insist on being heard, read. The gesture that is seen, enacted, and felt arouses analogies, associations, emotions. It makes sense. The meaning is what the dancer feels when he receives the symbolic gesture and then begins to incorporate it, to appropriate it, to embody it. The process leads to the gesture speaking to him; the dancer expresses corporeally and freely the emotion that the gesture has aroused in them, which will be different from the one in the neighboring dancer (Schott-Billmann, 2018).

PARKINSON'S DISEASE (PD)

PD is manifested by impressive and key motor disorders mainly in adults age 60, but younger subjects can also be affected. It is due to the disappearance, unexplained until today, of neurons in a brain area called the black substance. The function of these neurons is to make and release dopamine, a neurotransmitter essential to the control of the body's movements. Their necrosis show motors symptoms of the disease, which are called "Parkinson's triad." These are:

- Slowness (Bradykinesia) related to the difficulty initiating and coordinating movements. Patients feel fatigued, numbness or the feeling of being blocked. Blocking (akinesia) is when key motor skills, such as writing, which are semi-automatic actions are affected. In the case of walking, the blocking can manifest as dragging, fast and small steps (called festination) in front of an obstacle or even a stopping of the movement (called freezing).

- Hypertonia, muscular rigidity, muscular or tendinous pain, and a feeling of stiffness. This can be observed at rest with a posture that is clenched, arched forward, and the head bowed.

- Tremor: it is an involuntary tremor at rest; if the person initiates a movement it stops. As well as akinesia, Parkinson shaking is closely correlated to the emotional state of mind. A stressful situation or a strong emotion can make shaking considerably worse. Conversely, in comforting and safe situations, the shaking can be significantly reduced.

The degeneration of dopamine also causes non-motor symptoms, such as depression and fatigue, because it plays a role in the regulation of mood, psychic tone, and pleasure.

Dance, Rhythm, and PD

The treatment of PD is complex. It combines medication (L-Dopa Therapy) and supporting drug-free treatments: motor rehabilitation and physical activity. As PD is reflected mainly through motor disorders, the regular practice of physical activity is one of the pillars of its management (Rafferty et al., 2017).

Many studies (Hackney et al., 2007; Westheimer, 2007; Hackney & Earhart, 2009; Marchant et al., 2010; Heiberger et al., 2011), based on small groups, have shown the usefulness and benefits that the practice of dance could bring to patients at the motor, psychological, or relational levels. These observations were confirmed at the Congress of Neurology in Shanghai, where the positive effects of movement based on music, walking, and balance related to the symptoms associated with PD were shown (De Dreu, Van der Wilk, Poppe, Kwakkel, & Van Wegen, 2012).

Regarding dance-therapy, there are very few studies on the use of it for PD (Westbrook & McKibben, 1989). This study highlights the fact that dance-therapy improves the initiation of movement in people with PD as well as walking speed.

Much research has also been done on the use of rhythm in PD (McIntosh et al., 1997; Nombela et al., 2013; Pacchetti et al., 2000; Sacks, 2007). The research shows that the use of rhythm facilitates walking and helps patients overcome slow movements, freezing, imbalance, and lack of muscle control.

All of this research show us that Primitive Expression is an interesting dance-therapy method in the accompaniment of treating Parkinson's patients because it uses both danced movement and rhythm as specific tools to meet the needs and problems of participants.

That's why Doctor Fève, a Parkinson's expert at Bellan Hospital in Paris who knew the work of France Schott-Billmann, proposed to her in 2010 that she pilot a DRT workshop for a group of 12 Parkinson's patients.

Meeting the Patients

It is quite different to read descriptions of the disease and to be confronted with its manifestations in patients. When we met the 12 patients (five men, seven women, aged 28 to 72), their physical suffering struck us, especially that of the young Parkinson's patients.

As dancers, for whom the automatisms of the body are self-evident, this triggered in us a deep empathy, and we fully understood the complaint of patients about the psychological consequences of their motor disabilities. They talked about the difficulty of concentration and attention, loss of initiative, apathy, anxiety, memory loss, loss of self-esteem and in the majority, sadness, depression, or even despair due to the loss of quality of life.

At one of the first sessions, we proposed to the patients that they walk around while listening to the drum by moving their body freely (if we can say that, because we were struck by the stiffness of their movements) and singing all together. Despite reduction of the kinesphere,[6] the powerful effect of rhythm and song emerged: the disappearance of tremors and blockages, but more importantly, the group members' smiles, manifestations of joy and the desire to begin the process.

CREATION OF AN ADAPTED DANCE-THERAPY WORKSHOP IN COLLABORATION WITH PATIENTS[7]

The objective of this workshop was to give patients the benefit of both the regulating and stimulating role of rhythm in order to compensate for the dopamine deficiency that is at the origin of PD disorders.

Following this first session, we created and used an observation table (Table 13.1) in order to more clearly evaluate the impact of Primitive Expression on motor symptoms. However, this tool could only be used for a short period (four months). Indeed, it is very difficult for us today to be able to put in place tools to observe and evaluate our practice on PD in the institution where we work because the hospital lacks the resources, both financial and human, to support us in our sessions and in our research. However, it is important to note that the positive effects of the workshops felt by patients improved doctors' interest and confidence in our work. To be able to propose a therapeutic strategy to treat the different aspects of the disease, we base our work on our observations as dance-therapists and also on listening to the complaints, i.e., the needs of the patients. These needs made us broaden our objectives since, on the one hand, the symptoms that manifested themselves at the physical level were not only motor but also fatigue and pain as well as the disease's impact on the patients at the social and psychological levels.

At the Body Level

A DRT session begins by reconnecting the patients to their body through breathing and awakening their senses. Starting with a sitting circle we listen to the African drum (djembe) and then make slow movements of the arms (up-down, open-close) in connection with breathing and gentle stretches. This gradual entry establishes the first contact between the body, sound, external rhythm, and other participants. Work on motor and non-motor symptoms can begin.

Non-Motor Symptoms

There is much pain in PD: muscle, joint, tendons, visceral, and so on. (Moisan et al., 2018). Few studies were made on the effectiveness of dance to decrease the pain.

Note, however, the study of Berrol, Ooi, and Katz (1997) on the impact of dance/movement therapy in the elderly who have had neurological trauma. Berrol observed that participants had less physical pain after five months of participation in the workshops.

Table 13.1 Observation Table—Impact of Primitive Expression on Motor Symptoms

DAY:						*PATIENT'S NAME:*

Number of members in the group:
Number of patients present:
Number of patients absent:
Other members present:
Atmosphere of the institution (special event, and so on.):

GENERAL POINTS

SCORE (*)	1	2	3	4	5	*Comments*
Need help to initiate movement						Refused Reticent Accepted Requested
Tremor at the beginning of the session						
Tremor at the end of the session						

(*) Score levels: 1: very infrequent 2: infrequent 3: frequent 4: very frequent 5: always

SPECIFIC POINTS EXPRESSION PRIMITIVE

SCORE (*)	1	2	3	4	5	*Comments*
Pulsation with the feet						
Pulsation with the hands						
Use voice						
Combination feet, hands, voice						
Combination hands, voice						
Presentation Ritual						
Stop & go game						Rhythm increase: yes/no
Walking with opposition arm/leg						Rhythm increase: yes/no
Walking with bent knees						Rhythm increase: yes/no
Walking on half points						Rhythm increase: yes/no
Walking backwards						Rhythm increase: yes/no
Alternating slow/fast walking						Rhythm increase: yes/no
Statues dance						Rhythm increase: yes/no
Response to the drum						
Repeating movements						Rhythm increase: yes/no
Balance						Rhythm increase: yes/no
Bust twisting						Rhythm increase: yes/no
Isolations (head, shoulders, pelvis . . .)						Head: yes/no Shoulders: yes/no Pelvis: yes/no Bust: yes/no
Motion and sound proposals						
Presence of facial expressions						
Call/Response						
Final Choir						
Final Ritual						
Breathing Use						
Other observations						

(*) Score levels: 1: very difficult 2: difficult 3: fairly easy 4: easy 5: very easy

Additional comments:

Much research in music demonstrates the superiority of dance in physical therapy when the dance is, as in a tango, associated with the music. The music reduces the pain significantly after five minutes of exposure (Mitchell & MacDonald, 2006). Dance, which is usually pleasant, is a painkiller. Moving to music in a synchronized way, with a partner or group, makes it possible to better resist pain because the brain secretes endorphins (Tarr, Launay, Cohen, & Dunbar, 2015). These hormones have an analgesic role, and have an impact on the pain threshold of the participants. However, this happens on one condition: moving actively in rhythm with several people!

This is what we do in Primitive Expression to the beat of the drum. Indeed, bass and repetitive sounds, such as the sounds produced by the drum, promote muscle relaxation (Cungi & Limousin, 2003) and particularly affect the production of endorphins (Cardinale & Durieux, 2004). The state of well-being, strength, and effortless movement following the physical effort, is due to endorphins. Of course we do not ask for a performance from our disabled patients, but they may very well participate in the dance for 30 to 45 minutes at a pace of comfortable endurance.

Endorphins are also stimulated by laughter. It therefore seems essential to introduce an atmosphere of gaiety in the sessions, which is strongly supported by the humor of the patients and represented by an intelligent and effective defense system. For example, one day they sang, "We are Parkinsonians and we are not afraid of anything," to accompany a collective choreographic creation.

Non-motor symptoms are also defined by fatigue. Music has several relaxing effects (De Dreu et al., 2012), and rhythm is an important therapeutic factor. So from the beginning of the sessions, we are accompanied by the drum which supports the rhythmic warm-up and body percussion (i.e., produce a rhythm using our body as a musical instrument). We observed from the very first session (and what has recurred each time) how the rhythm stimulates patients, "taking them" quickly in it is repetitive flow, "as if we put us on a treadmill" they would say, and their tiredness is forgotten. The rhythm is a regulator that manages gestures, so it lessens fatigue. The percussionist takes on the role of a co-therapist who, in interaction with the dancers, slows down or speeds up the pace according to their shortness of breath. The session must remain constantly doable and enjoyable while also being active. One of our patients, Sophie, talks about feeling "good tired" at the end of a session.

The repetition of gesture was immediately popular with the first therapy group. It allowed for better control and increased endurance and strength. Both muscular rehabilitation and energy boost, the gesture renews itself like the beating of the heart. It recreates automatisms that facilitate movement, thus reducing both physical and mental fatigue.

Motor Symptoms

We can observe patients' PD motor symptoms in their walking and movements. We are not dealing with dancers; therefore the approach should be simple and promote awareness of their body by first separating the different parts of the body in a warm-up and then associating them again in dance movements accompanied by voice. Having a better awareness of one's body helps to fight against body stiffness. This increases both muscle and joint flexibility and leads to deeper breathing, which helps patients to relax. One patient, Laurent, said:

> This is an activity that I could never give up. In terms of pulsations, it allows me to better coordinate my movements and release any tensions.

In people with PD, deficiency of dopamine can cause an arrhythmia in walking. The walk of a Parkinson's patient is stiff, unstable, sometimes in small steps under the effect of bradykinesia, with a total and painful inability to move. Explaining or showing the gesture by breaking it down is ineffective. However, different studies have shown that the use of rhythm facilitated walking by synchronizing movement to a regular pulse (Nombela et al., 2013) helped patients to overcome slow movement, freezing, and imbalance and improved their muscle control (McIntosh et al., 1997; Pacchetti et al., 2000; Sacks, 2007).

In Primitive Expression, the rhythm of the drum brings on the beat, the sound is short and repeated; it is the pulse that pounds, which pushes and exerts a thrust on the body. The patient responds that it is as if he heard the drum tell him "go on" or "1–2–3 walk." The rhythm energizes the motor system.

"When I'm blocked, I put on some music and I walk. It releases me." We have seen repeatedly a blocked patient, both elongated and rigid, unlock himself on hearing the drum, his feet beginning to beat, then landing on the ground, he stood up and begin to walk. The rhythm, repeating the beat on a regular basis, allows one to rely on it and synchronize the different parts of the body, head to toe.

During the research done in the field of music, the comments and remarks from patients have encouraged us to use rhythm walks and stops in space to help restart patients' walking and decrease their apprehension of freezing, because they know how to identify it.

The feet take the beat proposed by the percussionist's various rhythms (slow, medium, fast), which are sometimes associated with hand clapping to enhance synchronization of different parts of the body. This also relies on the symmetric arm swings and laterality. The exercise to stop walking when the percussionist stops the music (which he does voluntarily by surprise) focuses the patients' attention on balance and body awareness. Then the music resumes and participants walk by taking large or small steps. During these sessions, we encourage walking by twos or threes, always in a playful spirit.

The work done on walking helps prevent falls, worry about which is part of the daily life of Parkinson's patients. With the rhythm and repetitive movements becoming more precise, detailed, and safe, patients learn to prevent falls by managing imbalances, by accelerating the speed of movement, and by anticipating their movements and potential obstacles. Thus, when we work the repetition of actions stand/sit, we are working on the transfer of weight which ensures better balance in a sustainable manner, as demonstrated by Louis: "Now I can get up and go to the toilet easier."

PD not only hinders the walking of our patients, but it also hinders their daily life movements. Therefore, we propose, through various dance exercises, to work on different aspects of movement such as amplitude, fluidity, coordination, tremor, voice, and facial expressions.

Amplitude is one aim of rehabilitation as the Parkinson movements are narrowed to a small kinesphere. Our way of expanding it, which has the advantage of being at the same time a source of pleasure, is the repetition of the gesture made on varying lengths of time (slow/medium/fast pace, or the execution of time in an 8, 4, 2, 1 time division). Repetition produces a resonance which results in an amplification and security, leading to gradual steps and movements, as if to loosen brakes because the apprehension of losing balance disappears, the movements "loosen up", expand, breathe.

The repetitive gesture leads to interaction between the protagonist/antagonist muscles: when one moves, the other, at the same time, relaxes. The repetition is automatic, the movement "walking alone", allowing for letting go, releases itself from tension and surrenders to the stream that spreads throughout the body, freeing the movement and steps which become gradually more flexible, more fluid. The result is fast: "It frees the body, these dance sessions," said Alice. It develops confidence in your own body, as Sophie pointed out:

> I practice the dance-therapy and over time I realize all the benefits I get from this activity. Indeed, it helps to improve Parkinson's symptoms by more flexibility, less pain and with a more secure walk. . . . This workshop gave me more confidence.

Having more confidence in her walk gives her more confidence in life. The body and the mind are linked. This is why, the Primitive Expression seeks to strengthen the supports of the body rather than relying on a partner as in couple dance. Symmetrical movement allows one to become aware of the body's axis and to focus its support on the spine, which offers structure both physically and psychologically.

Improving the coordination of movements is an essential to combat against disease. With repetition, movements become more precise, movements are better directed in body space and surrounding space where the dancer gradually feels at home. Synchronization by rhythm makes it possible to involve several parts of the body in the movement (e.g., feet, pelvis, and arms).

Stimulating, the rhythm is also an authorizing factor of movement: it organizes, structures, and makes it more solid—the dancer can lean on it like a railing. Coordination is also essential for another common disorder in PD, dyskinesia, abnormal and involuntary movements, which are uncontrollable and dangerous. "My dyskinesia tends to decrease or even disappear," said Laurent.

Before the workshop, some patients had hand tremors. These tremors were more or less strong and/or more or less wide. The movement attenuated tremors, and we were able to see that the use of rhythm accentuated this advantage: tremors decreased or even disappeared during the sessions. The presence of regular pulsations in auditory stimuli could increase the activity of basal lymph nodes affected by PD, thus compensating for the lack of dopamine stimulation that causes the tremors (Nombela et al., 2013). Here is an example with Paul:

> Paul has tremors in his right hand which are very frequent. These tremors constantly decrease in frequency at the end of the sessions. They will even disappear in the middle of a session during a workshop.

Another particularly disabling symptom of bradykinesia in the face is weakening of the voice and making the voice monotonous. The production of vocal sounds makes it possible to work out the phonation muscles, which are often affected by PD. In Primitive Expression, the chanted voice (ha-ha-ha-ha) or the voice linked in melody is part of the musical accompaniment. The dance-rhythm-therapist and patients sing while dancing. Also, voice and movement train each other: the volume of the sounds emitted influences the posture and movements performed by patients. On soft/low sounds, the associated movements are small, while on a loud sound, the postures rise and the movements gain in amplitude.

It is also emotionally liberating. The chanted or melodic voice awakens the emotion and gives it a sonorous expression. Moreover, through the vibrations of the vocal chords, patients participate in resonance which involves all parts of the body, extends to the brain and spreads to the cortical areas. The tuning of movement to the voice through sounds, vocals, and songs reinforces the physical action by giving it sense. It fights speech disorders and participates in the letting go process, which allows the patients to feel confident.

In PD, facial expressions disappear in part; the face becomes inexpressive. Parkinson's patients appear cold and scarcely smile. However, if in the playful atmosphere of Primitive

Expression, we "work" the faces through different choreographies, we notice that the muscles react. Moreover, this work on emotional facial expressions brings joy and laughter to the participants who forget all inhibition and have fun with each other.

At the Social Level

The Parkinson's triad (slowness, hypertonia, and tremor), the depression, and the fatigue caused by the disease are a social handicap for people suffering from PD. Anxieties about potentially falling cause the fear of going out of the house, and the difficulty in communicating one's emotions puts social bonds at risk. Patients isolate themselves and complain of solitude. For them, social and psychological suffering is more important than motor suffering.

The Group

A recent study by Johnson and Dunbar (2016) confirms the importance of group and social environment in the liberation of endorphins and therefore in the fight against pain and anxiety for the appearance of joy and well-being. DRT offers Parkinson's patients a group, as in traditional or tribal dances, which reinforces the social bond. Further, the cohesion of the group allow them to share a common rhythm. Synchrony, like sympathy, establishes attunement in the mother-child bond, the first interhuman bond (Stern, 1985). The sound space and rhythm that mark time not only have a container function but also give participants the desire to move and the pleasure of communicating. Every week they rejoice in the warmth of the group in dancing in unison. Their regular attendance is noticed by doctors who point out that it is a guarantee of success. Sophie confirms: "This workshop made me feel better; and it allowed me to meet again in a group where I have built relationships of friendship and solidarity." These friendships continue outside the session, particularly in the practice of other activities.

Communication

Parkinson's patients are often perceived as cold people because the disease freezes the muscles in their faces. We focus in our work on reviving expressiveness through the whole body. But it is also necessary to take patients out of their withdrawal from themselves and from disinterest in other persons. Thus, we multiply the interactions by creating two groups that dance face to face, thus allowing each one to see the other and to be seen.

Finally, the use of popular songs for circle dances makes it possible to identify with each other, to enrich oneself with the suggestions of others, and to share one's origins and culture with others. It is a way to keep the link with the outside world and the news.

The Expression of Emotions

To make up for the lack of expression of emotions that hampers communication, we stimulate the expressiveness of the body and voice. We offer patients eloquent gestures that we frequently borrow from the theatre to give them strong symbolism: give/receive, escape/attack, tear/repair, separate/unite. But we also utilize facial expressions, which are particularly important for these patients. Often this is successful, leading to "no more frozen faces." For instance, even Carole, whose face had lost all mobility, began to smile.

Quality of Life

Daily mobility is encouraged in DRT through space exploration exercises, movement management, self-confidence building, and relationships with others, therefore ensuring the body improves patients' autonomy and quality of life. We must therefore give them the tools to face the obstacles of everyday life. Thus, all these points converge to improve their quality of life.

At the Psychic Level

Body and psyche are in constant interaction. Thus, as we have shown here, work on the social and physical levels has an impact on the psychological level. Paul shares with us his feelings after several years of participating in the workshop: "I see a clear improvement on the clinical and psychological level during the "movement" and in particular during the dance-therapy sessions."

Self-Confidence and Autonomy

With the development of motor disorders, patients feel dependent on those around them to get out. This is very difficult for them to accept. Restoring self-confidence is essential. By repeating the same gestures over and over again, the patients gradually gain self-confidence.

When Paul first began attending the workshop, he would look at the dance-therapist to reassure himself about the movements and to keep the rhythm; for him, the dance-therapist was an important point of reference. As the sessions progressed, however, he no longer looked for the eyes of the dance-therapists. Instead he became self-confident, keeping the vocal and body rhythm on his own, even when there are several groups that make a different gesture and sound at the same time.

In group dances, everyone must anchor himself in the ground, and whether seated or standing,[8] find his own support, particularly in the axis of the spine. Finding one's axis and being able to rely on it, and therefore on oneself, is essential for autonomy. For example, the traditional dances based on "pas de bourrée," which is simple and close to the step of the walk, is a magnificent tool that can be used by the body to find its verticality and regain its support and self-confidence.

We also use the remarkable imagination and creativity of the patients. Indeed, physical and psychological relaxation linked to a greater sense of security and self-confidence is necessary to enable them to express themselves creatively, as we will see later. As the DRT sessions progressed, participants gained the self-confidence to propose new ways of expressing themselves in an atmosphere of benevolence and relaxation.

Depression

The decline in body functions leads to increased self-deprecation and depression. The DRT treats this suffering in different ways.

Each workshop proposes to get out of daily life. To get out of the gloom of a narrow life, we need strong, powerful proposals. The drum, the onomatopoeia and the proposed gestures refer to a primitive first register of an archaic and strong relationship with nature: hunting, fishing, picking berries, or cultivating one's field. "We don't feel like we're in Paris anymore," said the participants. We forgot the rain, the grayness and the cold to find the sun, the warmth, which was also mirrored in the relations of the group.

Primitive Expression strives not to put patients in a nostalgic mood that could reinforce their sadness. It can happen sometimes that a patient arrives at the workshop tired, angry, and sad; he doesn't want anything. In this case, the dance-therapist gives him personal attention before and after the session. She supports him more during the session, she proposes a theme or a rhythmic exercise that will allow him to express the emotion that manifests itself, to give meaning to what he is experiencing.

Music and songs used in Primitive Expression are joyful and invigorating. Rhythmic movements, shared with others, bring patients out of themselves and their sadness. This type of dance-therapy is based on the revival of the rhythmic structures of the transitional area that make the child discover that he is not fused to his mother but a person in his own right, and that by rhythm he can articulate himself to her in a playful way (Winnicott, 2002). Rhythm has an empowering "fatherly" function that frees the child from fusion. This makes him rejoice; joy always being the sign of victory in life. It is repeated in the sessions, and we see it appear in patients who "de-fusion," or free themselves, from their sadness. Dance brings a different type of joy than everyday pleasures. This is why joy is postulated in many traditional societies (in ancient Greece, in Africa, in shamanic societies) as coming from elsewhere, an extra-human gift. We call it enthusiasm, which means etymologically "possessed by a god." But the god in question is none other than the god of dance, the rhythm, which raises the body and makes it light. The pleasure of dance and communication is manifested in the collective joy and energy that the group multiplies as a sounding board. Lise said:

> Relations with the participants are very stimulating and warm. We conclude the session with a circular collective figure that brings together all the energies. Very beautiful!"

The dances, always playful, have the subjects "playing" in every sense of the word. With the help of the drum, the tribal imagination comes easily, and we solicit its expression in several situations, such as:

- The crossing of animals: each participant proposes an animal and an associated sound resulting from his imagination and adapted to his physical capacities. He finds a way to represent himself and to know himself, having recognized himself in a lion, snake, and so on and entering into a rhythmic and gestural dialogue with other animals. Every animal is played seriously, i.e., engaged and intense, without taking itself seriously.

- The "snake dance": the group walks in single file in the dance studio. Each of its members reproduces the movements proposed by the person in the lead. This can lead to surprising movements. Once when Paul led the group, he suddenly changed his forward gear for a reverse gear followed by a turn on himself. This is a movement rarely proposed by patients because of its difficulty in balancing and managing space.

- The two tribes: the group is divided into two clans, and each chooses its animal totem then invents gestures, movements, sounds related to this animal.

- Choreographies in small groups of four to five people, which encourage creativity and create a group dynamic, where we have to work together for a common purpose. In these choreographies, the patients stage their difficulties but in a disguised way, transposed into metaphors. For example, as a small abandoned bear or a cat that a mother stops from going out. These creations are accompanied by a text that tells the story of the situation in a "rapped" mode, that is to say, rhythmically scribbled and often humorous.

The reorientation from sadness to joy brings about a change of perspective that continues outside of the sessions. Nietzsche (2003) calls it "the yes to life." It is not an ad hoc adherence reserved for gratifying moments but an acceptance that life in all its moments, including the moments of suffering, is the affirmation of existence. Here is a clinical vignette to illustrate our words:

> A few days after the death of her father, Marion arrives at the dance-therapy session accompanied by her husband. At first sight, I find her slow, inexpressive in her face. "I'm not well," she says with a muffled voice and frozen eyes. I suggest that she settle down in a seated circle to begin the session with other patients, depending on her feelings and the possibilities of the moment. Soft music guides us through the breathing with slow arm movements. Marion follows the indications while remaining very slow. Then, the game of first names on a rhythmic pulse induces a movement of arms that twinkle towards a person called; everyone sends their attention to that person. Marion's face clears up during this exercise; she is happy to receive so much attention. We arrive to the second part of the session with a folk dance. It takes time to learn to greet each other, to make the appropriate polka steps in front of one's dance partner. Marion seems to enjoy herself and even sing the music of this little choreography. That day, Marion had to leave before the end of the workshop. She [got ready to leave] discreetly, and then suddenly started to jump around following the movement of the circle of dancers. Marion's departure was very joyful, full of good energy and smiles. "Time is moving faster and faster," her husband said when he left.

BRIGITTE, THE JOY REDISCOVERED

For the last two years, Brigitte has been participating in the dance-rhythm-therapy group. Her diagnosis with PD was 15 years ago. Lately, she has entered a phase of repetitive blockages and falls, which have negative consequences on her mood. This is a woman who has always been very active and involved in both her professional and private life.

The first year of dancing unveiled her main difficulties: trouble walking, loss of balance, freezing, difficulty with coordination, lack of self-confidence, self-judgment, and depressive traits. She also mentioned the disruption in her writing: "I can't read what I write . . . I hate this disease!" She often complained of the lack of understanding of her illness: "Sometimes people don't believe me when I say I'm sick. I have to fight in public transport, people push me when I'm blocked, or they don't offer their seat."

Having such blockages during the workshop annoyed her and made her vulnerable in her own eyes. She had been absent for certain periods, explaining that she was completely blocked and wasn't able to join the class as she was in so much pain. However, during an exercise she could tell another patient aloud: "You're blocked, you're having trouble doing."

This year the group has reconstituted itself within the hospital La Salpêtrière. Brigitte is with 14 other participants. After five months of work, she seems more motivated, more conscious, and less anxious about her motor difficulties. Her participation has become regular:

> Now, going to dance is my priority. I gave up a lunch I had been offered. I told my friends that they could wait and I'd see them after the dance.

Now, Brigitte is showing some improvements: the reduction of depressive symptoms, more balanced and tonic walking, resistance to fatigue and initiative. She is very enthusiastic. She even comes during her off period, when she can't handle the whole session because she is blocked by slowness or heavy fatigue. She adapts, accepts herself, observes others, accompanies us with her voice, and stays seated at the time of the blockages. "I'm proud of myself, I was able to outdo myself today." Currently, Brigitte shares a lot about her feelings; she tells me after each session. "You know, thanks to dance I feel alive and happy. My husband is surprised at home, how it changes my state. I love dancing!"

CONCLUSION

The "Parkinson Dance" experience shows us that the Primitive Expression method in Dance-Rhythm-Therapy effectively responds to the needs and difficulties encountered by participants. Indeed the use of rhythm, repetitive movement, and voice make it possible to act on the three levels affected by PD. The first, motor symptoms, allows mitigations of tremors, release of freezing situations, fluidity, amplitude of movements, and better balance. The second level includes non-motor disorders such as pain and fatigue. The third level is social-psychological and symptoms that impinge upon trust, expression of emotions, openness to communication relaxation, joy, strengthening of self-image, and creativity.

These experiences with Parkinson's patients also show how good dance is for our contemporary society. When we dance, our body informs us of the arrival of the joy, because dance is its privileged place, its instrument and its vehicle. It is the joy which announces to us that we live, that we create, that we advance far from death and the powers of inertia.

Dance-therapy by Primitive Expression gives rhythm a central place, which pushes the body beyond his limits and the dancer to a state called enthusiasm, or etymologically "possessed by a god" (in-theos). The god of life possesses our body with the rhythmic gods, Dionysus or Shiva, gods of life, vitality and creativity, because rhythm is the heart of humanity. The joy that dance gives to us is a presentiment of something beautiful and large that transcends human life: it is the Life, which will stop for each of us one day, but is immortal on the level of humanity.

NOTES

1. The abbreviation PD will be used for Parkinson's disease.
2. The abbreviation DRT will be used for Dance-Rhythm-Therapy.
3. Mediations means that rhythm and danced movement are tools used to foster a relationship and communication with patients, encourage and support creativity, facilitate transferential dynamics and access symbolization.
4. Parallel to the process by which the child comes out of fusion-nature, takes off from the mother, from the imagination and from the 'wild' impulse.
5. Verbal times are called raps; it is a method of putting rhythmic words to the aches of the body and daily life.
6. Kinesphere: the part of the space that can be reached by the extremities of the body's limbs. It is the space immediately accessible without moving by deployment of the body.

7. *Parkinson: de si fragiles danseurs.* (2015). Le Parisien. Retrieved from www.dailymotion.com/video/x2n5bs5.
8. It is possible to organize workshops for people in wheelchairs or who have difficulty walking. Other aspects can be developed: coordination, the amplitude of gestures, the precision of gestures, and of course, their symbolism.

REFERENCES

Berrol, C. F., Ooi, W. L., & Katz, S. S. (1997, Fall/Winter). Dance/Movement Therapy with older adults who have sustained neurological insult: A demonstration project. *American Journal of Dance Therapy, 19*(2), 135–160.

Cardinale, M. J., & Durieux, A. (2004). *Bien dans ma voix, bien dans ma vie.* Paris: Courrier du livre.

Cungi, C., & Limousin, S. (2003). *Savoir se relaxer en choisissant sa méthode.* Paris: Retz.

De Dreu, M. J., Van der Wilk, A. S. D., Poppe, E., Kwakkel, G., & Van Wegen, E. E. H. (2012). *Rehabilitation, exercise therapy and music in patients with Parkinson's disease: A meta-analysis of the effects of music based movement therapy (MbM) on walking ability, balance and quality of life.* XIX world Congress on Parkinson's Disease and related Disorders-Shanghaï (Chine), 11–14 December 2011. January 2012, pp. 114–119.

Dolto, F. (2013). Psychoanalysis and paediatrics: Key psychoanalytical concepts with sixteen clinical observations of children. London: Karnac Books Ltd.

Hackney, M. E., & Earhart, G. M. (2009, August). Short duration, intensive tango dancing for Parkinson's disease: An uncontrolled pilot study. *Complementary Therapies in Medicine, 4*(17), 203–207.

Hackney, M. E., Kantorovitch, S., Levin, R., & Earhart, G. M. (2007, December). Effects of tango on functional mobility in Parkinson's disease: A preliminary study. *JNPT, 31*(4), 173–179.

Heiberger, L., Maurer, C., Amtage, F., Mendez-Balbuena, I., Schulte-Mönting, J., Hepp-Reymon, M. C., & Kristeva, R. (2011, October). Impact of a weekly dance classes on the functional mobility and on the quality of life of individuals with Parkinson's disease. *Frontiers in Aging Neuroscience, 3*, 14.

Johnson, K. V.-A., & Dunbar, R. I. M. (2016). Pain tolerance predicts human social network size. *Scientific Reports, 6*, 25267.

Marchant, D., Sylvester, J. L., & Earhart, G. M. (2010). Effects of a short duration, high dose contact improvisation dance workshop on Parkinson disease: A pilot study. *Complementary Therapies in Medicine, 18*, 184–190.

McIntosh, G. C., Brown, S. H., Rice, R. R., & Thaut, M. H. (1997). Rhythmic auditory-motor facilitation of gait patterns in patients with Parkinson's disease. *Journal of Neurology, Neurosurgery, and Psychiatry, 62*, 22–26.

Mitchell, L. A., & MacDonald, A. R. (2006). An experimental investigation of the effects preferred and relaxing music listening pain perception. *Journal of Music Therapy, 63*(4), 295–316.

Moisan, F., Wanneveich, M., Kab, S., Moutengou, E., Boussac-Zarebska, M., Carcaillon-Bentata, L., . . . & Elbaz, A. (2018). Frequency of Parkinson's disease in France in 2015 and trends to 2030. *Bulletin Epidémiologique Hebdomaire, 2018*(8–9), 128–140.

Nietzsche, F. (2003). *Thus spoke Zarathustra.* London: Penguin Classics.

Nombela, C., Hughes, L. E., Owen, A. M., & Grahn, J. A. (2013). Into the groove: Can rhythm influence Parkinson's disease? *Neuroscience and Behavioral Reviews, 37*(2013), 2564–2570.

Pacchetti, C., Mangini, F., Aglieri, R., Fundaro, C., Martignoni, E., & Nappi, G. (2000). Active music therapy in Parkinson's disease: An integrative method for motor and emotional rehabilitation. *Psychosomatic Medicine, 62*, 386–393.

Rafferty, M. R., Schmidt, P. N., Luo, S. T., Li, K., Marras, C., Davis, T. L., . . . & Simuni, T. (2017). Regular exercise, quality of life, and mobility in Parkinson's disease: A longitudinal analysis of National Parkinson Foundation quality improvement initiative. *Journal of Parkinson's Disease, 7*(1), 193–202.

Sacks, O. (2007). *Musicophilia: Tales of music and the brain.* New York: Knopf.

Schott-Billmann, F. (2011). *The space between: The potential for change.* Plymouth: University of Plymouth Press.

Schott-Billmann, F. (2013). *Arts therapies and the intelligence of feeling.* Plymouth: University of Plymouth Press.

Schott-Billmann, F. (2015a). *Primitive expression and dance therapy.* London and New York: Routledge.

Schott-Billmann, F. (2015b). Mirror games in dance-therapy. In R., Hougham, S., Pitruzzela, & S. Scoble (Eds.), *Through the looking glass: Dimensions of reflection in the arts therapies* (pp. 54–64). Plymouth: University of Plymouth Press.

Schott-Billmann, F. (2018). Le rituel en danse- thérapie, symbolisation des émotions et connaissance de soi. *Art-Therapies and rituals. 18th Annual Colloquium of the French Federation of Art Therapists* (pp. 13–20). Paris.

Stern, D. (1985). *The interpersonal world of the infant.* New York: Basic Books.

Tarr, B., Launay, J., Cohen, E., & Dunbar, R. (2015). Synchrony and exertion during dance independently raise pain threshold and encourage social bonding. *Biology Letters, 11*, 20150767.

Westbrook, B., & McKibben, H. (1989, Spring/Summer). Dance/Movement Therapy with groups of outpatients with Parkinson's disease. *American Journal of Dance Therapy, 11*(1).

Westheimer, O. (2007). Why dance for Parkinson's disease. *Topics in Geriatric Rehabilitation*, April/June 2008, *24*(2), 127–140.

Winnicott, D. W. (2002). *Playing and reality* (2nd ed.). London: Routledge.

CHAPTER 14

DANCE MOVEMENT THERAPY AND PSYCHOSOCIAL REHABILITATION
Model Sampoornata

Sohini Chakraborty

INTRODUCTION

In 2004, Kolkata Sanved was formed by the author along with five survivors of sexual violence and sex trafficking. This organization is one of the pioneers in the field of Dance Movement Therapy (DMT) in India and uses DMT exclusively for psychosocial rehabilitation and reintegration. Kolkata Sanved's process has been drawn from the Western concept of DMT with Indian dance movements being incorporated into DMT processes developed in the West in order to create a successful model known as *Sampoornata*. The organization works in shelter homes, red-light areas, open communities, railway platforms, and hospitals. It must be noted that the core employee group of Kolkata Sanved were once residents of red-light areas themselves: they have been rescued from prostitution and other kinds of vulnerable situations (Kolkata Sanved, 2014).

Prior to delving into the core of this chapter, I begin with my connection to dance. Then, I introduce the formation of Kolkata Sanved and *Sampoornata* ('fulfillment'), the keystone of Kolkata Sanved's DMT program. After discussing the structure of *Sampoornata* as a DMT model, I reflect on its uniqueness and contributions to the field of DMT and social change. Transformation, empowerment, and social change are the three main elements of this model, while rehabilitation and reintegration into society are two important aspects and outcomes of it. Most importantly, after the healing and recovery process, survivors become healers and leaders. Finally, I discuss the academic research studies that have validated *Sampoornata* as an approach to healing and social change and have given DMT credence within India.

DANCE AND ME

At age seven I expressed my desire to dance, so my parents put me into a dance class. This particular setting was very restrictive, formulaic, and rigid, so I decided to leave. It was a big decision at the age of seven, but something was missing that I couldn't articulate. Therefore, my parents decided not to enroll me in any other course. However, my passion for dancing remained. The only channel through which I could express myself was free dance. When I was in fifth grade, there was a celebration in my school, and I wanted to perform with a group of older students. On the day of the celebration, I wore a plain sari to dance in, and so the senior students unceremoniously cast me away. They said that I needed a dance costume to perform. Their reactions left me devastated and filled my mind with many thoughts. It made me wonder why dance needed to be so decorative. However, that incident, like the previous one, did not dent my desire to dance. I continued to create dances to different poems and songs by myself and with friends at school.

When I was in ninth grade, it was my responsibility to organize a dance show that would be a part of a school event. The show had both Tagore Drama and contemporary dance components to it.[1] More than 50 students signed up, which was a very rare occurrence. It was saddening to realize that a few of them had never gotten an opportunity to dance on stage before, as they had been rejected for being unattractive or untalented. The dance show I organized did not have stage makeup or typical dance costumes; it was just dancing, in its truest element. The show received mixed reviews. While half the teachers were in awe of the performance, the other half was appalled. In the long run, it was the real legacy of the performance that was remembered. The joy and sense of achievement felt by the students who had never danced before was truly blissful to behold (Chakraborty, 2013).

I realized that dance, by itself, can contribute much more than the 'performances' with which it is normally associated. People assume that only those who are considered 'beautiful' by stereotypical social standards can become dancers. I noticed that in performances pretty girls with light skin would be asked to stand in front of the stage even if they weren't very talented, while many talented dancers were given positions in the back just because they didn't match with what society wants to see in a dancer. Therefore, I decided to search for the real meaning and process of dance, outside of what is taught in traditional dance schools and what is emphasized during show performances. In my search, I discovered that it is crucial to understand that movement, self-expression, ideas, and creativity are the actual gemstones of any performance (Chakraborty, 2004), which is often not understood because of societal obsessions with looks.

Studying sociology in college opened my eyes to how I could use dance differently. I created three small groups of non-dancers. One of these groups consisted of girls from a conservative Islamic institution. I persuaded the authorities of the institution to allow them to perform at cultural events. During this time, I also wrote a criminology paper on violence against women through which I began to understand that violence can lead to the formation of a negative image of the body and the self, which in turn affects people physically, emotionally, mentally, and socially. This eventually led to an epiphany: I began to wonder whether dance could help people recover after violence and improve their self-image in the process—just like it did for the girls from my ninth-grade performance. From the very day of this revelation, I knew what my purpose in life would be. My path ahead became a whole lot clearer. The path was: 'Dance Beyond Dance' (Chakraborty, 2013).

SEARCH: A NEW JOURNEY

I spent many a day thinking about the best way to implement my thoughts. In 1996, I was at the Kolkata Book Fair, and while I was moving from one bookstall to another, a poster mounted at one stall drew my attention. It consisted of a photograph of a girl, beneath which was printed this heartfelt poem: *"They sell me, my own blood for some gold and some silver, I rinse and rinse my mouth but the treachery remains. . . . I am no more mother to be, I am no more bride to be, I am no more future to be."* I stopped in front of the poster, and for a moment, my entire life stopped. I went inside to learn more about that girl and embarked on a new journey.

Armed with a master's degree in sociology and training in Bharatnatyam, Navanritya, and Theater,[2] I ventured into a Dance Movement Therapy program for children living at a care home. This shelter home was run by a Kolkata-based, anti-trafficking non-profit organization called *Sanlaap* and was founded by Indrani Sinha for the rehabilitation of victims of human trafficking and sexual exploitation.

Human trafficking is the third largest crime in the world, creating approximately $10 billion per year. The International Labour Organisation ([ILO], 2005) has estimated that the minimum number of persons in forced labor, including sexual exploitation as a result of trafficking, at any given time is 2.5 million. According to a United Nations UNITE report (2009), up to 70% of women experience violence in their lifetime (p. 1). The patriarchal social structure constantly teaches women and girls to normalize violence and take this as their fate. This leads to self-blame, resulting in a complete loss of self-respect and identity (Chakraborty, 2010). Dance serves as a powerful tool that helps these women and children overcome these feelings and develop a sense of comfort within their own bodies. Through dance, they begin a process of emotional and physical bonding with their own selves, releasing the limiting aspects of their trauma in order to recover and developing their confidence to start a new life (Chakraborty, 2011, 2012).

When I began working at *Sanlaap*, I was very excited. It seemed almost unreal because I had read so much about victims of violence in textbooks and newspapers, and now I was actually working with and for them. However, for the first two weeks I struggled to communicate with the children. Introducing unfamiliar movements was met by a lack of response and expression on their behalf. Therefore, I started my DMT sessions with physical exercises and story-based movements. Each activity was based on a simple theme such as movement of people walking on the street or movement around the home. We explored the body and space using various kinds of music, including Hindi film songs. The children eventually participated more actively, and I ended up spending more and more time with them. Some girls began sharing their life stories with me when we sat together after our sessions.

Each day became a learning experience for me, developing my understanding of how to deal with the participants. Every day I explored and discovered a new approach and path.

My experiences with the children at the *Sanlaap* shelter home made me realize that dance movement is therapeutic. With the progress of the sessions, the children's participation improved. They began to talk about their suffering and pain and used dance as a medium to express their feelings.

Working with them, I soon realized that my own position in society as a woman is deeply connected to them within the context of the patriarchal society that we all inhabit. I realized that my emancipation is incomplete without their emancipation. I also realized that dance movement, in its subjective interpretation, releases a person from various pressures imposed on them by society, and that I, myself, had become interested in this area because it had had a huge impact on me and my liberation. Through teaching, I realized that dance movement is almost like magic. It brings out self-confidence and creativity, empowering one to act as an active creative agent. Through dance, the girls living at the care home opened up physically and were able to articulate their thoughts. Soon enough, they developed eye contact, improved body posture, and moved through space with purpose and confidence, increasing their ability to focus in other areas of everyday life.

In 2000, I connected with the American Dance Therapy Association (ADTA). I acknowledge the importance of learning the fundamental theories developed in Western DMT practice, and thus continuously supplement my existing formal education by attending workshops rooted in Western knowledge. It helps me examine my entire process, while motivating me by showing me that I am on the right path of professional development and growth. However, I believe that it is imperative to modify the work so that it becomes appropriate for the Indian context; therefore, I have developed a model of DMT that is culturally contextualized and community-focused. I seek ways to incorporate the healing elements that have always been used in traditional Indian dances in a more systematic manner.

At the time that I connected with ADTA, it was difficult to find a community-focused DMT approach across the globe. I did not find any organization that used DMT as a core therapeutic intervention in psychosocial rehabilitation. Within India, dance is mainly seen as a form of entertainment, and in certain communities, it is even considered to be a taboo! This is true for therapy as well. Therapy is a resource that is unavailable to most Indian people, especially the underprivileged and marginalized. I wondered how I could break these barriers and take DMT programs to low-resource areas where the need is high. Keeping these gaps and cultural contexts in mind, I designed a curriculum that empowers the survivors themselves. It provides an innovative approach to psychosocial rehabilitation of survivors and gives them new options for their future. This curriculum was named *Sampoornata* and nurtured through Kolkata Sanved.

The curriculum explores the hidden and suppressed anger and guilt that lies deep within victims and helps them come to terms with themselves and their bodies. This is the key to psychosocial rehabilitation of victims of sexual violence (Chakraborty, 2019). Furthermore, the curriculum gives survivors a unique opportunity to interact with society. It also becomes a career option for them as performers, lobbyists, DMT practitioners, and peer educators.

FORMATION OF KOLKATA SANVED

In 1998, I developed a pilot project called *Rangeen Sapnay* ('colorful dreams') that combined movement and performance techniques from dance, music, physical theater, and miming. From 1999 to 2000, *Rangeen Sapnay* was supported by the government. During this time, it reached out to 120 children who were 6–14 years old and had been rescued from four red-light areas. The pilot project was a great success and marked the birth of *Sanved*—a platform for creative expression—in 2000. This started as a semi-autonomous program that advocated for children through performance, workshops, and regular sessions. It helped individuals identify their own potential as human beings rather than as victims. Since society tends to focus on class- and gender-based livelihood options, I attempted to break this barrier by thinking outside the box and taking risks. This led to the development of *Sampoornata* for women and children, who unfortunately, in most cases, do not receive the quality rehabilitation and reintegration services they need.

After formulating the rehabilitation methodology, I developed a model through which survivors can become healers and practice DMT in their communities. I trained ten survivors with no formal academic background to become DMT practitioners. DMT is not a field that is in high demand, so this was a challenge. However, I took these risks because my students agreed to start on a new journey with me and had the passion, body knowledge, and experience for the work. After a four-year rigorous training process, five of the original students and I founded Kolkata Sanved on April 29, 2004, with the mission of establishing DMT as a method for bringing about psychosocial rehabilitation and social change in South Asia.

SAMPOORNATA MODEL

Championing the arts and therapy as crucial aspects of social development is central to Kolkata Sanved's work. In the wider field of social development (World Bank OED, 2005), art and therapy remain sadly under-recognized and under-utilized. In that sense, Kolkata

Sanved is a pioneer in the field of DMT in India and South Asia. Developed in response to the communities Sanved serves, *Sampoornata* recognizes and explores dance as an art form and an experiential therapeutic tool. It has become the dynamic force motivating our organization and furthering DMT in the region (Rajan & Bhogal, 2017).

DMT is a tool that helps survivors, and subsequent practitioners, to connect and contribute to the lives of people from various backgrounds, age groups, and socioeconomic strata.

It is a creative process that emerges from the body through improvisation. The individual expresses their experiences with movement and verbally reflects on the process at the end of the session. Everyone's experience is different and unique. In the same group, DMT can make someone feel energized, another feel a sense of release and freedom, and yet another experience catharsis. Through DMT, we go on a journey through our body and learn from that experience in order to gain insights to implement in daily life (Bernstein, 1995). As a form of expressive arts therapy, DMT utilizes a natural skill: all you need is your body. It requires little to no investment in new infrastructure and thus can be utilized in almost all situations (Chakraborty, Mondol, Bhattacharya, & Chaudhuri, 2014).

THE PROCESS OF SAMPOORNATA

Sampoornata is a group process with two facilitators working with 20–40 participants at a time. The process is experienced mindfully in real time. It is a steady, consistent process that allows participants to take whatever risk they want within a safe space. What is beautiful about the process is that one learns from the journey of moving with peers while simultaneously going through the experience as an individual. In the group, participants often feel emotionally supported. They might break down because something deep is emerging, but they do not feel threatened while engaging with the group (Chakraborty, 2015, 2019).

The *Sampoornata* process comprises the following:

1. Needs assessment
2. Developing a plan of implementation
3. The DMT session (see Figure 14.1)
4. Documenting the process
5. Evaluation

What follows is the personal experience of a DMT practitioner who was once a program participant and who is now a senior facilitator in the organization:

What amazed me the most was that, at first, I was judging Sohini negatively. Sohini had not been talking much while facilitating. So, I thought this was not going to go well. Then, the space was transformed. On the first day, we did a warm-up with a piece of cloth. During this warm-up, there were individuals who were making use of the cloth. It was not the specific activity that affected me to such an extent, but the way space was held by Sohini on that first day. It became a very non-judgmental and safe space from the get-go. Even before we broke for lunch, the room had already been transformed. Later on, when I was reflecting, I understood that in reality, we all had co-created the space through our own creative experience.

Across the five days, each day there was a new discovery. On the first day, I felt that this was interesting. On the second day, there was a deeper reflection about myself through the process. I was able to partly share it with the group. Nobody judged. I took this back with me so

I could think and reflect about it. The main thing in the process was how the facilitator held her own being and how she held the space. Even without many conversations, teaching, or preaching, it was so deep. That was my memory of those five days. I was able to access deeper spaces within myself. I would not have done this before in a group, ever. The first five-day-long workshop pushed me to attend another one facilitated by Sohini.

Now, I have done many workshops with Sohini and am also a practitioner. Despite this, when I recently participated in a ten-day KS [Kolkata Sanved] workshop on a specific module, there was an activity that was particularly powerful to me. This activity was based on fear. Before the activity, everyone shared their stories through movement. It was like building blocks. I discovered that healing is a process. Prior to doing this exercise, I thought that I had healed. I thought that I had overcome it. I had spoken about it. . . . Yet, suddenly during that process, it all surfaced with great force. That day, I finally let it go. It was just gone.

After this activity, all of us shared our stories verbally. We did this with randomly chosen partners. I was able to share through movement such a deep thing that I had never thought I would share with somebody who I was not close to. This is one of my most powerful examples. There was also a balance activity that we did that was phenomenal for me. Different people shared different things. I was also taking on the role of the caregiver in the group, while also not taking space. I felt that that is how life is. People have to take and give. I felt and experienced it in that space. That balance to this date remains a very special memory. Each time that I do it now in the field I tell myself to not compare it with that time because my experience was very deep, and it is not necessary that in every group people would have the same experience.

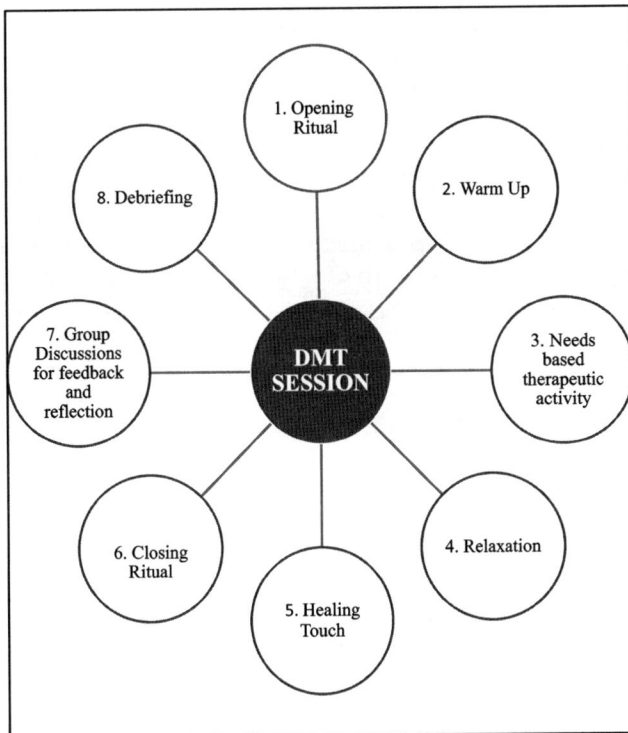

Figure 14.1 DMT Session Structure in the *Sampoornata* Process

DMT is a creative process, and the facilitators are like architects working with participants to design the process in real time. This is a step-by-step process wherein whatever emerges from the group's experience informs the next level of therapy (Fargnoli, 2014). Step one in the *Sampoornata* repertoire is a ritual and a warm-up. Rituals are predictable so that people feel safe: participants know what to expect. The facilitators co-create the rituals with the participants so that everyone owns that space. It is not a matter of everyone following what the facilitator does. This is about participants building ownership from the first session.

After the ritual, the session moves into a warm-up that engages all body parts. It is not an exercise class where you focus on specific movements. The practitioners get the participants to warm up through metaphors or creative ideas. Step-by-step, the body is prepared, energized, and loosened. Then the facilitator asks the participants about their feelings each time. Through this, the facilitator creates awareness for them. If participants are aware of every part of their bodies, then they can connect the center, ground, and body. That is the first building block.

After the warm-up, depending on what the objective for the session is, we take small steps towards that goal. For example, if the goal is to create focus, then we play with ideas such as 'following the finger' or using the image of the finger as a pencil. There are three stages: individual exploration, pair exploration, and group exploration. The facilitator first establishes a safe, therapeutic space through ritual. Then the facilitator does isolated body movements or uses a prop in a fun way to help the participants focus. After this, the main activity is introduced.

Without the conscious mind knowing, the subconscious comes out in the DMT process. Participants have a moment to reflect on the experience during the final stage of the process. Often, they realize that something that has been deep and suppressed for years has suddenly come out. Group DMT sessions use movement, props, music, and other means of creative experience to address challenges ranging from mental health problems to trauma. The *Sampoornata* model uses these creative tools as a means of learning to use one's voice and form cohesive, empowered communities.

Healing touch is also an integral part of the *Sampoornata* process. This is a touch the facilitator gives at the end of the process or when they believes it is required for a participant. The touch is on top of the head, and the facilitator ensures that everyone is comfortable with it. Its effect is very powerful and almost magical. Of course, this only happens at the appropriate time and only if a safe space has been created (Fargnoli, 2014; Chakraborty, 2019).

Facilitator's Role in the Process

The role of the facilitator is very important. If a safe environment has been established, there is a higher probability of participants opening up and sharing their feelings. Facilitators should be mindful of their body language, so that it is nonjudgmental, and they should aim to co-create a therapeutic space with the participants. If the facilitator feels burdened or negative, participants feel judged. This causes damage rather than leading to healing.

It is only once participants feel safe that they begin to experience the therapeutic process. Until this point, feelings are buried deep, but once a safe space is established, participants can bring their feelings out through movement. The process builds up step-by-step at each participant's own pace. They do not need to force anything. The movement that comes out of the body is authentic.

Facilitators need to know how to respect participants, hold the space, and not judge any movement as 'ugly' or 'beautiful.' A facilitator must compassionately allow for what is happening and let it be. Afterwards, participants can decide whether or not they want to take this process out into their everyday lives.

Settings of Kolkata Sanved's Work

The core of Kolkata Sanved's work takes place in community settings. This consists of DMT sessions for survivors of human trafficking, survivors of sexual violence, people living with mental illness, and other marginalized communities. Sanved's innovation—*Sampoornata*—not only makes DMT relevant to the Indian context but also makes it accessible to marginalized persons. *Sampoornata* has evolved from established DMT practice and has moved beyond the clinical structure to focus on the overall well-being of the participants. Though Kolkata Sanved's work results in healing, its aim is not restricted to this, unlike in the clinical setting. It is focused on removing systemic barriers from participants' lives that prevent attainment of optimal development.

As a result, the approach fits into a social development framework as contrasted with a clinical framework (Chakraborty, 2019; World Bank OED, 2005). This means that the model focuses less on treating an individual medically and more on the individual's needs within society (Wiese, 2017). This social focus has made *Sampoornata* successful in integrating participants back into society and preparing them to become leaders and healers themselves (UNICEF, 2016).

HOW *SAMPOORNATA* IS DIFFERENT FROM OTHER DMT MODELS

According to the ADTA (n.d.), DMT is the "psychotherapeutic use of movement and dance through which a person can engage creatively in a process to further their emotional, cognitive, physical and social integration" (para 1). DMT empowers individuals to find new means of communication, to explore ways of releasing the psychological and somatic impact of trauma, and to experience a greater sense of self-worth as they move forward (Bernstein, 2009).

Sampoornata adopts the four core principles of global DMT practice: (1) DMT as a creative methodology, (2) body-mind connection, (3) nonverbal movement beyond the hegemony of verbal creation, and (4) the experiential nature of the process. At the same time, it has emerged as a new model. *Sampoornata* focuses on integrating mental health, education, and employment using DMT (see Figure 14.2). Participants continue their healing journey not only through cognitive and emotional development in the therapeutic space but also as DMT practitioners, performers, and empowered community activists, thinking through and actively directing their own lives.

Specifically, Sanved offers professional DMT education to its participants through the DMT Leadership Academy. Students of the academy go through a rigorous, two-year academic training program and emerge as change leaders and DMT facilitators who can earn their livelihood (Chakraborty, 2019). Skilled practitioners can reach out to other individuals in vulnerable situations, creating a cycle of learning and development. DMT enables participants to make empowered life choices, such as pursuing a range of livelihoods or seeking

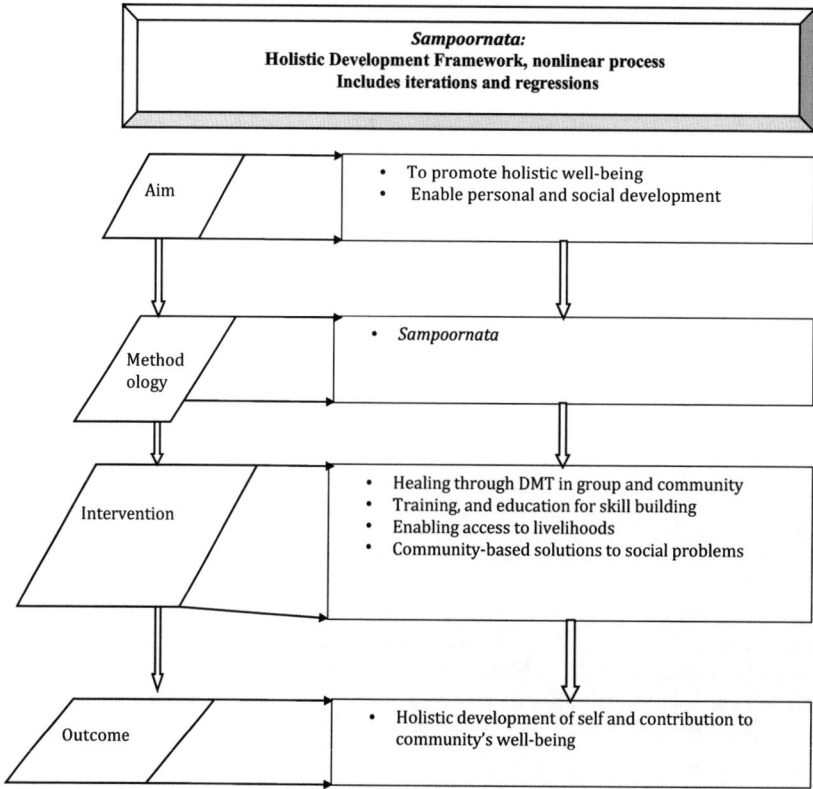

Figure 14.2 Sampoornata Development Framework
Source: Chakraborty, 2019.

an education to increase financial stability. Dance improves individuals' ability to express themselves powerfully and creatively, and it is a vital tool for giving marginalized individuals a voice (Wiese, 2017). Additionally, Sanved purposefully refers to its facilitators as 'practitioners' instead of 'therapists' to break the intrinsic hierarchy of that word. It indicates the ongoing 'practice' of the form and a deeper connection and openness to the larger community (Chakraborty, 2019).

MAIN CHARACTERISTICS OF *SAMPOORNATA*

Sampoornata Addresses Gender-Based Violence As a Social and Structural Problem

Sanved's work adds to the feminist movement and discourse both locally and globally; gender-based violence is supported and perpetuated by societal attitudes and structures. The *Sampoonata* model provides the opportunity for women and children to organize with other survivors and allies to combat these attitudes and structures. Sanved has reached a global audience by working with international partners such as One Billion Rising, Vital Voices, and many more women's rights advocacy programs. Further, Sanved has appeared in international documentaries and continues to work with international DMT practitioners and submit articles and research to international publications.

Sampoornata *Is a Community-Focused, Non-Medicalized Intervention*

Sanved's practitioners come from marginalized communities, and the process considers their life experiences and practical skills as important as their formal education in DMT techniques. Sanved has created a non-hierarchical model that is based on participation in a democratic process of healing. This model is culturally adaptable and does not rely on diagnoses, which may reduce human experience to a checklist of symptoms. It promotes skills for self-healing.

The *Sampoornata* Model broadens the scope of Dance Movement Therapy from a singular, isolated focus on mental and physical health to a broader, contextualized focus on the human rights of participants. This rights-based approach is new, and it actively encourages participants to address the social and structural determinants of health within their communities and in society at large. Sanved promotes this concept by training survivors to become practitioners in the DMT Leadership Academy and encourages them to set up independent units in their communities.

Sanved's Sampoornata *Model Goes Beyond Clinical Models of Rehabilitation*

Sampoornata provides an experimental space where participants can access personal freedom and explore themselves in a purposeful, non-hierarchical collaboration with others. The artistic practice of DMT challenges the status quo by acknowledging that all persons have a right to health, to bodily autonomy, and to the articulation of their own experiences. It also assists participants in developing self-confidence and independence. The artistic practice of DMT is sustainable: it is not limited to the therapeutic session. It has the potential to become a lifelong practice for well-being. The *Sampoornata* Model encourages participants to take lessons learnt within the session into their daily lives. It gives them the confidence to demand the same from their societies and peers and inspires participants to become agents of social change.

SAMPOORNATA IS AN EVIDENCE-BASED AND TESTED MODEL

Kolkata Sanved has conducted and published two studies (one qualitative and one quantitative) to generate evidence. The qualitative case study is called "Scripting Their Lives" and is a study of Dance Movement Therapy for children in a care institution in the Cooch Behar District of West Bengal. This study was conducted in March 2016 by Kolkata Sanved and the Paul Hamlyn Foundation (Chakraborty & Dasgupta, 2016). The case study method was used to understand the DMT intervention in a care institution for girls through which the *Sampoornata* model was used to overcome behavioral, psychological, and structural challenges faced by the children. The research study was conducted to measure and analyze the impact of our program so that we could replicate it and bring it to other shelter homes.

Challenges that Sanved faced while working with this care institution included stigma and discrimination faced and experienced by participants, issues in the structural organization of the shelter home—such as physical and emotional segregation of children according to whether they had a history of sexual abuse or not, and a generally negative attitude from the caregivers towards the DMT team. In order to address some of these challenges, we conducted a DMT orientation and workshops with the caregivers so that they understood the importance of healing. The outcome of this was that all the girls in that shelter were granted permission to attend DMT sessions, and some of the girls, who had not been able to access education before, even received school education within the shelter home. Further, the Survivor DMT Leadership Academy proved successful. Girls who left the shelter home after graduating from DMT academic training set up independent DMT units outside the shelter home and now work as DMT practitioners.

The second evidence-based study conducted by Kolkata Sanved was a randomized controlled trial. The purpose of the study was to assess the impact of DMT on the traumatic symptoms of survivors of trafficking and sexual violence. The quantitative research study examined the impact of DMT on trauma-related symptoms in a sample of 69 child survivors of sex trafficking and sexual violence living in childcare institutions (Dasgupta & Chakraborty, 2017). The participants, aged 15–16 years, were randomly assigned to a DMT treatment group and a waitlist control group.

Kolkata Sanved conducted a six-month-long DMT intervention module focused on self-image, anger management, and communication. Data were collected from government and NGO run childcare institutions in Maharashtra and West Bengal. Following a pre-test, mid-test, and post-test design, the Trauma Symptom Checklist for Children (TSCC) was used to measure the impact of DMT on psychological parameters. Results showed significant improvement in levels of anxiety, depression, posttraumatic stress, and dissociation in the group receiving DMT compared to those not receiving it at mid- and post-test phases. Sexual concerns among survivors attending DMT became clinically non-significant by the post-test, as well.

In light of the research studies conducted, Sanved's DMT intervention model appears to be successful for the following reasons:

1. It is viable in low-resource settings; two DMT practitioners can work with at least 20–40 children at the same time.
2. It has shown positive results in addressing behavioral issues of children. Often, care institutions resort to strict rules to control disruptive behavior. However, such behavior is often a cry for help and attention. DMT provides the safe space for children to express their fears, work on their insecurities, and develop positive coping strategies. The model results in a reduction of such 'deviant' cries for help.
3. It can lead to the positive personality development and can teach necessary life skills to children who will have to leave the care institutions and fend for themselves after turning 18.

Building Academic Credibility for Sampoornata

The work of Sanved has grown successfully, and just as with all developing professions, with ours there is a need to continue to build our knowledge. This is being done through evidence-gathering and a new academic program. While most art-based pedagogies for change remain in the informal domain, Kolkata Sanved has enshrined its DMT for Change curriculum into theoretical frameworks and grounded it in academia. The one-year diploma program in DMT held in collaboration with the Centre for Lifelong Learning Tata Institute of Social Sciences has gone a long way in building academic credibility for DMT. It is preparing DMT as a new, emerging profession in India by establishing its own principles and ethics of practice.

Steps Towards Quality Control Through Evidence Gathering

Kolkata Sanved believes that quality is maintained through effective monitoring and evaluation. We have generated credible evidence on the effectiveness of DMT with survivors of gender-based violence through rigorous research. We have developed a group DMT scale that measures the therapeutic processes. Use of qualitative data in the form of session reports is important. In addition, we have regular external evaluations to ensure accountability within the program.

CONCLUSION

Sampoornata has emerged from established DMT practices and has moved beyond these realms. It encourages participants to develop a range of life skills, most notably the ability to think creatively. It is inclusive and promotes tangible change. It encourages the coming together of mainstream and marginalized persons to create noticeable changes in the community as well as at the state and policy level. This has created a new perspective regarding both DMT and the field of psychosocial rehabilitation. This is an emancipatory model of DMT.

NOTES

1. Rabindranath Tagore is respected tremendously across the nation, especially among Bengalis, as he shaped Bengali music and culture with his sheer talent for music, poetry, and literature, giving it its own unique individuality.
2. Bharatnatyam is a major Indian Classical dance that originated in the southern part of India, and Navanritya is a contemporary dance language developed by Manjusri Chaki Sircar and her daughter Ranjbari Sircar that is based on a very feminist framework.

REFERENCES

American Dance Therapy Association. (n.d.) (para 1). Retrieved July 30, 2019, from https://adta.org/

Bernstein, B. (1995). Dancing beyond trauma: Women survivors of sexual abuse. In F. Levy (Ed.), *Dance and other expressive art therapies: When words are not enough*. New York: Routledge.

Bernstein, B. (2009). Survivors to healers: Dance/Movement Therapy and Expressive Arts Therapy in Kolkata. *Newsletter of the International Expressive Arts Therapy Association (IEATA)*, 4–7.

Chakraborty, P. (2004). Dance, pleasure and Indian women as multisensorial subjects. *Visual Anthropology*, *17*(1), 1–17. Retrieved from https://doi.org/10.1080/08949460490273988

Chakraborty, S. (2010). Dance as healing: Kolkata Sanved. In P. Chakravorty & G. Nilanjana (Eds.), *Dance matters: Performing India on local and global stages* (pp. 62–72). New Delhi: Routledge India.

Chakraborty, S. (2011). Empowering through Dance Movement Therapy. In U. Sarkar-Munsi & S. Burrige (Eds.), *Traversing tradition: Celebrating dance in India* (pp. 222–234). New Delhi: Routledge.

Chakraborty, S. (2012, August 13). *Dance a powerful tool to release trauma*. Retrieved March 2, 2016, from www.peacexpeace.org/2012/08/dance-a-powerful-tool-to-release-trauma/

Chakraborty, S. (2013). *Dance beyond dance.* Paper presented at the 48th Annual Conference of American Dance Therapy Association.

Chakraborty, S. (2015). *The implementation of Dance Movement Therapy and other creative therapies: Guidelines and strategies for working with government shelter homes in India.* Kolkata: Kolkata Sanved.

Chakraborty, S. (2019). *Transforming lives through Dance Movement Therapy* (Doctoral thesis). Tata Institute of Social Sciences, Mumbai, India.

Chakraborty, S., & Dasgupta, C. (2016). *Scripting lives: A case study of Dance Movement Therapy in a shelter home for children in Cooch Behar West Bengal.* Kolkata: Kolkata Sanved.

Chakraborty, S., Mondol, J., Bhattacharya, S., & Chaudhuri, P. (2014). *A journey of fortitude and discovery: The impact of Dance Movement Therapy on the participants of training of trainers.* Kolkata: Kolkata Sanved.

Dasgupta, C., & Chakraborty, S. (2017). *Impact of Dance Movement Therapy on trauma: A study of survivors of sex trafficking and sexual violence in shelter homes.* Japan: Kamonohashi.

Fargnoli, A. (2014). *Maintaining stability in the face of adversity: Self care practices of human trafficking survivor-trainers in India.* Chicago: Columbia College Chicago.

ILO. (2005). *A global alliance against forced labour: Global report under follow-up to the ILO declaration on fundamental principles and rights at work.* Geneva: International Labour Organisation (ILO). Retrieved September 10, 2018, from www.ilo.org/wcmsp5/groups/public/-ed_norm/-declaration/documents/publication/wcms_081882.pdf

Kolkata Sanved. (2014). *Impact report analysis: A compilation of two impact reports.* Kolkata: Author.

Rajan, A., & Bhogal, T. S. (2017). *Looking back and forward: Kolkata Sanved impact evaluation report.* Unpublished Report. Kolkata: Kolkata Sanved.

UNICEF. (2016). *Western regional consultation on strengthening restoration and rehabilitation of children under the juvenile justice system.* Mumbai: Author.

United Nations Secretary General's Campaign UNITE. (2009). *Violence against women.* Retrieved January 13, 2015, from www.un.org/en/events/endviolenceday/pdf/UNiTE_TheSituation_EN.pdf

Wiese, S. (2017). *Reframing rehabilitation of sex trafficked victims from the survivor's point of view.* Sweden: Lund University.

World Bank Operations Evaluation Department (OED). (2005). *Putting social development to work for the poor: An OED review of World Bank activities.* Washington, DC: The World Bank.

CHAPTER 15

ASIAN CULTURAL BODY, DANCE AND THERAPY

A Korean Perspective

Kyung Soon Ko

BODY AND MIND IN EAST ASIA

DMT uses body movement as a therapeutic tool. Although movement is a global language and 93% of communication is nonverbal (Mehrabian, 1972), for DMT to be effective, movement needs to be interpreted within a deep understanding of the unique cultural context of the client. DMT is uniquely positioned in this regard, because even though it is grounded in Western modern dance and psychology, its foundational emphasis on the body–mind connection echoes core components of many East Asian philosophies, which see a healthy mind and body as mutually interdependent.

This attitude towards the body–mind connection can be seen in the medical treatments that East Asian people have historically sought out, such as qigong, acupuncture, and herbal medicine. Haque (2010) stated that life energy (i.e., *Chi*) preserves not only the physical body, but also mental and spiritual health: "Thus, excessive, unbalanced, or undisciplined emotions are primarily the reason for any kind of illness" (p. 129). Tseng (2004) explains that people in East Asia tend to communicate their emotional, mental, and psychological problems through their bodies, instead of naming them verbally. Traditionally, the five emotions of joy, anger, worry, sorrow, and fear have been connected to the five visceral organs of the heart, liver, spleen, lungs, and kidney, respectively. This "may reflect that it is more acceptable in the Asian culture to communicate problems indirectly through the body, rather than directly through verbal and psychological expression" (p. 156). In Chinese medicine, these five organs are subsequently correlated with the five elements of nature: wood, fire, earth, metal, and water. These elements can then be easily transferred to movement qualities using Laban Movement Analysis (LMA) in DMT.

One example of this Asian style of manifesting distress is called Hwa-Byung in Korean, which is unique to Korea. This disorder is caused by the suppression of anger and is also known as "Anger Syndrome" or "Fire Disease" in the Diagnostic and Statistical Manual 4th ed (American Psychiatric Association: APA, 2000). A person with Hwa-Byung often complains of physiological symptoms which they describe as being like a fire or storm in their

Table 15.1 Connections Between the Five Emotions, Organs, and Elements in Traditional Chinese Medicine (Kuman, 2019)

Organ	Heart	Liver	Spleen	Lungs	Kidney
Associated Emotion	Joy	Anger	Worry	Sorrow	Fear
Associated Element	Fire	Wood	Earth	Metal	Water
Associated Saying	Hasty Heart	Elevated Liver fire	Losing spleen spirit	Full of air in the Lung	Exhausted Kidney

chest. They also often report generalized aches, indigestion, a feeling of a mass in the epigas-trium, palpitations, anorexia, dysphonic affect, and dyspnea (Min, 2009). This is because of the Korean culture's esteem of restraint and the established belief in the body–mind as one uni t, which in East Asia parallels DMT's core belief of a body–mind connection.

PSYCHOTHERAPY IN EAST ASIA

Psychotherapy is an unfamiliar concept in East Asia (Sue & Sue, 2008), as traditional mental health practices have instead focused on visiting a shamanistic healer, praying to Buddha, practicing meditation, or using herbal medicine (Tseng, 2004). The field of mental health in China has been shaped and influenced by the philosophies of Taoism, Buddhism, Con-fucianism, and traditional worship practices (Haque, 2010). The field of mental health in Korea was also originally heavily influenced by Shamanism. Psychotherapy was gradually introduced by the West after the Korean War in the early 1960s (Bang & Park, 2009).

Individual vs. Community

DMT in East Asia has grown rapidly under the influence of both local DMTs and visiting scholars from the West. However, there have been barriers and challenges in transferring DMT into places with different learning and teaching cultures (Ko, 2015). DMT in the West is deeply rooted in modern dance, which has promoted a nonjudgmental attitude, personally meaningful movement, individual self-expression, and emotional content. These elements align with Western values of individuation, self-actualization, and independence, which have become the core essence of DMT (Levy, 2005). In contrast, in the East, one's self is inex-tricably linked to one's society, neighbors, family, and friends. Sharing emotional difficulties and individual self-expression tend to be unfamiliar and difficult in East Asian cultures (Kim, Sherman, & Taylor, 2008).

The real difference here is on the importance of self-construal, focusing on the primacy of individual goals over those of others and groups. "Interdependent self-construal is char-acterized by a sense of connectedness with others, by attention to one's role in in-groups, and by the primacy of group goals over one's individual goals which can be seen in East Asians" (Cross, 2018, p. 1).

Dosamantes-Beaudry (1999) explained these divergent East–West cultural constructions of self by comparing the different ways that participants moved and interacted in a DMT workshop in the West versus the East. Participants in the Western group (which took place in Zurich, Switzerland) displayed a range of negative and positive emotions along with diverse expressive movements. In contrast, those in the Eastern group (which took place in Taiwan) hesitated to express emotion and performed only movements that were similar to those that others did.

Ho (2005) conducted a pilot study in which six consecutive DMT sessions were offered for patients with cancer in Hong Kong. Ho reported: "Chinese participants were not accus-tomed to moving and dancing in front of others" (p. 27) and recommended that DMTs working with Chinese people allow extra time for participants to gradually become comfort-able expressing themselves through movement.

Tepayayone (2004) investigated how cultural influences in attitudes, values, and biases play a role in how movement is assessed. Laban Movement Analysis (LMA) is an observation and assessment tool (Laban & Ullmann, 2011). Tepayayone found that cultural background influenced the way that movement was perceived and assessed. As a result of this study, it is recommended that the study and instruction of LMA include not only an awareness of body movement but also a consideration of historical, ideological, and cultural aspects in the analysis of human movement as well as the impact of the observer's cultural background.

When Voice Is Not Allowed, Dance

Korean shamanistic rituals involve mainly dancing and singing, and are primarily the domain of women. Ritual activity in Korean Shamanism provides an emotional outlet for people to share their pain with each other (Ko, 2006). Such ritual activity has much in common with DMT, as Levy (2005) argues that "body movement reflects inner emotional states and that change in movement behavior can lead to changes in the psyche" (p. 36). Two traditional Korean dances exemplify such healing practices: a group circle dance, Ganggangsullae, and a solo dance with a long silky scarf, Salpuri.

Ganggangsullae: A Circle Dance

This type of dance has traditionally provided a rare break from restrictive rules governing the behavior of young women, with free expression allowed within this sacred circle space (Kim, 2012). Simple movements are paired with songs and quickly create a sense of community, equality, and harmony (UNESCO, 2018). This dance is similar to some aspects of Marian Chace's DMT approach in that both involve forming a circle and sharing a rhythm or group rhythmic activity (see Figure 15.1, Ganggangsullae, 2008).

Salpuri: A Scarf Dance

The Korean scarf dance called salpuri usually takes the form of a solo dance with a white silk scarf as a key prop. It was originally a shamanist ritual that cleansed the spirit by portraying the "sorrow of human relationships and separations, the bitterness of unsatisfied desire" (Fong, 2011, p. 1). This white scarf is used as a symbolic prop with which to sweep away tears or wave goodbye to beloved persons who have gone away or died. This dance,

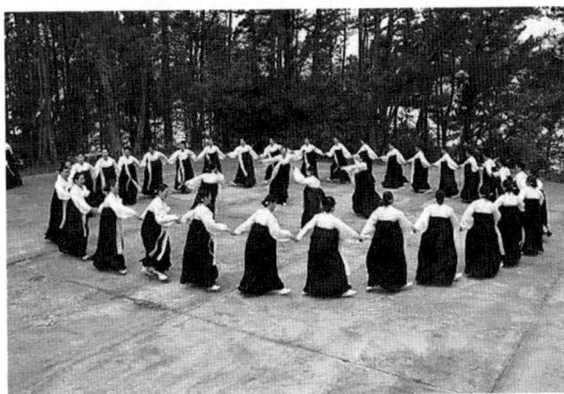

Figure 15.1 Ganggangsullae (Korean Circle Dance)

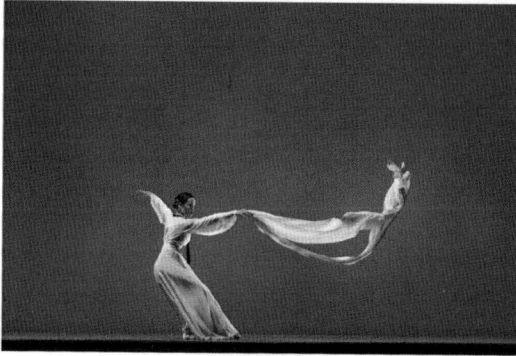

Figure 15.2 A Modernized Salpuri Dance Choreographed and Danced by Fong (2011)

combined with certain uses of the scarf, is used to symbolically express waving, flying away, shaking off, embracing, suppressing, folding, and spreading. Salpuri begins with a slow-paced rhythm, increases in speed as the dancer expresses her wishes, and then slows to a tranquil conclusion (see Figure 15.2). Using a scarf helps dancers to feel bigger and stronger and makes them more expressive. The physical and psychological key to the dance is a hold-and-release breathing cycle that generates energy and relaxation.

SPECIFIC KOREAN EMOTIONS

Haan: A Cultural-Psycho-Social Perspective

Korea's Confucian philosophical and cultural foundation supports rigid authority structures in the family, reinforcing the wife's submissive role and the husband's governing role (Lee, Wachholtz, & Choi, 2014). This expectation of self-effacement and nonentity can naturally lead many women to ignore their own wants and needs, and prolonged struggles with this conflicted female identity can lead to manifestations of haan. This culture-bounded syndrome may include mixed feelings of neglect, sorrow, and powerlessness; a suppression of feelings; a lack of self-identity; and a lack of a sense of belongingness (Min, 2009). Song and Moon (1998) described haan as a victimization-based syndrome resulting from perceived unjust treatment and the result of the lack of opportunity for self-actualization in a male-dominant society.

Haan as a Somatic Symptom and Cultural Syndrome

The expression of haan often includes psychosomatic pain, and it is related to another Korean-specific cultural syndrome known as *Hwa-byung*, an individualized expression of illness and a hallmark of haan (Min, 2009). Haan is a cluster of symptoms, and Hwan-byung is a diagnosed illness. Hwa-byung is described as a "cultural syndrome" that "manifests in the mixture of clinical depression, anxiety, and somatic symptoms characterized by the presence of a 'lump' and pressure in the throat or chest" (Kim, 2012, p. 237), feelings of heavy shoulders, a fire in the chest, difficulty breathing, floating without strength in one's lower body parts, a tight chest, a rapid heartbeat, or a lump in one's neck or stomach (Min, 2009).

Although haan has depressive overtones, it also features anger and rage, which tend not to be part of depression as manifested in Western cultures. These features explain why Hwa-byung is often referred to as anger disease or fire disease (Lee et al., 2014).

Haan and Generational Trauma

Haan is derived from prolonged intergenerational trauma beyond the individual personal level, a collective and national sorrow involving feelings of indignation and injustice that have been suppressed and endured. National traumas such as colonization by Japan, World War II, and the Korean War left deep scars of tremendous emotional suffering on the Korean people. Like any mental illness, this is a complex experience that should not, however, be thought of as completely negative, destructive, or without value: Kim (1998) emphasized that "Haan is not a passive process of suffering with acceptance and resignation, but an active process of suffering with a will to endure pain, to overcome and to triumph someday" (p. 219). Although several researchers have made excellent suggestions for using body-based expressive psychotherapy, research into these areas is insufficient.

CASE STUDY: BROKEN HEART FROM A WOUNDED LAND

This case study provides a description of Minji (a pseudonym), a Korean woman suffering from haan for whom ten sessions of Korean scarf dance were used as a DMT intervention. This case study took place through a nonprofit social service agency which mainly offers mental health services for Asian immigrants in the United States (Ko, 2006).

Description of the Patient

Personal details about Minji have been altered to protect her privacy. Minji was a 40-year-old Korean woman who had immigrated to the United States about two years prior to treatment after marrying a Korean-American man whom she had dated for six months. At the time of treatment, Minji was living alone in a small studio and working as a babysitter. Minji was in the process of obtaining a divorce due to domestic violence that began three months into her marriage. Previously, Minji had lived in a one-bedroom apartment with her husband and mother-in-law. Her husband discussed everything about Minji with his mother, blocked Minji from having social connections, and prevented her from attending English classes. During the initial intake, she complained of chest pains, headaches, muscle tension, and difficulty concentrating. Treatment goals established with Minji were to release suppressed feelings of haan by providing a space for emotional self-expression and to empower herself by finding her inner strength to build up her life in a new environment.

Summary of Sessions

Session 1: "I Cannot Breathe."

Minji walked into the office quickly and weightlessly. She looked nervous, with lots of tension in her shoulders; she made no eye contact and her hands shook. Minji did not say anything for a while. Suddenly, she took a deep breath and abruptly said, "I do not want to talk about everything all over again," and started to cry. I evaluated Minji's feelings and said, "You do not have to tell me." I then asked, "How are you doing?" Minji replied, "I don't feel good," and started to talk about her physical symptoms. "My shoulder is heavy," she added. I encouraged her to talk more about the pain in her body. Minji responded, "I cannot breathe; I do not have strength in my legs." This exploration of pain in the body extended to Minji's recounting her story of her abusive husband. Minji started to talk quickly without breathing, with many tangential run-on sentences and abrupt topic changes. Minji's verbal rendering of her story mirrored her movement of walking fast, with an indirect use of space and a lack of grounding. I encouraged Minji to bring attention to her body by touching herself where she felt pain. To ground her energy, I had Minji stand up, and encouraged her to feel the ground through her feet by pushing down through them and bending her knees. At the end of the session, Minji described her physical feelings as "I feel like something is going up and down in my body," and she gestured to her chest area. As her therapist, the impression I had was that Minji had many feelings bottled up and many unspoken stories.

Session 2: "A Quiet Voice."

Minji shared in a quiet voice how her husband had abused her verbally and emotionally, calling her names like "yellow cab" (a derogatory term for Asian women) or "prostitute," which made her feel very ashamed. Minji expressed very mixed feelings and described her somatic symptoms, such as difficulty swallowing or digesting food. I wondered if Minji's inability to swallow food symbolized her inability to accept the cruel things that her husband said to her.

I provided an empty chair for Minji and asked if she could express herself by saying what she wanted to say to anyone she chose. I did not specify to whom Minji might speak, as I did not want Minji to feel too pressured or directed. Minji hesitated for a long time, needing encouragement. I moved my chair to look in the same direction as Minji and stayed with the silence.

Minji started to talk, as if her mother-in-law was sitting in the chair, in a quiet, unassertive voice, like that of a little girl. She said, "You promised me life in America would be better than in Korea, and you lied to me." She looked down and did not look at the chair. Her body was very compressed, and she looked much smaller than she actually was, using a small Kinesphere (an LMA term denoting personal space that one can reach without moving one's feet). Minji then addressed her husband, maintaining the same unassertive attitude. Minji brought up the time that her husband had prohibited her from attending her mother's funeral in Korea, asking, "How could you do that to me? My mother was sick and you did not give me my passport." I could feel Minji's deep sadness and anger toward her husband.

When I encouraged Minji to talk to her mother who had passed away, Minji took a long pause. Minji said through tears, "I have haan when I think about my mother." I stayed with Minji's deep grief regarding her mother in silence for a while. When I asked Minji how she might be able to cope with her stress, Minji explained that she had limited relationships with other people in the United States, and was ashamed to talk about her problems with others. Minji had been surprised to learn that the scoldings her husband gave her constituted verbal abuse, because she had thought that only physical abuse could be serious. In response to this, I provided psychosocial education regarding domestic violence and types of abuse to Minji.

Session 3: "Korean Women Have Haan."

Minji was invited to write down her thoughts. Minji wrote that "all Korean women have haan," which is "a deep grief and pressure deep inside [my] heart where something is tangled and hard to release." Minji reported six different emotions making up her haan: "anger, sadness, powerlessness, anguish, loneliness, and frustration." When Minji talked about haan, she started to breathe and talk more rapidly. I then introduced the importance of breathing and did three-dimensional breathing exercises together with Minji, expanding outwards with her arms and moving her torso in a standing position. At the end of the session, I introduced both the ideas of DMT and of Korean scarf dancing. Minji agreed to participate in DMT through Korean scarf dancing because she wanted to explore her haan for "mental and psychological stability." It indicated she was engaged in a struggle against herself—she was desperate, stressed, and in need of help to survive in this abusive environment.

After the third session, I also created a tool to assess her level of haan, listing all of the six emotions that Minji described as contributing to her haan. I asked Minji to rate each emotion using a 10-point Likert-type scale from 1 ("not at all") to 10 ("a great deal") to help her track and clarify her level of emotion relating to her haan before and after each DMT session. The third data source consisted of Minji's written comments or drawings, for which a blank area on the bottom of the checklist was provided. I added this area because I believed that Minji's unspoken words and unexpressed emotions could not be captured in purely quantitative data.

Session 4: "More Haan."

Minji informed me that the breathing helped her to modulate her emotions, especially when she was angry. As a DMT intervention, Korean scarf dancing starts with the playing of traditional music and breathing from one's core. I provided an initial movement, and then Minji moved together with me, enhancing the therapeutic relationship by promoting attunement. The initial movement involved flicking back the scarf and pressing one's body down to the ground by bending the knees, as well as raising one's arms and enclosing the space. These are typical Salpuri beginning movements, as they can be easily followed and remembered. In her reflection after the session, Minji reported "feeling good, because while I am doing movement, I am not thinking." At the end of the session, in the blank area of her haan checklist, Minji wrote "happiness" and "future." She also said "It is weird, my haan is not decreasing, it is increasing." Minji reported feeling more haan after participating in the movement exercise, as indicated by the haan assessment tool. Her sadness, loneliness, anger, and frustration increased after the session, but her anguish and powerlessness did not increase.

I was troubled to hear that Minji's haan had increased instead of decreased. I talked about this with my supervisor, and realized that I had been focused on getting Minji to cast away negative feelings instead of containing her existing emotions. It is more important to help clients grow aware of existing emotions than to focus on getting rid of those feelings.

My clinical supervisor also explained the concepts of the old self and new self, emphasizing how difficult it is to experience the birth of a new self. Bergner and Holmes (2000) explained self-concept changes in psychotherapy. Many clients struggle with how to create a new, more adaptive self without letting go of and abandoning the sense of the old self. Minji's mixed and vague emotions now made more sense, and clinical supervision helped me to empathize deeply with Minji.

Session 5: "After Divorce."

Minji reported that she felt better, as her divorce had just been finalized. Her shoulders felt less heavy, and she felt less pressure on her chest. However, Minji looked angry to me, indicating a mismatch between what she was saying—that she was feeling better—and her facial expression and muscular tension. I then asked what coping skills Minji used for stressful situations, and Minji said that "listening to music helps [me] to calm down."

While listening to Korean traditional music, Minji and I reviewed the movements we did together in our previous session. I then added vocal attunement, such as rhythmic counting similar to the sound of a drum, sung to the tune to Minji's choreographed scarf dance. I asked, "What do you want to do for the next movement?" and Minji replied that she wanted to "move forward" four steps, so she did. Realizing that there was no space to continue moving forward, Minji said "no space!" I then asked her, "Where else can you go?" Minji paused for a while, then turned around halfway and moved back the way she had come. Minji moved on a diagonal rather than turning around and facing the direction she had come from because returning to the space where she had started reminded her too much of the past life she was not ready to face. Minji explained that stepping sideways on the diagonal was not about going back, but was instead about meeting people to ask for help. After the session, Minji noticed that the sound of counting was like the sound of a heart beating and that she had been able to match the movement to the beat. Minji also reported that "it made me focus on my body and these movements made me calm down and feel at peace." Minji drew a picture of a tree after the session and said, "It's about me without roots." She also wrote "change" (see Figure 15.3a). Looking at Minji's picture, I understood how difficult it would be to put down roots in a land with different soil and climate (i.e., a different culture), especially without any fertilizer (i.e., support). In this case, "change" might be necessary for this tree to survive in a new environment and situation.

Session 6: "No Place to Go."

Minji had been afraid to tell her family in her homeland about the divorce because it is considered shameful in Korea. For this reason, Minji did not want to go back there. The scarf dance movement started where the previous session had ended, going backwards four steps on a diagonal. Again, there was no space after Minji took four big steps: This was the second time she did not have enough space to move forward. Minji sniffled as she said, "I do not know where to go. No space." I encouraged Minji to take a couple of deep breaths, provided a little time, and asked again, "What can we do now?" Minji said, "Move back." I asked why she went back, and Minji replied that "Honestly, I had no place go to, so I went back." I then asked, "I wonder, why did you think that moving backwards was the only option?" Minji took a long pause and I stayed with her silence for a while. I encouraged her by saying, "Is there something in your life you want to change, just as you did in your movement?" Minji answered, "having met my husband" and continued talking about changing her arm movement. "I want to release. I feel like I have to move my left and right arms together because moving one arm is uncomfortable and difficult. . . . I want to go forward with two arms flapping lightly." When Minji opened both of her arms, it created more space in her core and allowed her to breathe more deeply. Minji wanted to change some of her arm movements to make her feel more comfortable. After she had verbalized that decision, her arm movement flowed from proximal to distal, which created more open space in her chest.

Then she started to talk. "I was a very shy girl, since I was young, and I tried to be a good daughter" who wanted to study more about "child psychology." I noticed that Minji was starting to bring up the hopes and dreams that she remembered from the time she lived in Korea. I hoped that as Minji noticed that she could move both arms, she would relive not only the abusive memories from her marriage but also positive memories about herself in Korea. Such memories could provide positive energy and strength to deal with difficulties.

Session 7: "No Way to See My Mother."

Minji complained of muscle pain on the right side of her shoulder. She explained that working as a babysitter was physically demanding because she had to hold the baby when it cried, which caused unbalanced shoulders. Then, Minji continued to talk about how a baby knows its mother. Minji said, "My mother's chest was so warm and cozy, I did not want to leave." I asked Minji, "Do you miss your mother?" She began to cry and said, "I had no way to see my mother." She then recounted a dream that she had had a couple of days previously. In this dream, her mother was very small, but she held Minji's hand and kissed her on the cheek with great strength. Minji said, "I want to see the future, not the past, because it [the past] makes me sad." For Minji, moving backwards in space reminded her of past memories. Her mother might symbolically represent strength, power, or life-force energy, as Minji's dream of her mother connected to a strong desire to move forward. Throughout multiple sessions, Minji repeatedly said, "No place to go" when there was no space to move forward. Her way of seeing space clearly represented her situation and feelings about life: with few real relationships to support her, Minji wanted to move forward to leave her current situation (see Figure 15.3b). I asked Minji, "What is it like for you right now?" Minji said "isolation." She then immediately sat down in a chair—which may have indicated resistance against further movement—and sat silently. Minji's reaction guided me to think about how to empower her: protecting the bruised ego of the current self while developing a healthy new self.

Session 8: "I Have to Move Forward."

Minji was clearly worried about being reductively labeled as a divorced woman, and considered halting the process of working to obtain citizenship because it was so painful to discuss her past. Minji started to talk about how the father of the baby she cared for treated his wife. His kind and respectful treatment of his wife made her feel "irritated and angry" because it was such a contrast to how her ex-husband had treated her, and it showed Minji what a good family and good husband could be like. She was very angry about having married her ex-husband, an "emotional burden" from the past that makes her "unable to move forward easily."

This invisible but emotionally and bodily felt burden extended to the session's movement work. I divided the space into the past, present, and future. I then encouraged Minji to stand in the present and asked her where she wanted to move; the scarf was wrapped around Minji's waist, symbolizing her emotional burden and making it difficult to move forward. I pulled on the scarf, and asked Minji to let me know when this sensation matched her perceived "emotional burden." Once Minji indicated that the resistance was correct, I asked, "What do you want to do?" Minji said, "I know I have to move forward but it is not easy." As Minji walked forward, the scarf tangled about her more and more tightly. She burst out crying, "I do not know where to go; this is the same as my situation." In this moment, she was trying to use her physical strength to overcome her emotional burden. Her repressed emotions were externalized through movement, making sounds and telling me how much she was suffering. To me, this was like a moment of opening up a boiling emotional container, which revealed Minji's internal strength (see Figure 15.3c).

Session 9: "Pushing Bad Energy."

Minji's dance started with the last movement from the preceding session. Minji did not have space in front of her, so she decided to step backwards. In Laban's theory, space is labeled based on where the person is headed, meaning that if Minji turned to face where she had started from, this would be considered her forward space. In past sessions, Minji had consistently maintained forward movement, clearly representing the strength of her desire to get away from her negative past. Session 9 was the first time she used the space behind her in her dance, by using a press movement; a press in action drive was also observed in her drawing (see Figure 15.3d). As part of the action drive, a *press movement* combines increasing pressure, weight, sustained time, and direct space (Laban & Ullmann, 2011); here, Minji's arms and hands moved along with the scarf as if pushing something back. This represented a clear moment of emerging new movement qualities, changing from flicking (characterized by accelerating time, indirect space, and decreasing weight) to pressing. Minji explained that her movement of pushing back the space behind her was related to "pushing bad energy . . . so it could not follow her." This moment demonstrated a new attitude of dealing with her past abusive memories by pushing against the violent memories, rather than avoiding or running away from them; here, her emotional strength was represented though her physical strength. I encouraged Minji's efforts and observed how this movement decision related to her life. Minji reflected on her dance, saying, "I cannot see any other space; I can only see forward. This was the same as when I danced." Minji reported that her strongest movement was when she stepped backwards, into the space that she had been avoiding. This felt like an important moment, in which Minji finally focused her courage and strength against the bad energy behind her.

Session 10: "Focus on Myself."

This session was the last session of the Salpuri. Together, Minji and I danced through all of the movements that Minji had previously choreographed. Minji looked shy but encouraged, and completed the dance herself. I suggested closing the Salpuri by pausing for one final

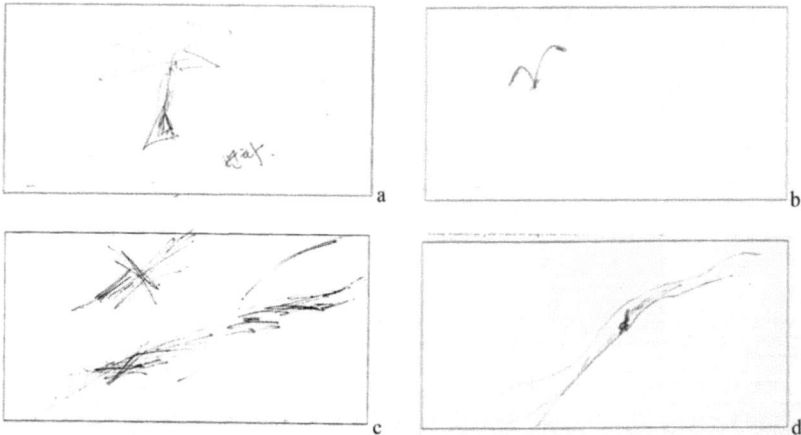

Figure 15.3a-d. Figures Drawn by Minji

moment. Minji then lightly hopped forward, with free childlike arm movements. Her arms moved up and down, a typical Korean arm movement of waving and flying. She opened both arms on a horizontal plane, advancing and spreading her chest forward as one would do upon reaching the summit of a mountain. This was the first time that Minji fully used her sagittal plane in her body posture. Minji shared her experiences with the scarf dancing by saying, "It was a great chance for me to understand myself better. The dance was not just about dance; it gave me more. I could see myself through dance. . . . When I am dancing I forget about everything. I am not thinking [of only bad things] and I can focus on myself."

What follows is my LMA-based interpretation of Minji's drawings (see Figure 15.3a-d). I used my own body movement as a tool to respond to each image and then described the movements that emerged according to LMA principles. I have also included my verbal therapeutic interpretation.

a. Float: A tree without roots represents the difficulty that she has had in becoming connected and finding nourishment in the United States. She reflected that perhaps it was time to adjust to a new environment in a new land, a step that requires "change" to survive.

b. Glide: The client drew a bird, symbolically representing her wish to fly away from her current situation on earth and take off to see her mother who had passed away. This drawing captures her loneliness, her longing to see her deceased mother, and a strong desire to move forward, because birds can only fly forward.

c. Slash: A boiling hot emotional container. This drawing made after Session 8 differs from all previous drawings: This drawing is abstract and expressed outward in rough way; it also uses much more space than the other drawings.

d. Press: Climbing a steep mountain alone. Unlike the drawings made in earlier reflections, this drawing expressed a mobilized quality, symbolically representing Minji's strength in standing her challenging situation, depicted as a steep mountain.

RESULTS

Data were gathered through the therapist's session notes, the patient's drawings, and movement observation, and they were analyzed with the help of NVivo.

Theme 1. Desire to Move Forward

Minji wanted to escape from her abusive marriage, which was symbolically represented by the space behind her. As a result, she was preoccupied by using only the space in front of her, and was unable to see other space. Minji had a strong negative emotional attachment to the space behind her, which was expressed through comments such as the feeling that "bad energy [was] dragging her down." The space before her symbolically represented the future, where she longed to go like "a flying bird" (Session 7), even though this was as difficult as "climbing [a] steep mountain alone" (Session 9). Although the room was large enough to create movement sequences, because Minji wanted only to move forward, she regularly encountered situations where she had no space in front of her. Minji's preoccupation with forward space limited her ability to see any other space, which decreased her options for spaces around her into which she could move. This reflected her difficulty in getting help, resulting in her social isolation and lack of support. In LMA, the sagittal plane represents intuition and decision making, It is lack of horizontal space representing relationship and resources around self. Here, Minji was able to intuitively use her body to make the decisions that she needed to survive her abusive relationship and environment.

Theme 2. A Boiling Emotional Container

The second theme, a boiling emotional container, symbolically represented Minji's emotional memories of the abuse she had experienced in her marriage. Min (2009) described haan as a mix of suppressed emotions that does not allow an outlet for the expression of emotions. Minji's identified haan was expanded to include 14 different emotions after Session 6. These increasing emotions were like bubbles that started to boil more once Minji was allowed to feel and express herself. When self-expression is not possible, this can lead to the suppression of anger, aggression, and other feelings and desires. This temporary increase in the emotions that comprised Minji's haan could have indicated that Minji's emotional experiences became deeper and clearer as she embodied and externalized them. While Minji wrote "I am angry and dreary" after Session 10, just being able to express her feelings clearly in writing, was a big step forward, and she reported feeling much more confidence.

Theme 3. Body in Pain and Shame

The third theme, body in pain and shame, encapsulated Minji's somatic distress relating to her emotions, many of which were linked to being a divorced Korean woman. In working with Minji, I found that the body was an easier place to start, as Minji was so reluctant to open up verbally about her emotional struggles. Minji often complained of physical pain instead of emotional pain. Allowing her to talk about these physical pains and sensations proved to be a good place to start to address emotional issues. Minji recalled being a "good daughter" before she got married but was now a "divorced woman," a shameful status in the Korean community that prevented her from returning to her homeland or talking about her current status to her family there. This fear and shame created social isolation and further prevented Minji from receiving support in either the United States or Korea.

Theme 4. Wisdom From Both the Moving and the Silent Body

The fourth theme speaks to the emergence of new movement, and to the moments of silence and pause. It explained how Minji used her body to understand herself and regain strength. She reflected on meaningful moments from her movements that connected to her life and helped her to find her own potential strength, asserting that "I have two arms" with which to fly. Minji also defined her movement of "pushing bad energy" from past abusive experiences as her most powerful moment in the scarf dance, while describing the moment of stepping backward. In later sessions, Minji engaged in new behaviors, taking time to pause and be silent. This more relaxed pace allowed her time to think and reflect, enabling her to gain insight and get in touch with her strength. Her new emergent movements, such as pressing, expressed hope that this "tree without roots" would put down roots in her new land, presenting more bodily grounding than at the beginning of therapy.

CONCLUSION

The world is incredibly culturally diverse; while this enriches culture and offers clinicians the chance to meet clients from various backgrounds, it also means that a competent and ethical clinician must learn and develop sensitivity to diversity (Chang, 2016). This study presents the use of traditional dance as a DMT therapeutic intervention, allowing an in-depth exploration of a client's psychological and emotional difficulties within her unique sociocultural context, thereby providing sensitive and effective treatment. This clinical case also represents, specifically, a cluster of emotions called haan that is unique to a Korean cultural context. Understanding haan gives a good example of how some cultures value containing emotions rather than expressing them. In these cases, it may be easier to approach treatment by talking about physical symptoms than to discuss emotional difficulties directly. It is hoped that this chapter supports dance/movement therapists' competency when treating clients from different cultural backgrounds, and offers inspiration as to how ethnic dance can be a resource with which to access embodied knowledge and to understand a client's unique context.

NOTE

The case study featured in this chapter was previously published in *Arts in Psychotherapy* (Ko, 2017) with the publisher's permission (#501388770). Modified portions of this article were also taken from a doctoral dissertation (Ko, 2015). Personal details about Minji have been altered to protect her privacy.

REFERENCES

American Psychiatric Association. (2000). *Diagnostic and statistical manual of mental disorders* (4th ed.). Washington, DC: American Psychiatric Association.

Bang, K., & Park, J. (2009). Korean supervisors' experiences in clinical supervision. *International Forum, 37*(8), 1042–1075.

Bergner, R. M., & Holmes, J. R. (2000). Self-concepts and self-concept change: A status dynamic approach. *Psychotherapy: Theory, Research, Practice, Training, 37*(1), 36–44.

Chang, M. H. (2016). Cultural consciousness and the global context of dance/movement therapy. In S. Chaiklin & H. Wengrower (Eds.), *The art and science of dance/ movement therapy: Life is dance* (2nd ed., pp. 301–318). New York: Routledge.

Cross, S. (2018). Self-construal. In S. Cross (Ed.), *Oxford bibliographies.* Retrieved from www.oxfordbibliographies.com/view/document/obo-9780199828340/obo-9780199828340-0051.xml

Dosamantes-Beaudry, I. (1999). Divergent cultural self construals: Implications for the practice of dance/movement therapy. *The Arts in Psychotherapy, 26*(4), 225–231.

Fong, J. (2011). *World arts west.* Retrieved from http://worldartswest.org/main/edf_performer.asp?i=187

Ganggangsullae. (2008). Cultural Heritage Administration. Retrieved from https://ich.unesco.org/en/RL/ganggangsullae-00188

Haque, A. (2010). Mental health concepts in Southeast Asia: Diagnostic considerations and treatment implications. *Psychology, Health & Medicine, 15*(2), 127–134.

Ho, R. (2005). Effects of dance/movement therapy on Chinese cancer patients: A pilot study in Hong Kong. *Arts in Psychotherapy, 32*(5), 337–345.

Kim, H. S., Sherman, D. K., & Taylor, S. E. (2008). Culture and social support. *American Psychologist, 63*(6), 518–526.

Kim, L. I. (1998). The mental health of Korean women. In Y. I. Song & A. Moon (Eds.), *Korean American women: From tradition to modern feminism* (pp. 209–224). Westport, CT: Greenwood Publishing Group.

Kim, Luke I. C. (2012). *Beyond the battle line: The Korean war and my life.* Bloomington: Xlibris.

Ko, K. S. (2006). *A case study: The use of Korean scarf dance as a dance/movement therapy intervention for a Korean woman with hann* (Unpublished master thesis). Columbia College, Chicago, IL.

Ko, K. S. (2015). *Asian dance/movement therapy educators' experiences of teaching dance/movement therapy in East Asia after training in the US* (Unpublished doctoral dissertation). Lesley University, Cambridge, MA.

Ko, K. S. (2017). A broken heart from a wounded land: The use of Korean scarf dance as a dance/movement therapy intervention for a Korean woman with haan. *The Arts in Psychotherapy, 55*(4), 64–72.

Kuman, M. (2019). The true meaning of the law of five elements (organ's reciprocal dependences and their practical use). *International Journal of Complementary & Alternative Medicine, 12*(3), 110–113.

Laban, R., & Ullmann, L. (2011). *The mastery of movement.* Hampshire, UK: Dance Books Ltd.

Lee, J., Wachholtz, A., & Choi, K. H. (2014). A review of the Korean cultural syndrome Hwa-Byung: Suggestions for theory and intervention. *Journal of Asian Pacific Counseling, 4*(1), 49–64.

Levy, F. J. (2005). *Dance/movement therapy: A healing art.* Reston, VA: National Dance Association and American Alliance for Health, Physical, Education, Recreation and Dance.

Mehrabian, A. (1972). *Nonverbal communication.* Chicago, IL: Aldine Atherton.

Min, S. K. (2009). Hwabyung in Korea: Culture and dynamic analysis. *World Cultural Psychiatry Research Review, 4*(1), 12–21.

Song, Y. I., & Moon, A. (1998). *Korean American women: From tradition to modern feminism.* Westport, CT: Greenwood Publishing Group.

Sue, D. W., & Sue, D. (2008). *Counseling the culturally diverse: Theory and practice* (5th ed.). New York, NY: John Wiley & Sons.

Tepayayone, W. (2004). *Culture, perception, and clinical assessment in dance/movement Therapy: A phenomenological investigation* (Unpublished master's thesis). Drexel University, Philadelphia, PA.

Tseng, W. S. (2004). Special section: Cultural issues in mental health services and treatment: Culture and psychotherapy: Asian perspectives. *Journal of Mental Health, 13*(2), 151–161.

UNESCO. (2018). *Ganggangsulle.* Retrieved from https://ich.unesco.org/en/RL/ganggangsullae-00188

CHAPTER 16

DANCE/MOVEMENT THERAPY IN JAPAN AND ITS CULTURAL ROOTS

Yukari Sakiyama

As dance movement therapists, we try to understand our clients. In this context, there is no difference between Western and Japanese DMT. The following sentence reflects our universal beliefs: "Every little movement has a meaning all its own, every thought and feeling by some posture can be shown" (Hauerback, 1910). DMT also reflects each culture, especially through their dances and attitude toward the body. I have had numerous and varied experiences of DMT within different cultures. When I attend annual conferences of the American Dance Therapy Association (ADTA), I learn many things from my DMT colleagues from Western countries and other Asian countries as well. I appreciate both the wonderful diversity of DMT and the similarities we share, although our history and cultures are quite varied. The differences are hard to clearly explain, but this chapter will attempt to do so through a description of Japanese DMT history and our DMT features that reflect our body culture.

GENERAL HISTORY OF DANCE/MOVEMENT THERAPY IN JAPAN

Japan has a background of various types of dance, just as every country does. Our distinctive and traditional dances are *Kagura* (sacred Shinto dance with music) and *Shimai* (*Noh* dance). Some trials using dance/movement for therapeutic approaches with psychiatric patients were reported in a research journal of the Japanese Society of Psychopathology of Expression & Art Therapy. They made use of such traditional dances such as *Shimai*, (Nogawa & Murai, 1979), *Kagura, Oni kenbu*, and *Shika odori* (Ban, 1981). *Shimai* is rather grounded and has steady steps with sliding feet.[1] They tried to apply the slow and steady steps for clients in a psychiatric hospital, and it enabled them to concentrate on the movement. *Shimai* is a solo dance, and a good example of introspective movement. *Kagura, Oni kenbu*[2] and *Shika odori*[3] are rhythmic and extroverted group dances. They include jumping and sometimes spreading energy in order to bless all the gods and goddesses. Ban utilized these local dances for groups, particularly for the use of symmetrical movements. Members of the group had to be aware of each other in order to follow the same choreography. The leaders were not dmts, but a psychiatrist and a clinical psychologist who tried to apply Japanese traditional dance forms. However, these trials did not continue, unfortunately.

Butoh, a specific type of dance created by Tatsumi Hijikata, is now being used by professional Butoh dancers working as dmts. Their DMT has been established gradually through their work with clients within psychiatric hospitals. Officially they aren't trained in DMT, but one has been working with a psychiatrist and nurse, and the other is a psychology professor. Other types of dance are traditional dance forms for rituals or related ritual community performances like *Bon dance*. Historically, Japanese DMT pioneers often utilized dance forms with people who were not used to physical expression and without dance experience. By comparison, Western DMT was started by modern dancers, and modern dance emphasizes creativity for free expression. There was one research paper using modern dance in a Japanese psychiatric hospital (Sakata & Shimoyama, 1970), but the practice was not discussed.

In the 1980s, Machida (1999) tried to gather all possible information about dance therapy in Japan by personal communications, attending conferences and meetings, or searching research papers and worked toward creating a large network for DMT all over Japan. In 1984, an American dance therapist, Sharon Chaiklin, was invited to a Japanese psychiatric hospital and gave some sessions for the staff there (Momonoi & Matsubara, 1985). Beginning in 1988, Amy B. Wapner was invited to another psychiatric hospital in Tokyo and taught DMT to clinical psychologists and nurses (Ogiwara et al., 1993). Finally, the Japan Dance Therapy Association (JADTA) was established in 1992. In the 1990s, some Japanese who had studied DMT in the United States or the United Kingdom came back to Japan as registered dmts and started working in different regions, such as Okayama and Gunma.

An interesting difference to note is that when compared with Western countries, males (9) were almost the same number as females (8) actively working in 1970s and 1980s in the aforementioned research papers (Nogawa & Murai, 1979; Ban, 1981; Sakata & Shimoyama, 1970; Momonoi & Matsubara, 1985). They were DMT practitioners and clinical psychologists (Shimoyama) or psychiatrists (Murai). Additionally, the first Japanese registered dance therapist (DTR) by ADTA, Motohide Miyahara, is male.

One reason there may have been more men in the field may be related to applied dance forms of DMT used in clinical settings. Many dance forms were performed by men who are closely connected to Shinto or Buddhism. Not only religious ceremonies but also other traditional art forms such as *Noh* and *Kabuki* are performed by men. Also, Butoh is a unique Japanese dance form that in its beginnings was performed only by men.

Several features of Japanese DMT outlined by previous JADTA president Machida (2012) are as follows:

- It reflects Japanese culture.
- Group sessions are more popular.
- Massage is often included.
- Verbalization is not often required.

The following sections will discuss these features.

TRADITIONS OF THE BODY

Dmts recognize the importance of the integration of body and mind. Which body parts do you point to when you say "mind"? Japanese take it for granted that our body and mind are not separable. Western people have different ideas about this, so they point to the head when they say mind. Many Japanese put their hands on their hearts, despite knowing the brain controls the body. In our cultural context, the body includes a spiritual aspect and that cannot be separated. (Sakiyama, 2000)

Bathing Culture

The Japanese *Onsen* (natural hot springs and public bath)[4] is frequented by families and by unrelated people who bathe together. All who bathe in the *Onsen* together, whether related or not, are equally touched by the waters that comfort and soothe, creating a collective body

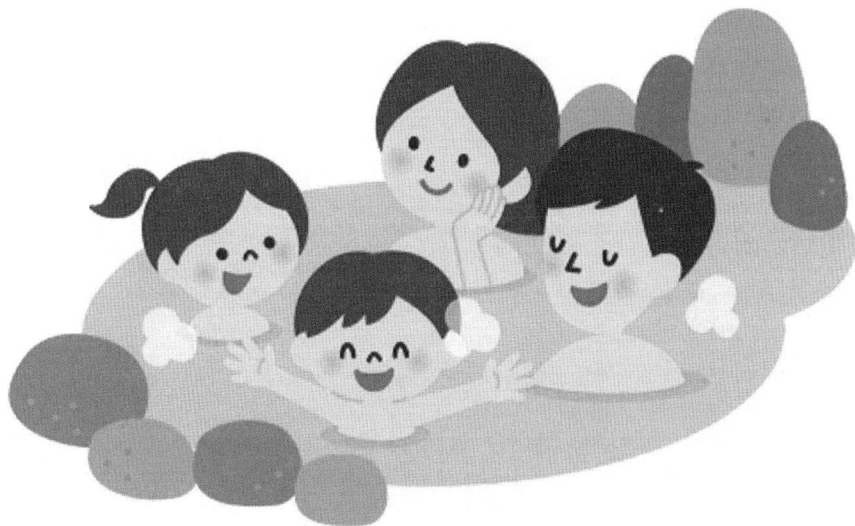

Figure 16.1 Family Enjoying *Onsen*

sense (see Figure 16.1). In addition, the act of bathing with others at the *Onsen* provides children with a venue in which to learn how to negotiate personal space and to support the development of the body sense within the public context. (Sakiyama & Koch, 2003). Dmts use the image of *Onsen*, since we have a pleasant association with it. It is "more than a bath". Kitajima (2012) gave her session participants an image of soaking themselves in *Onsen* together by using a giant stretch band. She used a Japanese onomatopoeia, *hokkori*, which means warm and fluffy. Hirai and Sakiyama (2016) also used the image of *Onsen* at a workshop at the International Association for Analytic Psychology to introduce Japanese body culture.

Broderick and Moore (2010) state that this bath is not only for cleaning but for relaxing and getting rid of the day's worries. Merry (2013) explains Japanese bathing culture as follows:

> Japanese bathing culture is a phenomenon remarkably different from most traditions in the modern Western world. To many, the concept of stripping off one's clothes and bathing communally is foreign. However, in Japan, this accepted and loved convention permeates society, transcending generational, social, economic, and geographic barriers. The sheer number of hot springs and baths in Japan attests to their cultural significance and importance. Due to the great degree of variance in the types of baths and the rituals surrounding them, an understanding of their distinctions is critical to interpreting their individual societal functions and implications.
>
> (p. 1)

The Image of bathing may be part of dreams and may be used as a therapeutic image. (Ohnuma, 2012) Mostly, we shower and take a bath alone. However, we still keep the experience of taking a bath together in our memories of our daily life or of leisure with family or friends or even unknown people when visiting *Onsen*. Sharing the same hot water in the tub at the same time is a good opportunity for communication, as it is a shared experience.

Use of Touch and Massage

The Japanese are accustomed to "indirect" touch through sharing the same tub to bathe as mentioned earlier but we don't hug much in salutation. However, in child–parent relationships, we have experiences of direct touch through playing (see Figure 16.2). As an example, there is a traditional nursery song when children give shoulder-tapping massage (*Kata Tataki*) to their mothers.

The translated English lyrics are:

Mommy, shall I tap your shoulders and ease your stiffness? Tap, tap, tap, tap, tap, tap, tap

Mommy, you have some gray hairs, did you know? Tap, tap, tap, tap, tap, tap, tap

Our veranda gets plenty of sunshine Tap, tap, tap, tap, tap, tap, tap

Bright red poppies are smiling at you Tap, tap, tap, tap, tap, tap, tap

Mommy, are you feeling so much better now? Tap, tap, tap, tap, tap, tap, tap

(Original lyrics by Saijo Yaso Music by Nakayama Shinpei,
English Translation by Yamagishi Katsuei ©)[5]

Japanese children who are Westernized still know *Kata Tataki*. This suggests that massage is not done only by specialists. Sakiyama and Hirai (1997) showed how to use touch in psychiatric settings during relaxation and mentioned the importance of rhythmical touch that includes an image of progressiveness and moving forward. Through rhythmic active stimulation, as the massage goes on, clients can feel the tension in the muscles being released. The lyric, *tap, tap, tap, tap, tap, tap, tap* easily gives us the image of rhythmical shoulder tapping. When doing this massage, we sing along with the original lyrics. It is *tan ton tan ton tan ton*

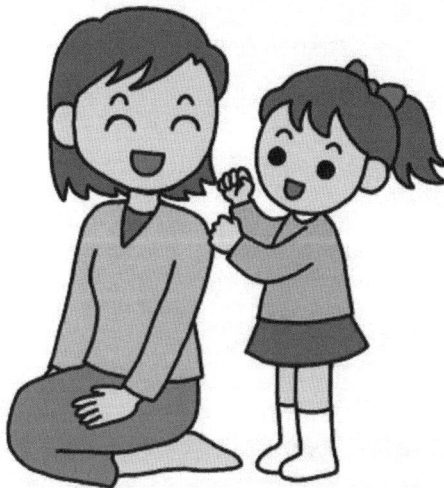

Figure 16.2 Kata Tataki

ton, an onomatopoeia which means "light touch with tapping" and promotes an intimate contact. Touch exists within the daily lives of families and friends just like *Kata Tataki* (see Figure 16.3).

Included with these kinds of rhythmical touch, we often use the word, "*Karada Hoguchi*". *Karada* means body, and *Hogushi* is a noun meaning disentangle, straighten out, and relax the tension. The concept of *Hogushi* is not active but rather being passive in order to allow the body to be just the way it is naturally. The concept of *Karada Hogushi* is officially adopted in physical education.

Kata Tataki is not done by facing your partner. Every child stands behind their mother, father, or grandparents. They all face the same direction. The back is left defenseless because they trust their children and grandchildren and there is affection between them. Japanese body culture embraces this defenseless back. Here is a vignette:

> K (male, 25, mentally handicapped, epilepsy) initially could not participate in group DMT sessions. At first, he disliked entering the room. When the session started, he would run away and each time I would run after him. It became a game to him, and the "game" seemed to be a way of starting a relationship with me. It was then that I noticed he always stood with his back toward me. It seemed completely defenseless to me. I also stood with my back toward him. This appears to be a common body position among Japanese.

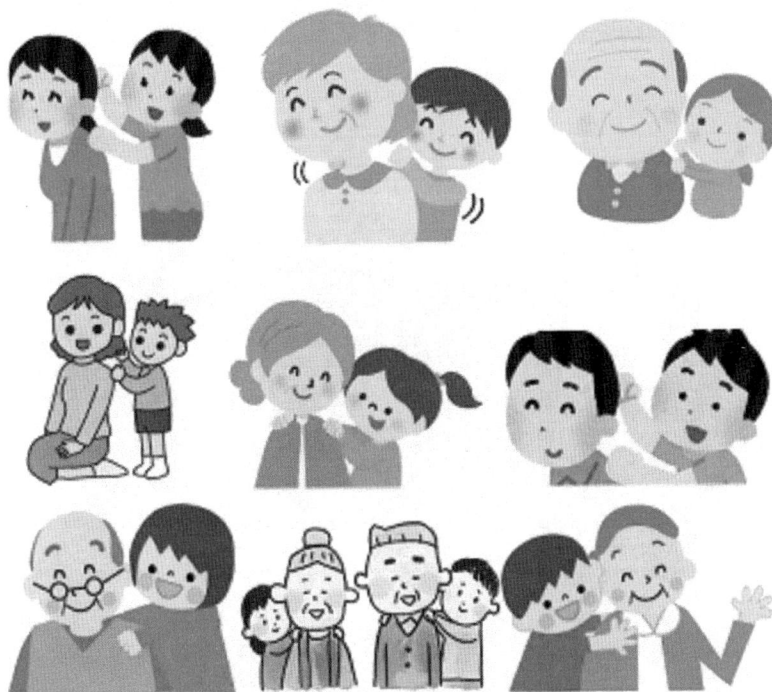

Figure 16.3 Examples of Google Illustration Search of *Kata Tataki*

K and I have since developed a good relationship due to, in part, the "defenseless back" position. Perhaps a lack of eye contact helps most Japanese feel comfortable. Possibly, most Japanese unconsciously develop relationships through their "defenseless backs" that are open to the world. These ways of communication give us some information which is useful for DMT in Japan (Sakiyama & Hirai, 1991).

American dmts who had several experiences providing sessions in Japan understand our body culture. Appel (2005) introduced the Japanese concept of the body through personal communications with Chaiklin and Koch as follows:

> Japan is open to the use of the body through such things as martial arts and an understanding of the body through meditation and other Buddhist influences. There are many rituals and ways of doing things and no one wants to be embarrassed in having [to] "lose face," but these are choices that people make. In Japan, the body has not been repressed. . . . The Japanese did not have the perspective that we inherited from the Puritans about the body being a source of sin. It is rather a source of pleasure and accomplishment, i.e., martial arts, noh, kabuki.
>
> (personal communication, 1999)

The body is not sinful but respected. Therefore, we can share spaces with others even while naked in *Onsen*. It is a great advantage and historical treasure.

In Japan, as is true of Eastern thought, the mind and body are seen as one. This idea, distinctly different from what has been perceived as a split in the West, gives the Japanese a particular openness to using dance as therapy (personal communication, 1999).

TRADITIONS OF IMAGERY FROM FOUR SEASONS

Other cultural images are closely related to climate and the school year. Japanese culture is full of traditional seasonal events related to nature. They are cherry blossoms in spring, *Bon dance* in summer, red leaves in autumn, and *Kotatsu*, a Japanese foot warmer with a quilt over it in winter. Figures 16.4–16.7 show us these typical images of each season.

The Japanese school year begins in April. Families celebrate the entrance to schools for children. The timing is just the same as with beautiful cherry blossoms, Sakura. In spring, images of cherry blossoms are sometimes utilized in psychiatric hospitals. I gave my sessions at a psychiatric hospital for the first time more than 30 years ago. It was located in a rural place in Nara prefecture, close to Mt. Yoshino,[6] famous for beautiful cherry blossoms and registered as a world heritage site in 2004. At that time, inpatients had the opportunity to go out and enjoy the beautiful cherry blossoms on an excursion (see Figure 16.4).

Many Japanese people enjoy *Bon dance* in summer. *Bon* (or *Obon*) is a Japanese Buddhist custom to honor the spirits of their ancestors in mid-August. *Bon dance* (or *Bon Odori*) is a style of dancing performed during *Bon* period. Originally a *Nenbutsu Odori* is to welcome the spirits of the dead. The style of celebration varies in each region. It was established more than 800 years ago.

In summer, all the patients and staff danced *Bon dance* together in the courtyard at the hospital. I didn't know the local *Bon dance*, so a patient who loved *Bon dance* taught me how to dance before the event. At the event, it didn't matter if we were a psychiatrist, nurse, or patient. Sharing the same time and space and enjoying the same rhythm and choreography allowed all the participants to feel that they belonged to the same community (see Figure 16.5).

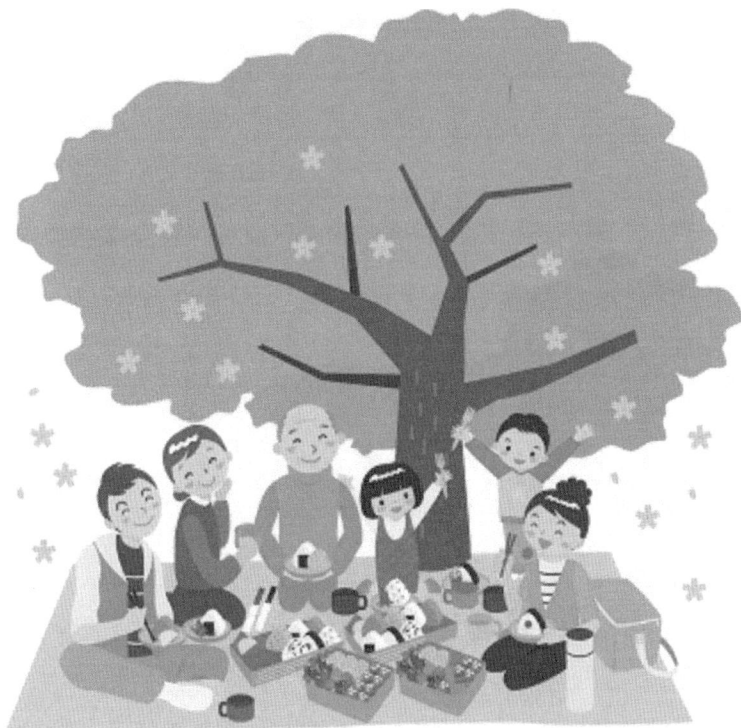

Figure 16.4 Family Enjoying Cherry Blossom Viewing Picnic in Spring

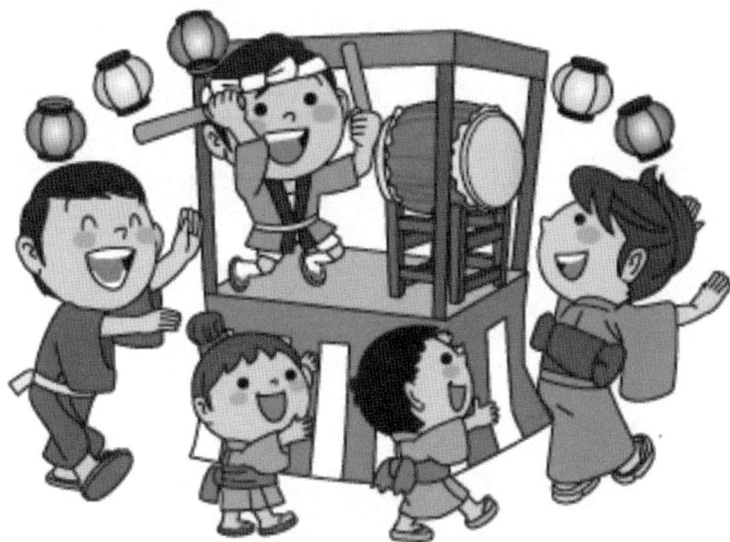

Figure 16.5 Family in *Bon Dance* in Summer

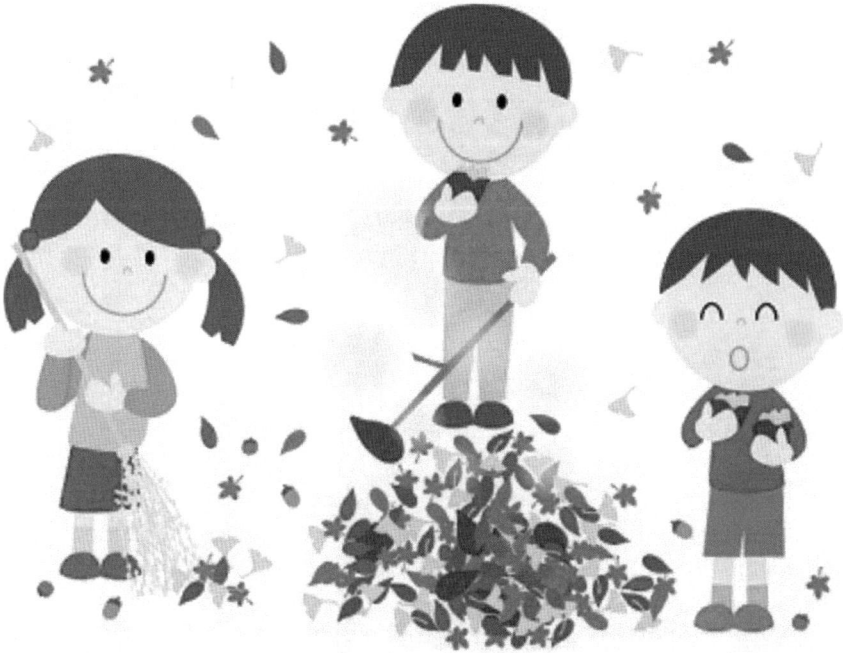

Figure 16.6 Children Baking Sweet Potatoes in Autumn

In autumn, Japanese people can enjoy beautiful red leaves just as they love cherry blossoms in spring. Children often play with red leaves. In kindergarten, occasionally many red leaves are gathered in order to bake sweet potatoes outside (see Figure 16.6).[7]

Japanese dmts apply these ideas in various ways in their sessions. These drawings of Japanese images are sometimes utilized for encouraging people to move. Here is an example of playing with red leaves presented by Yo Teruya in 1993 (Machida, 2012):

Teruya showed many red leaves which he picked up during an autumn morning. He asked participants to pick a favorite one and to examine it and then to feel it with eyes closed. After that he asked them to walk slowly with the leaf on one's hand and then, to exchange it with someone else and put the new red leaf on another body part . . .

Teruya always gave suggestions to all the participants such as this, to facilitate their movement exploration. These intimate images are appropriate for many Japanese who do not feel comfortable with free expression. These seasonal images come from experiences in daily life. They are concrete and easy to reflect upon. Japanese collective cultural images support clients' expressive movement and are a key to communicate with others in DMT sessions.

Kotatsu is a traditional heater in Japan. Each family shares this heater together and spends their own time as they choose. The heat from the bottom is quite comfortable so people often fall asleep (see Figure 16.7). When winter came, inpatients enjoyed the *Kotatsu* in the recreation room in the hospital. Some read books or newspapers, some enjoyed talking with friends, and others did nothing but just take a nap just as shown in the figure.

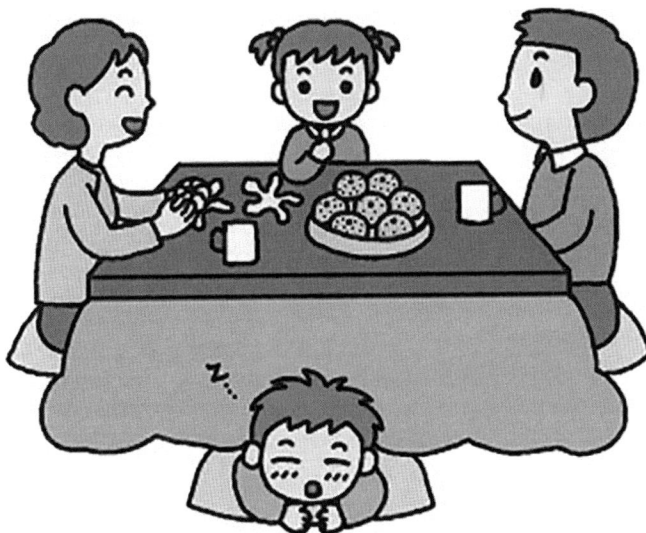

Figure 16.7 Family in *Kotatsu* in Winter

Many Japanese share the same images of the four seasons because these experiences exist in our daily life from childhood to adulthood. Such concrete images are easy to transfer to physical movement. People recall what they did in their past with others. The concrete suggestions by dmts often work well for clients without confidence to explore movement.

INFLUENCES OF WESTERN DANCE/MOVEMENT THERAPY

Kayoko Arakawa and Kyoko Jingu are both pioneer dmts in Japan who graduated from an approved course in the United States. Their explanations about DMT illustrate the importance of approaching one's inner world and the use of improvisation. Arakawa says that based on the idea that "the mind and the body are connected and interact with each other" through improvised movement, it is possible to reach deeper parts of the self, namely, through freely associative movements and images, iconic languages, physical sensations, and so on. .[8]

Ogiwara et al. (1993) describe their group sessions at psychiatric settings in Hasegawa Hospital. At one session, a dmt tried to reflect one client's fear through vocal sounds and then added movement related to fear. The other clients shared the same voice sound and movement. As the session progressed, angry feelings gradually came up. The therapist used imagery to help them verbalize and use movement to symbolize the feelings that arose and were thereby supported by this process. This example is similar to the Western DMT approach. An American dmt, Wapner had visited Hasegawa Hospital many times and taught these approaches that were adapted to Japanese clients. In Ogiwara's article, a dmt picked up an image from a client's gesture/posture to activate his movements. She suggested appropriate words that clarified the movement for that person. These sessions focus on the importance of free expression or improvisation, and after that their reflection through verbal sharing.

AN INFLUENCE OF BUTOH IN JAPANESE DANCE/MOVEMENT THERAPY AND *NOGUCHI TAISO*

Butoh is a worldwide famous post-WWII Japanese original dance form originated by Tatsumi Hijikata. (Jones, 1992)

With a number of collaborators, including Kazuo Ohno, Hijikata developed a style of choreographic extremism designed to startle the Japanese into recognizing unpalatable truths about their society. The name given to their movement was *Ankoku Butoh*, which can be translated as "dance of the dark soul." Butoh has since evolved a more flexible aesthetic that makes room for lyricism and even humor alongside grotesquerie (p. 236).

Hijikata and Ohno are the most famous Butoh dancers. Fraleigh and Nakamura (2006) analyze these Butoh dancers' ideas and spiritual darkness. In *Ankoku Butoh*, the dancer's body is always shrinking and full of tension. It sometimes looks like spastic paralysis or cerebral palsy. It has no lightness in Effort, no gentleness in precursors of Effort. It looks grotesque, just as we view a human's dark side (see Figures 16.8 and 16.9). Figures 16.8 and 16.9 show us these aspects.

Sometimes people confuse Butoh and *Ankoku Butoh* because of the historical background from Hijikata and Ohno. However, when we use Butoh in DMT in Japan, dmts don't focus on the dark side of human nature as *Ankoku Butoh* which is full of shrinking shape flow and High Intensity of Tension Flow Attributes.[9] Japanese dmts who use Butoh methods also don't focus on clients' inner worlds. Instead, they try to focus on the body itself for body awareness and relaxation.

Iwashita and Hashimoto (2004) named Iwashita's sessions as *Iwashita-Konan Method* after 14 years of practice. Table 16.1 describes a workshop given by Iwashita (see Figures 16.10 and 16.11). We can see how the session was divided, and many parts had specific suggestions to move. This means the session progressed step--by--step with easy movements and clear instructions. The most important thing is to be free little by little.

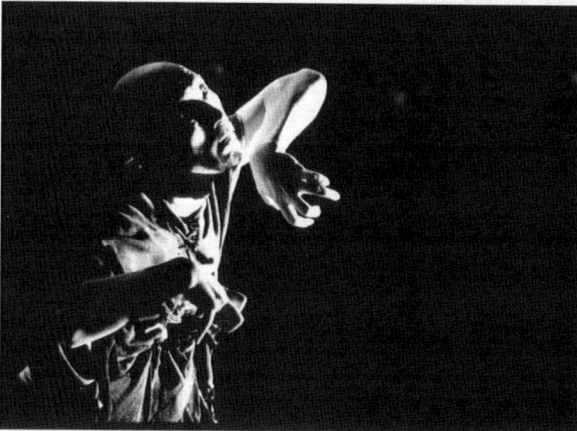

Figure 16.8 Performed by Itto Morita, *Goo Say Ten* Dancer

Photo: Katsumi Takahashi, 1999.

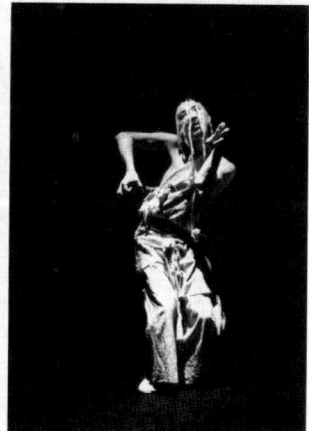

Figure 16.9 Performed by Itto Morita, *Goo Say Ten* Dancer

Photo: Katsumi Takahashi, 1999.

Table 16.1 Group Session Example of *Iwashita-Konan Method*

1	Salutation
2	Lying on the floor to find comfortable state
3	Turning over with a clap
4	Waking the upper body with a clap and smoothly lying again
5	Lying on the floor to find comfortable state again
6	Standing slowly
7	甩手 *suwaisho* from Tai Chi movement
8	Lying on the floor to find comfortable state again
9	Standing slowly again, walking around and making a various pose with a clap
10	Making some relations with someone by movement
11	Lying on the floor to find comfortable state
12	Tea break with masala tea
13	*Karada Hogushi* by oneself
14	Pair massage
15	Improvisation of pair posing
16	Improvisation of group posing
17	Interactive start-stop movement between two groups
18	Corporative wall posing with all the members
19	Lying on the floor to find comfortable state

Translated by Sakiyama from Iwashita and Hashimoto (2004)

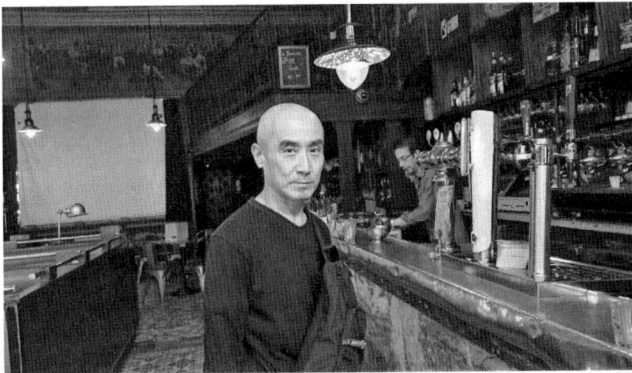

Figure 16.10 Toru Iwashita, *San Kai Juku* Dancer

Reiko Shiga, 2015.

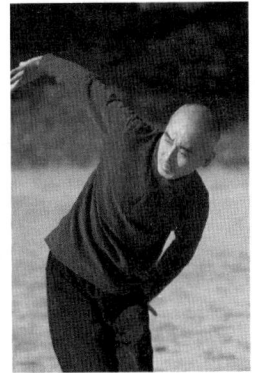

Figure 16.11 Toru Iwashita, *San Kai Juku* Dancer

Toshihiro Shimizu, 2012.

Kayo Mikami, who is a Butoh dancer and researcher, described the connection between Butoh and *Noguchi Taiso* (1998). *Noguchi Taiso* is an original gymnastic exercise created by Michizo Noguchi. Since the 1970s it has been the most well known of Japanese exercises for relaxation. It focuses on the body–mind connection, especially the importance of loosening rigidity and tension. Butoh dancer, psychologist, and researcher Toshiharu Kasai mentioned the connection of Butoh and *Noguchi Taiso* with Esposito (Esposito & Kasai, 2017) and also described the connection with Butoh as follows:

> The following are central principles in Noguchi taiso: a) It is important to pay attention to passively induced movements; b) the muscles should be regarded as sensors rather than effectors when controlling the body; c) the heightened sensory awareness leads to movements performed with the minimum amount of energy. Noguchi taiso shares with butoh a concern for enhancing bodily sensitivity and responsiveness through a focus on gravity, inertia, the principle of an equal and opposite reaction for each action and the use of imagery.
>
> (Esposito & Kasai, 2017)

Kasai has been working with psychiatric patients for a long time as a dmt. He focuses on the importance of slow and small movements. Kasai (2015) wrote:

> . . . small or slow movements are not always regarded as "non-expressive" but "significant" because most traditional indoor dances in Japan use delicate movements mainly because they tend to avoid rude movements and the resultant air turbulence and dusts in a small room with a tatami mat floor. The small and slow movements and peripheral vision exercise have been utilized for Japanese clients in dance movement therapy. They often induce a different and meditative mental state when they are extremely slow, as described "painfully slow" in Butoh dance.

He concludes that their effect enabled change in thinking and creativity. He often describes it as body-oriented psychotherapy (Kasai, 1999). He introduces his work in video clips with his colleague, Butoh dancer, Mika Takeuchi. They demonstrate seven kinds of movements which you can observe.[10] One of the famous movements is *Nenyoro*. It is body-waving movement for relaxation in pairs. One of the pair lies on his/her back. The other holds their partner's ankles softly and shakes them side to side on the floor. If one can loosen tension, the body waves smoothly from the ankles to the head. Kasai pointed out his concept for body relaxation by referring to *Nenyoro* as follows:

> A basic idea of *Noguchi Taiso* is that our body is not a skeleton with muscles and flesh on it, but a kind of water bag in which our bone and viscera are floating. He also places great emphasis on the significance of the weight of our body, saying "listen to the god of weight," and appreciates most efficient movements with minimum muscle tension and instant tension release. (p. 309)

> On the other hand, Ohnuma (2014) thought that restricted non-free movement is also good for her psychiatric patients as a challenge for new movement experiences. Butoh has various styles and movements created by each Butoh dancer. The idea of focusing within the body itself can be applied to DMT and other dmts often use some of the same concepts: The body has its own language and its movement describes how it feels.

CULTURAL SENSE OF BELONGINGNESS AND VERBAL SHARING

Japanese dmts, including me, have been learning DMT from the United States or European countries. They influence us as they do with other psychotherapeutic approaches. One Western idea is the importance of verbalization, especially from the DMT psychoanalytical approach, where the talk about what is felt after movement is quite central.

Though verbalization is important, it was hard for me to find a way to incorporate it when I started learning DMT in the United States. Sharing was done in pairs, small or large groups, and it was too much for me. Expressing my feelings in English was difficult, but beyond my language skills, I felt overwhelmed by speaking about unformed feelings. I needed more time to notice, feel, and hold it before verbalization.

However, in my many years of clinical experience in Japan, after a movement session, I often experience, together with the participants, a peaceful and quiet time of being together in the present moment. All is calm, and clients seem satisfied without verbalization. It is not meant to avoid confrontation against unsolved emotions which are hard to express. When the time for verbalization comes, we can share our feelings.

The experience of moving in a group and sharing space and time is sometimes therapeutic enough. Even if one doesn't express his/her feelings verbally, the other group members recognize, through the movement, both the emotions and the sense of belonging.

Sometimes we cannot verbalize our feelings in the same session, but we can hold on to them. We can express our feelings in drawing or painting or singing. We might use these kinds of creative ways of expression. We also need to feel empathy with other group members. This is important for a sense of belonging. Just to be there is OK. This is not only for clients who cannot express their feelings in words such as small children or people with intellectual disabilities, but for all of our clients. All dmts understand that as a profession, we need to wait for clients' words, and they should not be rushed. It is best for clients if their feelings come up like a spring and they speak of them naturally. Verbalization puts some meaningful words on emotions.

Psychoanalysis and psychotherapy originated in the Western world. There is some discomfort about verbalization among Japanese psychotherapists. Clinical psychologist, Tanaka (2011) summarizes her ideas on the importance of careful and cautious verbalization. She also insists that it is not necessary to replace experience with words and says experiences will naturally be condensed into words if necessary. Finally, she concludes that the experience may be enough. She also points out:

> In countries where multiple ethnic groups are gathered, they don't have a shared agreement or understanding. Therefore, they must build a consensual foundation to avoid ambiguity. Since Japan is a homogenous nation, it makes it more possible for the Japanese to figure out meanings from feeling and to understand through atmosphere than replacing feelings into apparently clear words. Our country has been putting more values on understanding ambiguous atmosphere than clear verbalization.
>
> (pp. 14–15 Translated by Sakiyama)

Jacobs (2005) pointed out some issues to consider:

> One root of the problem, I believe, stems from the historical fact that although Freud was a keen observer of nonverbal behavior in his patients, he did not elaborate on or develop this aspect of analytic work.
>
> (pp. 166–167)

Despite the clear evidence that nonverbal transactions are of the greatest importance in analysis, instruction in this aspect of clinical work remains minimal. In many institutes, in fact, it is nonexistent.

In the training analysis, too, the nonverbal dimension of communication is often overlooked. Many senior analysts, though highly experienced in other aspects of analysis, have had comparatively little experience in the decoding and interpretation of nonverbal data. Often uncomfortable in working with this mode of expression, they tend to slight it in favor of the more familiar and more congenial verbal material. As a consequence, communications that are conveyed through posture, gesture, movement, and other bodily means often go unrecognized (p. 185).

Stern (1995) criticized traditional psychoanalysis and the intellectual tendency against placing action at the center in understanding human behavior.

As Eugene Gendlin states the problem:

> Many people conclude that anything human *depends entirely* on language, concepts and history. Nothing of human animal seems to remain. As Foucault (1977) puts it: our erstwhile animal bodies were "utterly destroyed" by history. History and language seem utterly to determine what we will perceive, what we will distinguish as touched, seen or heard.
>
> (Gendlin, 1992, pp. 341–342)

Gendlin focused on the *Felt Sense* of the body and Stern worked with infants and caregivers whose primary way of communication is nonverbal. Dmts are always aware of body knowledge and have an understanding that we can wait patiently to "listen" to what our eloquent body will have to say.

Japanese say that they always live in relationships and the importance of *WA* (good harmony in human relationships) is often emphasized in social life. In a sense, Japanese have a tendency to compare with others in their belongingness at home, school, neighbor, society. People who need psychotherapy are troubled with or worried about such relationships around them. As a dmt with a Japanese cultural background, I always take special care not to force something in sessions. Japanese often make great effort not to give offense to others. Tactfulness and concern for the other group members are not required, but we tend to "read" the atmosphere and think what to do for *WA* in the groups to which they belong.

PERSONAL DEVELOPMENT AS KMP ANALYST INTEGRATING WESTERN AND JAPANESE INFLUENCES

The advantage of learning LMA (Laban Movement Analysis) or KMP (Kestenberg Movement Profile) is having a universal language with which to observe and manifest qualities of movement. KMP language in particular gives many possibilities to express tiny nuances so that we can understand the features of our clients' movements. Being able to share this information enables useful feedback for further approaches.

Japanese dmts who only study in Japan don't have many opportunities to study Laban or Kestenberg observational techniques. This doesn't mean Japanese dmts don't have words for expressing quality of movements. Instead, we make use of onomatopoeia.

The Japanese language has a lot of onomatopoeia, and it is natural to use it in our daily life. When we go to *Onsen*, we will be *hokkori*, which means warm and fluffy. When children tap their mothers' shoulders, the shoulder tapping rhythm is expressed by *tan ton tan ton* just like an old song. Even in *Noguchi Taiso*, *Nenyoro* is one famous movement for relaxation. *Ne* means lying on the floor and *nyoro* is an onomatopoeia which means curvy and soft movement like snakes. We can describe various qualities of movement by using onomatopoeias. To my advantage, I have two languages to express and describe movement.

SUMMARY

DMT is still developing in Japan. As ever, there shall always be four seasons in Japan. There is a bathing culture where many Japanese people share the same tub. DMT cannot ignore the view of our body culture which includes our spiritual selves and experiences fundamental to our development. Many of these characteristics may already be shared in other countries, as DMT always considers what the client requires and should keep in mind their cultural background.

It is hard to simplify Japanese culture. However, the author has tried to illustrate influences related to culture which would affect DMT in Japan. Attention to the Butoh method, touch and massage and further awareness of the body, bathing and the importance of the seasons are all considerations.

NOTES

1. Pasochan (2017) *Wanobutai Daisyugo Noh kanzeryu Shimai Kasanodan* [video file]. 2017 July 19. Retrieved from www.youtube.com/watch?v=tshF1DR5RO0.
2. Area mj (2019) *Futago Onikenbai Iwate Kizuna Matsuri in Miyako 2019* [video file]. 2019 July 15. Retrieved from www.youtube.com/watch?v=-E7hoISRSNo.
3. A. Kawata (2012) *Kokoro o Furuwasetsuzukeru ShikaOdori digest Michinoku Geinou Matsuri2012* [video file]. 2012 August 13. Retrieved from www.youtube.com/watch?v=rIE_RLWiSfI&t=98s.
4. Japan National Tourism Information; Things to do hot springs (Onsen). 2020 April 18. Retrieved from www.japan.travel/en/things-to-do/relaxation/onsen/.
5. maniwa menuet (2014) *Kata Tataki* song [video file]. 2014 April 17. Retrieved from www.youtube.com/watch?v=hMr80bx5X48.
6. Mt. Yoshino Tourist Association (2009) Cherry, autumn leaves and hydrangea of Mt. Yoshino. 2020 April 18. Retrieved from www.yoshinoyama-sakura.jp/english/.
7. Kibogaoka Bunka Koen (2015) 2015/12/23 Ochibade Yakiimo Zukuri[video file]. 2015 December 25. Retrieved from www.youtube.com/watch?v=cj8IRx-X2Iw.
8. Arakawa, K. Founder of Body Mind Health Center. Retrieved from http://bmh-c.org/ Sakiyama translated Arakawa's explanation of DMT in Japanese in her website into English.
   Jingu, K. Founder of DMTLab. Retrieved from https://dmtlab.net/. She also explains what DMT is in her website.
9. Tension Flow Attributes is one of technical terms of Kestenberg Movement Profile (KMP), consisting of six factors, such as Even Flow-Flow Adjustment, High Intensity-Low Intensity, Abruptness-Graduality
10. P. Esposito & T. Kasai (2017) Butoh Dance, Noguchi Taiso and Healing. 2020 April 18. Retrieved from http://relak.net/butoh_us/paola_book2015/.

REFERENCES

Appel, C. (2005). International growth of Dance Movement Therapy. In F. J. Levy (Ed.), *Dance Movement Therapy: A healing art* (Rev. ed., pp. 263–272). Virginia: American Alliance for Health, Physical Education, Recreation and Dance.

Ban, T. (1981). Ancient Japanese ritual dancing and principle of symmetry and autogenic psychodrama. *Japanese Bulletin of Arts Therapy*, 12, 53–57.

Broderick, S., & Moore, W. (2010). *Japanese traditions rice cakes, cherry blossoms and matsuri a year of seasonal Japanese festivities*. Vermont: Tuttle Publishing.

Esposito, P., & Kasai, T. (2017). Butoh Dance, Noguchi Taiso, and Healing. In V. Karkou, S. Oliver, & S. Lycouris (Eds.), *Oxford handbook of dance and wellbeing* (pp. 255–272). New York: Oxford University Press.

Foucault, M. (1977). *Discipline and punish: The birth of the prison* (A. Sheridan, Trans.). New York: Pantheon Books. (Originally published in 1975, French version, *Surveiller et Punir-nassance de La Prison*. Paris: Éditions Gallimard.)

Fraleigh, S., & Nakamura, T. (2006). *Hijikata Tatsumi and Ohno Kazuo* (Routledge Performance Practitioners). New York and London: Routledge.

Gendlin, E. T. (1992). The primacy of the body, not the primacy of perception. *Man and World*, 25, 341–353.

Hauerback, O. H. (1910). *Historic sheet music collection359*. Digital Commons @ Connecticut College. Retrieved from https://digitalcommons.conncoll.edu/sheetmusic/359

Hirai, T., & Sakiyama, Y. (2016, August). *Dancing moving images in nature-focusing on Japanese body culture.* Paper presented at the 20th International Congress for Analytic Psychology. Retrieved from https://iaap.org/wp-content/uploads/2019/01/images-and-texts-IAAP-2016-Kyoto-Pre-Congress-Compendium-Workshop-Authentic-Movement-May-31th-2018-Unlocked.pdf

Iwashita, T., & Hashimoto, M. (2004). Seishinbyouin niokeru dance therapy no kokoromi [A trial of dance therapy in psychiatric hospital in Japanese title]. In M. Iimori & S. Machida (Eds.), *Dance therapy* (pp. 11–33). Tokyo: Iwasakigakujutsu syuppansya.

Jacobs, T. J. (2005). Discussion of forms of intersubjectivity in infant research and adult treatment. In B. Beebe, S. Knoblaunch, J. Rustin, & D. Sorter (Eds.), *Forms of intersubjectivity in infant research and adult treatment* (pp. 165–189). New York: Other Press Inc.

Jones, G. (1992). *Dancing the pleasure, power, and art of movement.* New York: Abrams.

Kasai, T. (1999). A Butoh Dance Method for psychosomatic exploration. *Memoirs of Hokkaido Institute of Technology, 27,* 309–316.

Kasai, T. (2015, September). *Significance of slow and small movements in Japanese Dance Therapy.* Paper presented at the 13th European Consortium for Arts Therapies in Education.

Kitajima, J. (2012). Kyoikugenba niokeru dance therapy [Dance/Movement Therapy in educational settings in Japanese title]. In Y. Ohnuma, Y. Sakiyama, S. Machida, & Y. Matsubara (Eds.), *Dance Therapy no riron to jissen karada to kokoro eno healing art* [Theory & practice of dance therapy healing art for body & mind in Japanese title] (pp. 285–298). Tokyo: The earth kyoikushinsya.

Machida, S. (1999). Nihon niokeru dance therapy no 30 nen [30 years of dance therapy in Japan in Japanese title]. *Japanese Bulletin of Arts Therapy, 30*(1), 24–32.

Machida, S. (2012). Dance Therapy no Gaiyou, Teruya Yo no "Watashi no kobeya" [Outline of dance therapy My Cubicle by Yo Teruya in Japanese title]. In Y. Ohnuma, Y. Sakiyama, S. Machida, & Y. Matsubara (Eds.), *Dance Therapy no riron to jissen karada to kokoro eno healing art* [Theory & practice of dance therapy healing art for body & mind in Japanese title] (pp. 20–21, 344–349). Tokyo: The earth kyoikushinsya.

Merry, D. M. (2013). More than a bath: An examination of Japanese Bathing Culture. *Claremont Colleges Senior Theses,* Paper665. Retrieved from https://scholarship.claremont.edu/cgi/viewcontent.cgi?article=1593&context=cmc_theses

Mikami, K. (1998). Noguchi Taiso no shakaiteki eikyo—Butoh group wo chushin ni- [Social effect of Noguchi Gymnastics-Focusing Butoh Group in Japanese title]. *Journal of Health, Physical Education and Recreation, 48*(2), 134–138.

Momonoi, F., & Matsubara, T. (1985). Dance therapy at a private psychiatric hospital. *The Official Journal of the Japan Association of Group Psychotherapy, 1*(2), 203–208.

Nogawa, T., & Murai, Y. (1979). The use of Noh Play in Art Therapy: An attempt of therapeutic approach to chronic schizophrenics by the use of Mai(dance) training. *Japanese Bulletin of Arts Therapy, 10,* 7–12.

Ogiwara, M., Hatanaka, W., Komori, C., Sawamura, K., Matsuo, T., Kouda, M., & Akiyama, T. (1993). Technique and application of group Dance Movement Therapy. *The Official Journal of the Japan Association of Group Psychotherapy, 9*(2), 136–140.

Ohnuma, Y. (2012). Seishinkaryoiki niokeru kojinheno dance therapy [Individual dance therapy in psychiatric fields]. In Y. Ohnuma, Y. Sakiyama, S. Machida, & Y. Matsubara (Eds.), *Dance Therapy no riron to jissen karada to kokoro eno healing art* [Theory & practice of dance therapy healing art for body & mind in Japanese title] (pp. 227–240). Tokyo: The earth kyoikushinsya.

Ohnuma, Y. (2014). A study on release of the mind and body energy by the Butoh dance. *Japanese Journal of Dance Therapy, 8*(1), 31–41.

Sakata, S., & Shimoyama, T. (1970). A trial of dance therapy. *Japanese Bulletin of Arts Therapy, 2,* 39–44.

Sakiyama, Y. (2000). Meaning of the integration of body and mind in dance therapy: As a conceptual pilot study for analysis, evaluation and diagnosis of movement. *Japanese Journal of Dance Therapy, 1*(1), 22–29.

Sakiyama, Y., & Hirai, T. (1991). A study on Dance/Movement Therapy and Japanese body communication: Through defenseless back with the mentally handicapped. *Japanese Bulletin of Arts Therapy, 22*(1), 124–130.

Sakiyama, Y., & Hirai, T. (1997). A study on touching in Dance/Movement Therapy. *Japanese Bulletin of Arts Therapy, 28*(1), 113–120.

Sakiyama, Y., & Koch, N. (2003). Touch in dance therapy in Japan. *American Journal of Dance Therapy, 25*(2), 79–95.

Stern, D. N. (1995). *The motherhood constellation: A unified view of parent—infant psychotherapy.* New York: Basic Books.

Tanaka, C. (2011). *Play Therapy eno tebiki: Kokoro no aya wo douyomitoruka* [Guide to play therapy: How to read & understand Japanese mental fabric in Japanese title]. Tokyo: Nihon Hyoronsya.

CHAPTER 17

DANCE MOVEMENT THERAPY AND FLAMENCO
Relationships through Traditional Rhythms

Elena Cristóbal Linares

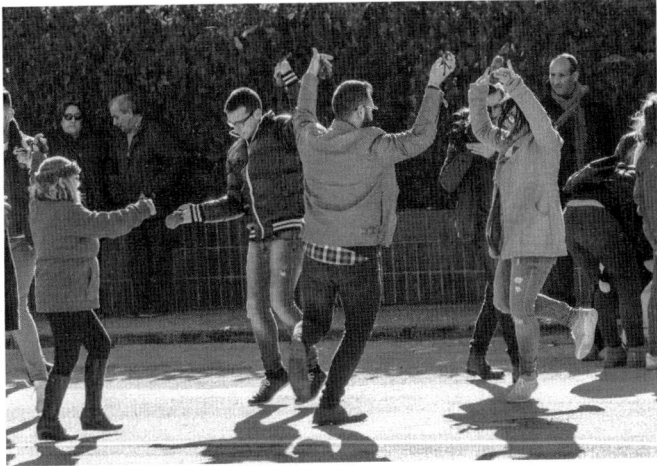

Image 17.1 Flamenco in the community

INTRODUCTION

This chapter will:

1. Introduce to the reader an experience of Dance Movement Therapy (DMT) in which flamenco was part of the methodology.
2. Delimit the opportunities that flamenco can provide for people with severe mental disorders who have difficulties with introspection and a limited and/or distorted knowledge of their bodies.
3. Present an empirical study that collected objective measures of the effectiveness of a treatment integrating flamenco into DMT.

ASPECTS OF FLAMENCO THAT CONTRIBUTE TO THE HEALTH OF PEOPLE WITH SEVERE MENTAL DISORDERS

Flamenco reflects all the vital experiences and the emotions of a people through its songs, touches and dance, from passion to death, hence its cathartic function. It has an enormous wealth of musical forms and rhythms and is a powerful channel of emotional expression, so it can be used as a tool in social intervention developed through art.

(Grötsch, 2012)

While recognized throughout the world as a dance of the Iberian Peninsula, flamenco can be adapted to the possibilities, tastes, abilities, and preferences of individuals and groups to meet their situation and needs as they can work from the creation of rhythms or melodies with different instruments (including the palms of hands), lyrics, dances, and use of accessories (fans, flowers, shawls, handkerchiefs, and so on). The history of a people and the events that took place around the formation of flamenco—art, photography, architecture, poetry—can also be implemented in DMT.

In this chapter I will present some aspects of flamenco that align to principles of Dance Movement Therapy (DMT) as outlined by the pioneer Marian Chace. It will be shown how these aspects of flamenco can contribute to the treatment of people with severe mental disorders. Although presented separately, the different aspects interact simultaneously.[1]

Expression and Communication

Chace's foundational concept is that dance is communication. Since flamenco is a dance genre that privileges expression of feeling and communication, this form is well suited for use in DMT. It is this aspect that has become basic for the application of flamenco in our workshop experience. It has allowed us to use, in a dynamic and relational way, the different resources of flamenco art, thereby tuning the DMT workshop to the needs and circumstances of those who attend it.

Flamenco is part of a ritual that, along with singing, guitars, and percussion instruments, occupies circular spaces to facilitate intercommunication, coexistence between groups, mutual learning, the exchange of roles, and so on. It is capable of giving structure to a space, providing it with order and also with timing, rhythm, and silence (Cruces Roldán, 2002a). When flamenco is used within a group model, it enables the sharing of experiences and knowing of other people directly, allowing participants to acquire a more realistic experience of themselves and the others in the group (González de Chávez, 2008).

The basic structure of flamenco dancing allows for three main elements of flamenco art—dance, song, and guitar—to be integrated in a harmonious way. Through this structure, there is communication in the group. Similarly, in DMT, there are also fundamental elements that provide structure: rhythm, as a special way of connecting movement in space, time, music, as well as the body in relation to weight and gravity. In the structured space of DMT, the person who dances realizes that their dance is understood up by the therapist (Fischman, 2008).

This communication between dancer and therapist in DMT gives further credence to the use of flamenco in Dance Movement Therapy. Flamenco allows for the interaction between individuality and group experience. The participants in a group are encouraged to be aware of their sensations and emotions in the present moment. Further, while its execution is individual, flamenco is also a collective art that acquires meaning through the forms of sociability in which it is inserted (i.e., parties, meetings, and other social events). During these social events, all present are participants. Thus, when integrated into DMT, the communicative aspect of flamenco laid onto the structured space can enable therapeutic processes to be carried out.

Time and Rhythm

Time is fundamental in flamenco—an art full of rhythm, tempo, and speed. The rhythm is the arrangement of musical time and indicates, through a numerical expression, the sequence in which the accent of a melody falls. The tempo is the metric entity composed of several units of time that are organized in groups in which there is a contrast between stressed and unstressed parts. In flamenco music, accents are especially important since the metrics of the different flamenco styles or musical forms (palos) rest on those accents, which gives them their characteristic rhythm. The regularity of these accents is one way to indicate the corresponding palo.

Time in flamenco includes the time within oneself, in the world, the natural succession of natural events. The emphasis on time is rooted in the history of the dance, for flamenco resulted from historical processes in continuous formation, change, and consolidation. The notion of temporality, as a result of experiences and the behavioral expression of it, becomes a marker for organization of the self. Temporality, then, becomes important not only to individual development but also to the field studying and helping those with mental disorders. Concepts, such as impulsivity, passivity, or tolerance of frustration, are determined by a temporal aspect that marks the appropriateness of a behavior (García, 2010).

In psychosis, a person is broken and their story is interrupted. It is the job of therapists to help an individual rebuild it in some way. During this time, a person has to reinvent their self to be able to live. Rhythm, a fundamental component in the temporal aspect of dance and music, is a vital element that awakens in every human when in the womb and accompanies them throughout life in the heartbeat, in the circulation of blood, in breathing, in marching, and in conversation.

The innate predisposition towards rhythm is one of the aspects that allows for empathizing and connecting with others, speaking, walking, dancing, or making love. However, urban life and the processes of mechanization force people to adapt, in many cases, to external rhythms opposed to their internal ones (Reca, 2007). To facilitate the recovery of rhythmic experience, diverse strategies exist. For example, activating the voice by singing or reciting song lyrics while listening to music and dancing. These strategies favor the integration of movement, music, and words, which helps to express emotions, to release tension, and to focus a person or group through external rhythms (recorded music and instruments) and/or internal rhythms (breathing, heartbeat, voice). All of this helps the breathing to be deeper and improve the body-mind connection (Fischman, 2008).

In flamenco, following the beat with the feet, clapping, or using another part of the body as an instrument helps to focus attention on the rhythmic structure and allows an individual to become more aware of their self. Emotions become conscious and are communicated through shared, symbolic rhythmic action (Chace, 1975).

Flamenco within DMT, then, has an effective integrating capacity. In the sessions, rhythm can be used as a communicative force between therapist and patient and among patients. An example of this can be found in the following quote:

> In their daily life Gypsies take the different rhythms of flamenco, manifesting them with their hands, feet or sounds, until the moment comes when their breathing becomes one with the rhythm. Thus their actions are transformed into small dances. By keeping the rhythm of their lives, they reach a state of connection with their being, where everything is and turns in harmony with nature, "a long sustained movement leads to trance."
>
> (Garaudy, 1987)

Body Action and Body Awareness, Movement, and Dance

Our body image, the mental representation of the body, is formed through the integration of information coming from the different sensory modalities, the history of interpersonal relationships, and the influences of the environment/culture. Body image is fundamental for the development of the concept of oneself. People with psychosis have limited and distorted knowledge of their bodies. The stormy and apprehensive self can often be observed as these individuals move with great tension, with a limited range of movement variation, and have a reduced use of space. Often, their posture is rigid and passive, lacking in relaxation (López, 2014). They may make unnecessary, jerky movements due to the secondary effects of neuroleptics, such as agitations, strange hand gestures, or rigid postures.

Another key aspect of individuals dealing with psychosis is how the sensory aspect affects body image. Usually this information is congruent, and our brain combines it effectively. That integration makes us perceive a coherent world and ourselves in it. Psychosis involves a certain disorder in the field of the senses that leads the person suffering from it to have a distorted images of things, including their self. When the information is received in an uncoupled way between some senses and others, the brain warns that an incongruence is taking place, which, at least, produces a sensation of strangeness. In people with psychosis, there are situations in which there is a lack of concordance between the senses, that is, they may hear something that does not match up with what they see.

An important step to redefine body image is in the kinesthetic identification of the different parts of the body, its joints, and the constructive use of the muscles—an aspect absent in most people with psychotic disorders. An improvement in these individuals' situation may come from identifying body parts and being aware of how they use or used them. In DMT integrating flamenco, to establish body boundaries—that is, where the body ends and where another's begins—some simple experiences of contact with one's own body are proposed, such as stroking, applauding, clapping, and stomping. Working with weight (moving, grounding) and the use of forward and backward movements, push and stretch, join and separate help to establish awareness of those limits through moving in and being aware of space.[2]

DMT workshops using flamenco among people with severe mental disorders have proven effective in helping them to establish a sense of weight since, when striking the feet on the ground in a progressive way, one is able to feel presence, rootedness, connection with the ground (grounding) and with the "here and now." In this movement, thinking ceases and one can connect with what is happening, with reality. While this population may have trouble concentrating on the sequence of movements, on both feet and palms, being part of the group as one in the production of the rhythm is a difficult, but highly rewarding, task.

For example, in some of our sessions, the break from isolation to group integration was easily observable. Some participants began the sessions disconnected from the group as if they weren't there. Sessions would begin with a simple rhythm and synchronous handclapping. The structured sound produced by this body action/dance then facilitated connections between the others in the "here and now." After several minutes, those who had isolated themselves would yawn and stretch, establish visual eye contact, and even greet others in the group.

In flamenco, the feet are fundamental because of the importance allotted in this dance to keeping beat, which contributes to its energetic aspect and makes it so appealing. "The tap of the foot" is perhaps the most insistent and particular aspect of flamenco dance and requires having the legs bent, which gives it a terrestrial and undulating sense (Cruces Roldán, 2012b).

The upper part of the body moves freely with the melody and lower part with the rhythm (Lowen, 2006). Earth provides support, a ground to be experienced and moved on, as through gravity Earth is literally our support and flamenco becomes Earth. Simple and adequate movements to stimulate the experience of contact with the ground and the group are proposed by the therapist and prove useful in DMT groups: pelvis, legs, feet pressing the floor according to the beat and the rhythm.

At a certain stage, introducing castanets to the DMT integrated with flamenco sessions adds an element of concentration and group cohesion. Using castanets requires unusual gestures that need much effort of coordination but achieve the isolated movements of the fingers and strengthen the torso, specifically the pectoral, dorsal, forearm, and solar plexus. Thus, the addition invites innovation to the posture.

These creative and integrating experiences help participants become aware of their body and their potential and reinforces their personal identity within the group. Being aware of how we move, how much space we use, and the personal and social distance we need are fundamental aspects in DMT interventions. As participants grow in understanding and gather insight, they are more prepared to establish contact with others and simultaneously acquire new information about the self.

The use of images in DMT provides a means through which a patient can remember, create, and reexperience. Some problems can be overcome at a purely symbolic level. A Dance Movement therapist accepts the symbolic meanings of the patient. Both the patient with a severe mental disorder and the dancer use symbolic body actions to communicate emotions and ideas. While the dancer can voluntarily choose bizarre and exaggerated postures to communicate with the public, the patient's gestures communicate their internal emotions and convey feelings that cannot be verbalized. The dance therapist not only reacts to the symbolic expressions but also creates new symbolic interactions with the patient.

Thus, flamenco can be particularly useful toward this end goal. For example, if a patient feels anger, then the dance therapist may suggest that they stomp on the ground (*zapateo*) as if they could drill into it with their feet. This strong movement may then begin to unearth further feelings of anger or hostility or possibly evoke further memories.

In summary, DMT offers patients with severe mental disorders the possibility to express, reflect, and respond to emotional material. Put another way, to the extent that the subject shares individual emotions, the possibility of a feeling of belonging and being recognized is strengthened within a DMT group (Capello, 2008). When flamenco is integrated into DMT, it adds further benefits by offering the possibility of self-control, strengthening listening abilities, improving concentration and attention, and increasing organization of cognitive capacity. It can encourage verbal and nonverbal interaction and allows patients the experience of singularity (González de Chávez, 2008).

SPECIFIC DMT GROUPS INTEGRATING FLAMENCO IN TENERIFE, CANARY ISLANDS, SPAIN

Context

The following discussion is based on Dance Movement Therapy workshops carried out in the Canary Islands, specifically the Island's Plan of Psychosocial Rehabilitation for people with Severe Mental Disorder in Tenerife, Spain. One of the objectives of the DMT workshops was the rehabilitation of psychic functions, physical health, interpersonal relationships, performance of roles, and coexistence in a normalized environment. A set of complementary resources was implemented to cover the needs of the patients and their family members.

Within this context, there are two kinds of housing solutions. The first is protected dwellings, or "sheltered apartments," that are distributed throughout the territory of the island to facilitate patients' accessibility and contact with their families. Patients with less deterioration live there and are supervised by a multidisciplinary team. The author worked there with the support of a nongovernmental organization (NGO). The second housing solution is the "miniresidences" where treatment is more personalized. It is in the miniresidences that persons with greater cognitive deterioration live.

DMT was provided to both populations, and during the sessions, flamenco dynamics were used as a socio-affective experience that facilitated body expression.

Patients/Groups

For the intervention integrating DMT and flamenco, there was a total of 42 participants with severe mental disorders who belonged to the Insular Plan of Psychosocial Rehabilitation of Tenerife, Spain. The control group was created with the 37 persons who participated in the workshop of Occupational Therapy for Activities of Daily Living (ADL).

In the DMT workshops, participants were distributed among four groups in the miniresidences and one group in the sheltered apartments. In the latter, patients came to the space where the DMT sessions were held and offered by a town hall. With the other groups, the sessions were held in a structured space created in the same center (the miniresidences) where the patients lived. Participants signed a consent form at the beginning of the intervention.

The members in the DMT workshops presented differences in levels of cognitive deterioration, little autonomy, and little verbal and nonverbal interaction; they also had tendencies to social isolation. The sessions were adapted to the patients' characteristics. The more independent patients and groups tended to make more use of the space, while the more deteriorated preferred to stay seated and responded better to structured sessions.

We offered those in the miniresidences groups of ten participants, realizing that dropouts could occur at any time, and we also formed an open group in which patients were free to attend or not. On average, each group was comprised of seven to eight participants with the number varying by day.

For the persons coming from the sheltered apartments, a setting of a closed group with an average of seven participants that ran for a three-month period was chosen. After a three-month period, an assessment of the process was made since the DMT offer was in high demand.

All group sessions took place twice a week for a duration of 45 minutes per session. We were clear that the work focused on the person who moved, not the disease or the symptom, but this does not mean that we did not know the characteristics of each individual's pathology.

METHODOLOGY

The therapeutic objectives were established after evaluating the characteristics of the users. The majority were found to have a lack of body-mind integration, an absence of corporal limits, and a lack of gestural unity (twisted, sporadic, irregular movements, and so on). Once these baselines were established, the therapeutic goals were established. Examples of thera-peutic goals include:

- To promote the integration of the body and reinforce the real sense of the body image of each participant. That they were able to recognize it, feel it, and differen-tiate it from the environment.
- To promote trying different movement patterns since having more freedom to move could foster autonomy and experience of other ways of being (Wengrower, 2008).
- To assist in the control of impulsive behavior and stereotypes.

After several sessions of DMT, a movement profile of each user was generated that gave us information about the body, the movement, the coordination, the use of rhythm, and rela-tional aspects like proximity, visual contact, and presence towards the group, the therapist, and the accessories (see the Appendix).

Development of the Groups

During the development of the sessions, it was very important to create a ritual that would be repeated each time. We started with some rhythmic songs from the collections of Solo Compás, Rumba de los Chichos ("Libre quiero ser") and Tangos de Camarón ("Como el agua"). The musical activity diminished the patients' negative symptoms and improved their interpersonal contact, while the compass of flamenco helped them to find structure and stay calm (López, 2014).

Most of the DMT flamenco-based interventions were carried out in the free move-ment segment within the sessions where there were improvisations of flamenco movements accompanied by the recorded music of Camarón, Solo Compás, and Enrique Morente. On some occasions, after a closing verbalization, the group improvised, moving to various flamenco rhythms, like tangos, soleá, rumba, and so on, by forming a "flamenco group" where each individual entered into the center of the group and danced. Reinforcing "jaleos" were used, that is, each person who entered the center of the group received from the other patients a word to bolster their self-esteem, such as "Ole!," "You are beautiful!," "How brave you are!," and "You are so worthy!"

Jaleos are part of the flamenco culture; participants encourage and celebrate the dance of each one in the group's center. There are infinite expressions in jaleos, which are said following the beat and express respect for the performance. The jaleos were so effective that in one of the groups it was used as a farewell ritual for almost a year of therapy. This was done with the aim of helping the process of internalization and to verbally share moments that had happened in the round of "jaleos." In these improvisations, the movement patterns were extended. We began to realize how important it was for the identity and self-esteem of the participants that they receive a compliment, a show of affection, admiration, and so on.

The work was progressive, moving from a simpler to an advanced use of space, body, and timing-rhythm. Here is the progression we followed:

- Perform exercises to basic flamenco rhythms (clapping, foot tapping on the floor, beat-palm combination, and so on) toward the creation of a common rhythm (group cohesion).
- Perform exercises to everyday and easily identifiable rhythms (ticking of the clock, the waves of the sea, a dripping tap, the ring of a telephone, and so on).

- Perform improvisation exercises of rhythms with music.
- Introduce some flamenco beats and rhythms (tangos, soleá, bulerías, and so on).
- Move and improvise with these rhythms as a reference.

On some occasions, games were introduced to stimulate expression, communication, and mitigate the patients' tendency to self-absorption. The most cognitively impaired patients had more problems creating cohesion and recognizing themselves as part of a group. In this case, it was through the game that they managed to stay attentive and focused. They played to reproduce sounds or sang, imitated others, made faces, and so on and thus released tensions. Some of the games offered were change of expression of the face and body, pass the ball between the group members, mirror the movements of a partner and exaggerate them, or even playing pretend, such as pretending that one individual was a sculptor and another a piece of clay.

Other interventions introduced were based on the integration of color and emotion and the clock wheel, which is commonly used in the teaching of flamenco.

Color and Emotion

Colors are able to stimulate joy or sadness, they can make us feel energetic or relaxed, they favor sensations of cold or heat, and they make us perceive order or disorder. Although the perception of color is an individual and subjective process, cultural factors also influence how color affects us. For example, some colors are identified with the masculine and with the feminine, and others with the romantic, but this differs by culture (Heller, 2004). What follows are some associations made about color in the flamenco-based DMT interventions:

- Patients were told to associate each emotion with a color (red-passion, blue-loyalty, black-sadness, orange-joy) which is then materially shown through a colored handkerchief or fabric. In this game, everybody would choose a handkerchief according to its color and their personal association with the mood they felt, and then they improvised flamenco steps alone or interacted with one another. At the end of the session there was a verbal sharing of the experience.
- In another game, patients were told to associate a color with a flamenco rhythm (palo) (red-passion, blue-loyalty, black-sadness, orange-joy).
- A third activity was pretending to "paint colors on the canvas" as a metaphor that involved the creation of choreographies that start from within the group itself.

There were differences between groups and between individuals in the capability to engage in imagination and symbolization. For example, one of the miniresidence groups that worked very well with the rhythm was unable to get out of the everyday, the common, and demanded a rigid structure and containment. For that reason, in the free movement segment of the sessions there was hardly connection or participation. Therefore for them, verbalizing aloud in unison a rhythm by soleá or counting the numbers that represented time was much more satisfying than working in free movement.

Clock-Wheel for Learning the Compass by Soleá

The group with the least cognitive impairment learned through this mnemonic rule to recognize the rhythm and measure of the flamenco palos soleá and bulería. They first learned

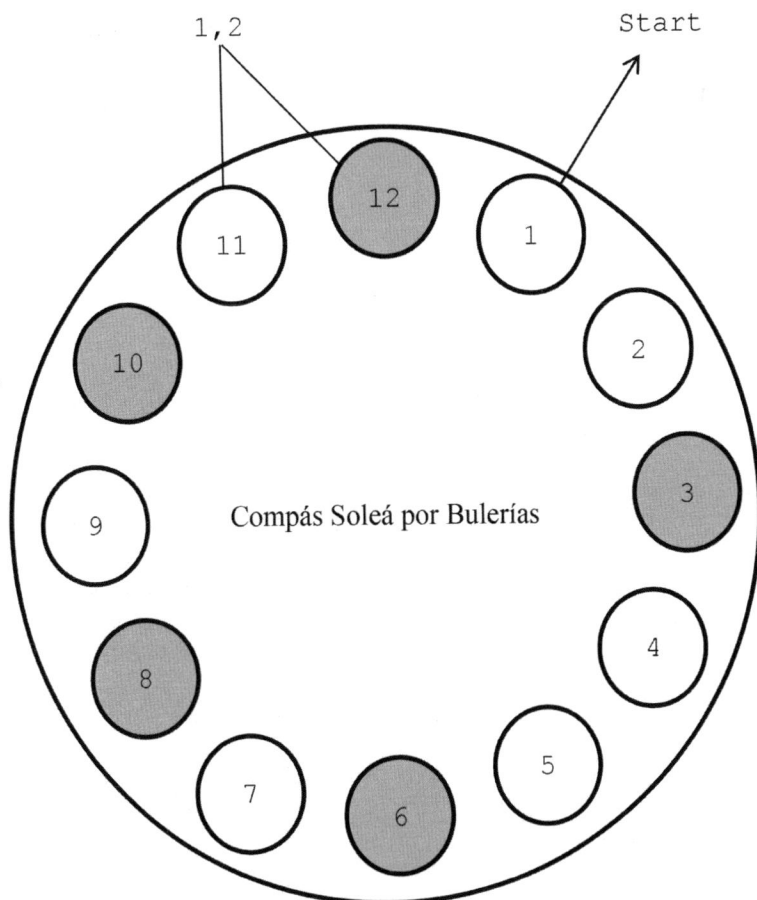

Image 17.2 Clock-Wheel for Learning the Rhythm for *Soleá* by *Bulerías*

through the word, naming in unison each number and time, and progressively added palms with hands and feet. In time, the participants marked with the voice and palms the 12-beat time in *soleá* and were even able to memorize it (Image 17.2).

Process

After a period of approximately six months, users recognized the purpose of the DMT groups and the space where the sessions were held as well as established trust with the therapist and the other participants. In all the groups, the movement patterns were widened and self-absorption diminished, thus increasing group interactions. The group setting allowed each user the opportunity to receive from the other participants a recognition and feedback on their actions.

After six months, the first physical interactions and emotional expressions began to appear: touching hands, hugging, crying. During this time, the patients began to recognize the effects of the disease on themselves and others. They began to have expand movement capacity. This differed from how they had started with rigid bodies and mechanical movements that gave the feeling of being protected by a shield, containing emotions inside. Flamenco requires work on posture, and it is effective when the patient acquires greater body awareness and therefore greater autonomy. The postural change, slow and progressive, made people need more space in the sessions, and in some groups, this was an obstacle in terms of the workplace but it was a reward to be able to observe these bodies "larger" and exhibiting more autonomy.

Using Marian Chace's DMT model as a reference, we structured the sessions into different phases. It was in the central part of the session where different types of dynamics were carried out. Depending on the group or the circumstances, this middle section was free or guided and based on different creative proposals (plastic, musical, body, moving, and so on). On some occasions, the initial proposal led to other spontaneous actions generated by the participants, and it was therefore very important to observe carefully and assess their interventions and motivate their autonomy.

In this phase, the majority of the flamenco dynamics took place: improvisations, use of castanets, photo visualization of flamenco artists (i.e., Carmen Amaya, Camarón de la Isla, Paco de Lucía) so that patients could know about and learn from these inspirational figures. To know and recognize the flamenco compass, we clapped with our hands, feet stamping against the ground, and used a metronome. Thus, the memory capacity was also enhanced by repeating a sound or a movement proposed by each one of the members of the group and joining them all in a wheel with greater or lesser speed, thus producing an improvement in coordination and perception of space. Using flamenco art at specific times enriched the sessions because of the great variety of resources it has.

Evaluation Study

In the following sections we shall discuss the evaluations carried out to check if the DMT flamenco intervention affected the interaction and cohesion of the groups.

The objective of the study was to verify the effect of a DMT treatment using flamenco on the interaction behaviors of the participants over a two-year duration. More specifically, we compared the level of verbal and nonverbal interaction that occurs spontaneously in the DMT group versus a control group that participated in an occupational workshop. The global level of interaction was compared between both groups.

For the study, a double-blind methodology was used. Videos were recorded in situations of spontaneous interaction before beginning a session of the different therapies in which the patients participated. Patients did not know that they were being observed in their interactions, nor did the observers have information that the people they were observing were mental health patients, much less that they belonged to different treatment groups.

Method and Procedure

A video recording of three minutes was taken with each one of the DMT groups and the control groups while they waited for the beginning of a session. They were unaware they were being filmed and did not receive specific instructions on what to do. The only instruction they received was that they should wait in the space at the beginning of the session. The objective of this instruction was that the possible interactions produced would be spontaneous and not induced by the researchers, and that differences between both groups would not be established. During this time, no researchers, therapists, or center staff were present.

Table 17.1 Register Sheet of Interaction Behaviors During Videos

Behavior Record Sheet—Interaction
Age: _____ Gender:_____
Verbal interaction level
nothing 0-1-2-3-4-5 a lot
Nonverbal interaction level
nothing 0-1-2-3-4-5 a lot
Global interaction level
nothing 0-1-2-3-4-5 a lot

One three-minute video of a DMT group and another three-minute video of the control group were chosen at random to be evaluated by observers. In the instructions given, observers were asked to assess the participants' levels of interaction in each video in three categories: verbal, nonverbal, and global or general interaction. Evaluators indicated their observations on a Likert scale of six levels (0–5) in which the 0 was labeled as "no interaction" and 5 as "a lot of interaction."

The DMT group in the video consisted of five patients (one woman, four men, ages 35–55), and the video of the control group consisted of eight patients (five women, three men, ages 34–59). Evaluators were either fourth-year psychology students ($n = 35$) or sixth-year medicine students ($n = 17$). The total sample of observers ($n = 52$) had an average age of 23 years (the age range was from 21 to 56 years), and 77% of the sample were women.

The videos were projected without sound, so that both verbal and nonverbal interaction could be evaluated from exclusively visual information. Each observer filled out the form anonymously, only indicating his/her age and sex. After the sheets were delivered, the purpose of the study was explained as well as what type of patients participated in the research.

The image of the videos was distorted to guarantee the confidentiality of patients' identities. As previously stated, each participant signed an informed consent document prior to entering the study.

Results

Three analyses of variance (ANOVA) were carried out using IBM's Statistical Package for the Social Sciences (SPSS). Each of the ANOVAs compared the score assigned by the students on the Likert scale to the DMT group and the control group. The students noticed more interaction in the DMT group than in the control group (Figure 17.1).

For nonverbal interaction, greater interaction was seen in the DMT group than in the control group (see Figure 17.2).

Regarding general interaction, the video of the DMT group was rated higher than the control group (see Figure 17.3).

The Pearson correlations between the categories was significant in all cases ($p < 0.001$). Within the DMT group, for verbal and nonverbal interaction, the value was 0.45, between verbal and global 0.67, and between global and nonverbal 0.63. In the control group, for verbal and nonverbal interaction the value was 0.63, between verbal and global 0.56, and between global and nonverbal 0.80.

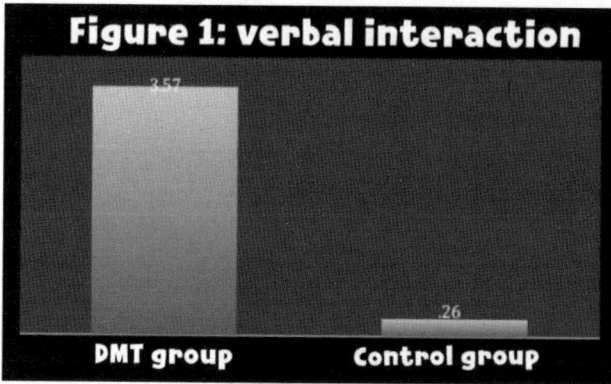

Figure 17.1 Average of the Verbal Interaction Level Estimates Provided by the Evaluators

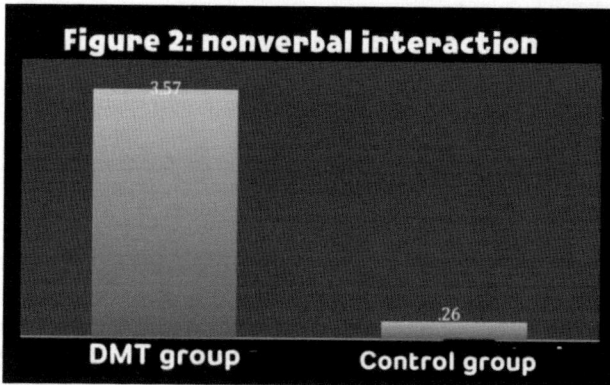

Figure 17.2 Average of the Nonverbal Interaction Level Estimates Provided by the Evaluators

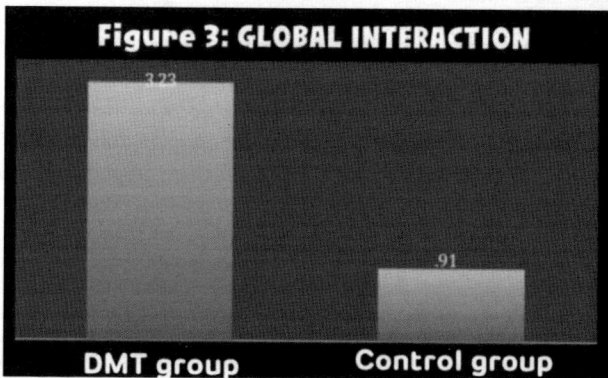

Figure 17.3 Average of the Estimates of the Level of global Interaction Provided by the Evaluators

Discussion

The DMT group was rated by the observers as more interactive than the control group at all levels. We could say that the results of this study support the idea that the treatment developed based on the principles of DMT and the use of flamenco during two years of intervention promoted interaction among users and therefore could be related to a reduction of some of the negative symptoms of their disease, or at least with an increase in group cohesion and reduction of the isolation felt and experienced by this type of patient (see Image 17.3). We should not consider that our results are in any way definitive and significant since there were few patient groups analyzed and we do not have evaluations/measurements of the patients prior to the beginning of the treatment. Additionally, the patients were not randomly assigned to the treatments of the different occupational workshops; they voluntarily enrolled in the groups. Despite these limitations, we can point out that the findings presented in this work are very encouraging.

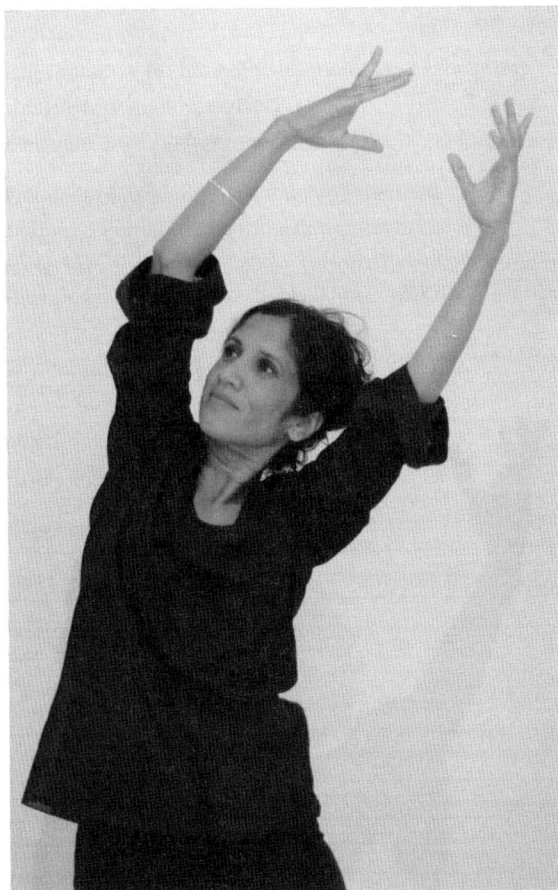

Image 17.3 Participants experience reaching outwards towards others through their enhanced presence.

Photo courtesy of Keren Yehuda. Photographer: Svetlana Oltzblat Taub.

CONCLUSION

From our experience, we can say that flamenco art enriches DMT sessions due to its great variety of resources. Following the rhythmic structure requires great attention and the ability to listen in order to perceive the nuances of the accents and to mark the times, the offbeats,[3] and the syncopates. Thus, the memory capacity of patients is enhanced by repeating a sound or movement proposed by each of the members of the group and joining them all in a continuous wheel at a higher or lower speed, which thus produces an improvement in coordination and perception of space.

The results of this study showed the intervention appeared to have a good effect on the interpersonal relationships of participants. It allowed the expression of emotions and feelings in a creative way. Flamenco art shares musical, verbal, and gestural language and common signs in the culture of large areas of Spain. Its elements complement, enrich, adapt, and support each other without losing their identity. The common denominator to all of them is the rhythm. Therefore, it is ideal to use as this communicative form for DMT interventions in Spain, for, in addition to the work presented here, flamenco is integrated into working with people in other therapeutic, educational, and social settings.

APPENDIX

Observation Sheet. Based on Laban's Movement Analysis (White, 2008)

Movement Observation Sheet Date_____

Therapist's Name_____

Date of the Observation_____

Context of the observation: what is the participant doing, where, with whom . . .

1. The general impression the therapist has from the patients (metaphors, images)
2. Body:
    2.1 Posture: rigid or tense, relaxed, curved . . . Is there tension in any part of the body?
    2.2 Do all body parts move equally? What body parts are most active? Body parts that lead the movement.
    2.3 Physical contact: with himself, with members of the group.
    2.4 Breathing (deep, shallow, sighs . . .)
    2.5 Sense of one's own body, grounding.

3. Actions: Frequent movements, tics, touching themself
4. Temporal aspects: Preparations, transitions, accents
5. Spatial aspects: Use of the general space. Personal kinesphere (near, medium, far) Levels preferred (high, low, medium) Planes (table—horizontal, door—vertical, wheel—sagittal)
6. Efforts

    Flow: Free—bound

    Space: Direct—Indirect

    Time: Sudden—sustained

    Weight: Firm—light—passive

7. Relational aspects
    _____

    How the Patient Contacts with the Therapist, Other Participants and Props

    Proximity
    Eye contact
    Grounding, presence
    Verbal communication
    _____

8. Use of the voice and verbal communication
    _____

    Voice Volume
    _____

    Intonation
    Vocabulary
    Phrase construction
    _____

9. Comments regarding coordination and rhythm

NOTES

1. For more information about the Chace approach, see S. Chaiklin & C. Schmais (1993) The Chace approach to dance therapy. In S. Sandel, S. Chaiklin, & A. Lohn (Eds.), *Foundations of dance/movement therapy: The life and work of Marian Chace* (pp. 75–97). Columbia, MD: Marian Chace Memorial Fund.
2. For more examples on DMT work with persons with severe mental disorders, see Capello (2008, 2016), Wengrower and Bendel-Rozow (in press).
3. An offbeat is the accent shifted between two times: clapping exactly between two times. That is, the notes played or sung in the weak parts of the measure are preceded by a silence located in the strong part.

REFERENCES

Capello, P. P. (2008). Bascics: Un modelo intra/interactivo de DMT con pacientes psiquiátricos adultos. In H. Wengrower & S. Chaiklin (Eds.), *La vida es danza: el arte y la ciencia en la Danza Movimiento Terapia* (pp. 101–128). Barcelona: Gedisa.
Capello, P. P. (2016). Bascics: An intra/interactional model of DMT with the adult psychiatric patient. In S. Chaiklin & H. Wengrower (Eds.), *The art and science of Dance Movement Therapy: Life is dance* (pp. 77–102). New York: Routledge (First edition, 2009).
Chace, M. (Ed.). (1975). *Marian Chace: Her papers*. Columbia, MD: American Dance Therapy Association.
Cruces Roldán, C. (2002a). De cintura para arriba. Hipercorporeidad y Sexualidad en el Baile Flamenco. In *Comunicación en congreso. Seminario Internacional de Estudios De las Mujeres*. Sevilla: Signatura.
Cruces Roldán, C. (2002b). Más allá de la música (I). In *Antropología y Flamenco*. Sevilla: Signatura.
Cruces Roldán, C. (2003/2012). Más allá de la música (II). In *Antropología y flamenco*. Sevilla: Signatura.
Fischman, D. (2008). Relación terapéutica y empatía kinestésica. In H. Wengrower & S. Chaiklin (Eds.), *La vida es danza: El arte y la ciencia en la Danza Movimiento Terapia* (pp. 81–96). Barcelona: Gedisa.
Garaudy, R. (1987). *El Islam en Occidente. Córdoba, capital del pensamiento unitario*. Madrid: Editorial Breogán.
García, E. (2010). La vivencia del tiempo en la psicología normal y en la patológica II. *Revista de la Asociación Española de Neuropsiquiatría, 30*(1), 137–143.
González de Chávez, M. (2008). *Psicoterapia de grupo y esquizofrenia. Abordajes psicoterapéuticos de las psicosis esquizofrénicas: Historia, desarrollo y perspectivas*. Madrid: Fundación para la Investigación y Tratamiento de la Esquizofrenia y otras Psicosis, pp. 293–312.
Grötsch, K. (2012). Génesis de un patrimonio. El caso del flamenco. *La Nueva Alboreá, 23*, 56–61.
Heller, E. (2004). *Psicología del color. Cómo actúan los colores sobre los sentimientos y la razón*. Barcelona: Ed. Gustavo Gili.
López, L. S. (2014). Efectividad de la expresión corporal para la mejora de la capacidad expresiva en el Trastorno Mental Grave. *NURE Investigación: Revista Científica de Enfermería, 11*(73), 6.
Lowen, A. (2006). *The language of the body: Physical dynamics of character structure: How the body reveals personality*. Alachua, FL: Bioenergetics Press.
Reca, M. (2007). Danza/movimiento terapia en la reconstrucción del mundo del sobreviviente de tortura por razones políticas. *Hologramática, 6*(4), 49–65.
Wengrower, H. (2008). El proceso creativo y la actividad artística por medio de la danza y el movimiento. In H. Wengrower & S. Chaiklin (Eds.), *La vida es danza: el arte y la ciencia en la Danza Movimiento Terapia* (pp. 39–58). Barcelona: Gedisa.
Wengrower, H., & Bendel-Rozow, T. (to be published). Integration in motion: Dance Movement Therapy. In U. Volpe (Ed.), *Arts-therapies in psychiatric rehabilitation—evidence and experience*. New York: Springer.
White, E. Q. (2008). Las teorías del movimiento de Laban: la perspectiva de una danzaterapeuta. In H. Wengrower & S. Chaiklin (Eds.), *La vida es danza: el arte y la ciencia en la Danza Movimiento Terapia* (pp. 239–258). Barcelona: Gedisa.

CHAPTER 18

TIME, SPACE, AND AN AESTHETICS OF SURVIVAL
Dance/Movement Therapy and Embodied Imagination after Unimaginable Loss

David Alan Harris

Each art has its own imbricated techniques of repetition, the critical and revolutionary potential of which must reach the highest possible degree, to lead us from the dreary repetitions of habit to the profound repetitions of memory, and ultimately to the [symbolic] repetitions of death, through which we make sport of our own mortality.

Gilles Deleuze, *Répétition et différence*[1]

INTRODUCTION

Dance/movement therapy (DMT)—imbued with the vital energies of dance itself—exhibits an unusual capacity for fostering resilience, restoration, and recovery in the aftermath of severe traumatic suffering, including that associated globally with the atrocities of war and organized violence. Deconstructing what dance means in relevant sociocultural contexts, as in the war-torn West African region highlighted in this chapter, may help gauge this healing modality's value in such settings. As experienced virtually everywhere, dance is both a visual and a temporal phenomenon; it invariably entails witness of the human body, in space, as in time, deliberately transformed. Cultures worldwide consecrate a range of human experience through dance—often by sacralizing spaces and in them marking a rhythm in time's passage, manifest through human bodies moving: These are processes that dance/movement therapists may usefully replicate.

If prepared to investigate dance and dance aesthetics with an awareness of context through an analytical lens borrowed from cultural anthropology, DMT's practitioners may engage with the art form's elemental components of time and space. Doing so can foster insight and well-being in the face of debilitating illness, mental torment, and mortality itself.

In 2005, as a newly registered dance/movement therapist, I relocated from the United States to Sierra Leone for a couple of years in order to supervise paraprofessional counselors in a nongovernmental torture rehabilitation program across four towns in the rural Kailahun District. At the millennium's start, Sierra Leone was perhaps the world's least developed country—with the highest infant and child mortality, and lowest life expectancy, at only 38 (UNICEF, 2000). Kailahun was then not only the nation's remotest district but arguably its most war-ravaged as well. My arrival there came four years after a demilitarization that officially marked the end of a ruthless conflict characterized by massive violence against noncombatants. In the capricious course of its 11 years, the war had decimated almost every sector of Kailahun society, cruelly uprooting nearly the entire local populace—with the vast majority of survivors eventually fleeing for refuge in nearby Guinea. While most of Kailahun's refugees had been repatriated by the time of my arrival, across the district practically no shelter of any kind remained intact and rare were the survivors unaffected by the ubiquitous physical traces of terror. During wartime, corrugated zinc roofs had been melted down for munitions, and few houses had been repaired five years after the war's end. In Koindu, a town where I conducted much of my work, huge craters in the central mosque's minarets reminded everyone daily that the war had left unscathed not even the sacred house of Allah.

My role in training and supervising Kailahun's paraprofessional psychosocial counselors for the Center for Victims of Torture entailed helping them upgrade services to recently returned war refugees and developing programming to facilitate recovery. In four towns across the district, we launched community healing initiatives and conducted public health workshops, among them trainings designed to inform local leaders about the impact of violence on vulnerable populations. In addition, while running four DMT groups for adolescents and young adults, I supervised nearly 100 short-term counseling groups that addressed a range of ages.

DESOMATIZING MEMORY

Developing a DMT practice for 21st-century application in developing world contexts with people who have endured the worst of war and organized violence may necessitate taking an inclusive approach to what constitutes dance, as well as what constitutes healing, and reframing their merger. The discipline of DMT was first fashioned in the middle of the 20th century by creative women in the United States and countries in Europe whose understandings of both psychotherapy and dance as an art form were intrinsic to the cultures in which they lived and worked. In the intervening decades, the prevailing definition of dance has expanded exponentially, even in the global North's art dance venues. After U.S. composer John Cage (1961) had produced a score that consisted entirely of "silence," and his partner, choreographer Merce Cunningham, had divorced dancing from music entirely, it did not take long for dance practitioners in many places to redefine their work as something of any possible scale involving human bodies of any kind moving—or remaining motionless—in time and space. Dance/movement therapy has evolved along with broader multicultural developments, and contributions to DMT from the rich dance and movement practices of Africa and its diaspora have grown increasingly pervasive as well. It is in this deliberately inclusive spirit of the meaning of dance that this chapter incorporates description of ritualized acts, including private ceremonies performed in secluded spaces, as well as vast choreographed processions that fill entire streets for transformative ends.

In recent decades, evidence has likewise grown that healing the psychological wounds of war and organized violence depends in part on facilitating embodiment of a revitalized imagination. Survivors of war crimes and egregious human rights violations may carry in their musculatures and nervous systems the imprint of that abuse—potentially until the end of their days. It is not uncommon for survivors, especially those who have faced the threat of extinction, to undergo frequent reliving in mind and body of the horrifying events that they had witnessed or endured. The central goals of therapy in the aftermath of such life-threatening incidents, as leading psychotraumatologist Bessel van der Kolk (1996) has cogently explained, are "taming the associated terror and desomatizing the memories" (p. 205).

Advances in neurobiological research in recent decades are constantly reshaping understandings of how memory functions and what such posttraumatic recovery entails. Psychological theorists have differentiated two types, or systems, of memory, each associated with a discrete part of the human brain: (a) implicit memory, linked to the amygdala, and (b) explicit, or declarative memory, linked to the hippocampus (Ogden, Minton, & Pain, 2006). *Desomatizing*, a notion that van der Kolk apparently coined, inherently involves integrating the two systems, such that memories stored, not as lucid and logical narratives, but in fragmented traces of sensory information, may "collaborate" (van der Kolk, 2014, p. 176) in generating a coherent, balanced response to even threatening stimuli. Research underscores the possibility that such integration, letting survivors "feel fully alive in the present and move on with their lives," can be accomplished from the "bottom up," that is, by enabling "the body to have experiences that deeply and viscerally contradict the helplessness, rage, or collapse that result from trauma" (van der Kolk, 2014, p. 3). It follows that dancing can play a significant role in such a process, as is documented in the narratives in this chapter.

SUSTAINING RHYTHM

During my Kailahun tenure as trauma clinician and trainer, on numerous occasions I joined our psychosocial counseling team in facilitating community discussions about the recently concluded war and its impact. On an airless morning in March 2005, in Koindu, an outpost within walking distance of the Liberian and Guinean borders, we gathered a group of some 50 primary school students in a central schoolhouse to speak about a video we had screened for them the day before. The documentary, produced in tandem with the country's Truth and Reconciliation Commission, shared findings from the Commission's investigation into the fighting, its origins, and its aftermath.

On this occasion we drew the classroom's backless benches closely together in a circle in the hope that intimacy might help contain and hold difficult emotions. The facilitating counselor began by affirming the normalcy of feeling upset about the cruelties witnessed in life, especially of the kind suffered during the war. He then opened the floor to the children's comments on what they had seen in the video. Early on, a small girl of around ten put up her hand and timidly asked to speak. Grasping her green school-uniform skirt in one hand, she rose to her feet, and in a rambling dissertation on events that had taken place some years before, told her peers about her wartime ordeals. Captured with an uncle by rebels in Liberia, she had witnessed them stage a sort of lottery for him—writing three possible modes of execution on slips of paper, dropping them into a pot, and forcing the man himself to draw from the vessel the slip with his inscribed destiny—as if his fate had been preordained by an avenging deity. Rather than being shot blindfolded, she said, or drowned in a nearby stream, the kindly man who cared for her after her parents' killings was scalded to death with boiling oil. Quietly sharing her inescapable memories with us, this little child, who would not have been older than six or seven at the time of the events she narrated, had been forced to watch it all.

Like her peers, we counselors were shaken by the little girl's indelible images of horror. Working to counter the collective impulse to dissociate in response—to drift away from the classroom and begin to revisit mentally the terrors of the recent past, perhaps in the process to fall prey to utter and unending hopelessness—we opted to introduce a technique that encourages grounding in current bodily reality. I whispered to staff a common DMT adage, "Rhythm creates a holding environment," a principle, echoing Winnicott's (1971) landmark formulation, which I had shared with the counselors for application in our groups and community events of all sorts. Hoping to ease a return to the present moment, we urged all of the children to come to their feet and to sing a familiar song, knowing that when singing together the pupils would unite in clapping, swaying, and stepping to the music of their own making. In sensing, as they sang, the floor's solidity under their feet and the very resonance of their own vocal cords, they would perhaps be equipped to evade momentarily the perilous siren call toward an inward journey back to a space and time of omnipresent danger. Instead, they might find in their own bodies a place of safety, surrounded by friends and caring adults. It was clear that as survivors of horrific atrocities, these children would have to learn to live with what could never be forgotten. Moving together to music may have provided at best an impermanent solution, yet the emotional regulation it afforded them in this particular moment was undeniable and swift—and as such may have furthered another day's survival.

DMT WITH ADOLESCENT FEMALES

Fourteen months later I sat on the floor in a dingy secondary school classroom in Kaila-hun town. A woman and a man—both DMT/counseling trainees—joined me on woven-plastic prayer mats spread over the cement floor. Shutters were closed tight to keep out the blazing midday heat, and the room's rough-hewn wooden benches and tables had been pushed to the darker peripheries. We were co-facilitating the eighth of ten DMT sessions, and on this occasion we had already improvised together with our clients in a circle to some of their favorite Sierra Leonean hip-hop. Now we would wait in quiet expectation as three of the group's six members (all female, aged 14 to 16) were about to bring to life challenging scenes from their personal histories. Joined by a couple of their peers, we formed their audience.

As survivors of the war, these teens might well have chosen to depict vicious acts of violence that had undoubtedly shaped their early childhoods. But as the scenes unfolded before us, it was clear that more recent events were on their hearts: deaths of family members, events that had repeatedly stolen these group members' homes from them, along with their sense of safety and belonging. A 14-year-old orphan had already chosen from among her peers the actors to play the roles in her family drama. (Here I will call her "Siawoh"[2]—in remembrance of another of my paraprofessional counselor trainees who left psychosocial work and entered nursing only to become among the first fatalities of the Ebola outbreak that ravaged the district in 2014.) In this session, Siawoh had tears in her eyes while witness-ing the actor who portrayed her uncle drive the peers playing her aunt and herself from their home.

At the role-play's end, Siawoh arose quietly, ready to assume a part in another group member's very similar story. Siawoh knew the scenario, and despite a tendency to hide her emotional life, she had been cast as the lead by her peer, "Aminata," a friend who had taken a place among us to watch. Three times in recent years, Aminata, too, had been driven from her home, and before that she had surely joined the refugee caravans to Guinea and back. Accordingly, in the drama's first scene, Aminata's elder sister, desperate and unable to feed and shelter one more dependent, kicked the young protagonist out of the house. When in the next scene the child went to live with her father, he died suddenly, leaving her bereft and subject once more to immediate dislocation. For Aminata at this juncture, being made home-less persuaded her elder sister to shelter her again. In the subsequent scene, though, the sister unexpectedly grew ill and perished, leaving the child permanently on her own.

Tasked with portraying the enormity of the grief inherent in this daunting succession of losses, Siawoh, who minutes before had tears in her eyes while watching her own recent history, stunned her audience with an improvised response. With no hint of physical prepa-ration, she catapulted herself into the air and crashed hard onto the cement floor—missing entirely the portion covered by prayer mats. It is the single most violent movement I have ever encountered in the context of DMT, and in that moment it knocked the breath out of us spectators. Shuddering, we felt then as if we too had plummeted without a net into this cold, hard reality, and maybe risked dashing our brains out upon impact.

Dance/movement therapists comprehend such identification with the performer, in this case the moment's perception that we share in Siawoh's risk of serious injury, as indicative of what we term *kinesthetic empathy*—an empathy experienced through witnessing another's body movement (Berger, 1972). This phenomenon is now widely considered hard-wired by mirror neurons (Berrol, 2006) and thus is unlikely to be culture-bound.

In the moment of Siawoh's dive, I shuttled in my mind back to fourth grade: When looking the wrong way while running fast through a gym, I had snapped my right clavicle against an interior brick corner. The collision in fact had propelled me onto my back unconscious, and this bodily memory in the Kailahun classroom signaled to me strong evidence of somatic countertransference with my therapy client, the performer sprawled on the floor in front of us. At the same time, I recognized the need to resume my professional monitoring role. Making eye contact with my supervisees, I joined them in surveying the frightening scene and quickly forming a nonverbal consensus not to stop the action but instead to let the powerful narrative unfurl without pause.

In embodying her friend at a moment of tragic loss, Siawoh transformed herself entirely from the member of the group who most typically shied away from showing authentic feelings to a virtuosic performer capable of using her body to convey extreme emotional pain—undoubtedly, her own, as much as that of her friend. Upon learning of "her" sister's death, Siawoh threw herself onto the unyielding floor, and wailing there, rolled in Kailahun's omnipresent dust. Her crying looked as real as the fresh dirt stains that appeared on her clothing, and she seemed to hold nothing back. Performing this role apparently enabled Siawoh to vent emotions associated with her own story, which she had been holding inside for a long time.

REINVENTING RITUAL PROCESS IN DANCE

It remains remarkable that Siawoh was uninjured, despite the treacherous improvised dive. Surely, her daring as a performer was attributable in part to the impetuosity of adolescence, for in her own daily life, recklessness was indeed an issue. There are a number of plausible explanations, moreover, for the apparent absence of physical consequences from her crash onto the unforgiving floor. Csiksentmihaliyi's (1975) notion of "flow" may plausibly explain the apparent absence of physical consequences. Siawoh had entered a zone of total involvement where "[a]ction and awareness are experienced as one" (Turner, 1977a, p. 47). In an ultimate state of flow, she proved impervious to bodily pain, even while portraying agony to the audience: Flow, and the fearlessness she embodied in that state, allowed her to repudiate the very prospect of fragility. It was as if denial itself, of such mundane realities as bruised muscles and fractured bones, offered her an otherworldly power to survive, as if not giving into mortal fears afforded a protective amulet to shield against injury. Likely, the body–mind warm-up she had undergone in the course of all-out dancing to Sierra Leonean popular music minutes before primed her to manage this uncalculated risk. In turn, it enabled her crossing into a liminal space where she might defy the bounds of quotidian reality.

That afternoon, like everyone in the darkened, dusty Kailahun classroom, I was aware of the pivotal ritual process to which Siawoh's perilous dance alluded. The previous year, just weeks after my arrival in Kailahun, I had joined co-workers in traveling over nearly impassable roads to a tiny village deep in the forest—a trek made to honor a recently deceased staff member on the occasion of a pivotal funeral commemoration, his 40-day ceremony. Upon reaching the village, our crew walked solemnly past its collection of mud and thatch huts. People of all ages had positioned themselves, barely mobile—standing, sitting, squatting, or crouching—on a hard-packed earthen yard in front of one of the houses. There we noticed a very thin woman, one of the older people present, and as we discovered, elder sister of the deceased. She abruptly rose up into the air, slammed her body hard onto the dirt, and pulsed there in sobs. As she cried out, her wails turned first into keening, and then to a repeating phrase, piteously sung in her tribal language. I was mesmerized and somewhat stunned by the mourner's performance, but no one else appeared to pay her the least attention. The entire village seemed instead to look away as she bore the sorrow for everyone and all alone let grief's gaping wound bleed in public.

There is a widespread assumption that such performative rituals in traditional cultures function conservatively as phenomena that enable humans to endure time's passage untrammeled by change. But this view is problematic. Indeed, Victor Turner (1977a), a prominent anthropologist of ritual (1920–1983), illuminated cultural rites' transformative capacities. Countering views of ritual as inflexible containers for upholding the status quo, he indicated that "tribal rituals are anything but rigid. . . . [W]hile there are fixed, stereotyped sequences of symbolic action, there are also episodes given over to verbal and nonverbal improvisation" (p. 35).

Turner (1977a, 1977b) thus highlighted aspects of the ritual process in which imaginative experimentation emerges. He drew significantly from van Gennep's (1873–1957) analyses of three distinct temporal phases in rites of passage: (1) separation from society, (2) transition through the threshold, or *limen*, into an otherworldly space/time where possibilities seem endless, and (3) reaggregation into society with revised status following the transition. In particular, the second, liminal phase—for Turner a gateway to social reversal and transformation—allowed for the possibility of significant innovation, and potentially, utter communal joy. Moreover, he deemed "the liminal in socio-cultural process . . . similar to the subjunctive mood in verbs—just as mundane socio-cultural activities resemble the indicative mood," (Turner, 1977a, p. 33). Hence, liminality, or "being-on-the-threshold," constitutes a playfully subjunctive space/time *as if* apart from daily reality, and the sacralized borders of liminality frame a potentiality for "enchantment, subversion, and change" (Harris, 2009, p. 97).

Within the safe therapeutic container of our DMT group, Siawoh's dramatic abandon enlivened for all of us present her people's funeral tradition. In the process, while risking nothing short of fatality in a place lacking even emergency medicine, she created a *meta*-performance. Indeed, her startling physical portrayal, as understood within the context of a country still in mourning five years after the end of a decade's ruthless civil war, inhabited multiple valences of meaning. Siawoh not only powerfully transformed the distress over her own personal history of significant losses while evincing at once her friend's grief, but simultaneously danced an image that made for a resonant symbol of her entire people's survival in the midst of unspeakable devastation and despair.

Nearly every person we encountered in our Kailahun outreach had named the inability to perform the obligatory rites for deceased loved ones as the bitterest experience of their lives—more horrible than even the butchery they had witnessed. In the absence of these vital ceremonies, the deceased forever lacked what was needed to transition from this brutal world to the kinder next one. Lyotard (1977), dissecting Freud's corpus, identified the unconscious as stage director (*metteur en scène*), mounting public performances. In replicating a funeral rite, Siawoh may well have assumed a role staged by the *collective* unconscious of her people. Whether or not she engaged the strategy deliberately, she appropriated a performative ritual movement idiom from the public square and privatized it for a small coterie of spectators, thereby advancing a critical symbolic purpose, the fulfillment of duties required throughout Sierra Leone for passage from this world to the next. She thereby achieved a level of impact sought by choreographers everywhere and likewise brought to our DMT group session the liminal possibility of healing, our core therapeutic enterprise.

Rituals, in Kailahun and globally, buttress cultural understandings of mortality and not only represent but become the continuity of the life-force in the face of death. Siawoh's breathtaking choreography—including her virtuosic, head-first dive into oblivion—illustrated the reflexivity through which, as Turner (1977a) put it, "a group or community seeks to portray, understand, and then act on itself" (p. 33). Her performance was at once an intimate improvisation and a timeless expression for herself and her grief-struck friend alike of their people's faith that death is but a pause in an endless flow of being.

WHAT THE BODY REMEMBERS IS PARADOX

Dance, at its most essential, is a culture's embodied barter with human finitude. Invariably, dance practitioners must face the invincible fact of dance as entropy, the truth that what is done in dancing exists only to disappear. To dance is to acknowledge, implicitly, that everything about this form vanishes, just as all human bodies eventually decay, dissolve into dust, and disappear from the face of the earth. But dancing in many cultural contexts is likewise quintessentially an enterprise for undoing the ephemeral, for suspending disbelief in immortality. Virtuoso dancers in many cultures create "lasting impressions" that raise the bar on human attainment. While it is a truism that dance is the most ephemeral of art forms, dance truly makes the transitory something to be remembered.

Responding to this paradox, in practically all cultural contexts, more or less inevitably involves engaging with repetition as an artistic strategy. Working in dance means constantly repeating oneself in order to bring solidity to bodies that are mutable and movements that are fleeting. In building dances, choreographers repeat or interpolate images, gestures, or phrases of movement, thus affording audiences multiple viewings of body motifs in space/ time. Without such direct repetitions or variants, spectators would be less apt to "see" the dance, to recognize and engage with its craft and meaning, either in the passing course of its performance or afterward in recollection.

Memory, time's shadow, is equally fundamental to dance's creation through the medium of human bodies: the practice of shaping the body into purposeful expression, as tutored through the rigorous execution of movements deliberately patterned onto the skeletons and sinews of living organisms with minds of their own. Decades ago I visited the Kerala Kalamandalam, a renowned training academy for practitioners of various classical Indian dance forms. In a dirt-floored hut I watched as a crew of male elders drilled barefoot boys in the intricate percussive footwork of what I took to be *kathak*. Without a break, the young trainees in short pants thrust their heels into the dust at high speed, beating out elaborate rhythms with unexpected syncopations. The effect was heart-stopping—especially given the tendency of our circulatory systems to synchronize with the speed of these tiny legs moving in brilliant unison. Moreover, the boys' exacting rigor was not unlike that of young ballerinas at the barre. Indeed, in similar fashion within widely differing cultural contexts dance has been handed down meticulously, body-to-body, for centuries. A relentless regime of repetition prepares novices to assume the expressivity of their progenitors, in effect enabling the most evanescent of art forms to outlast the corrosive effects of time as dances move from generation to generation. And as dances survive through the centuries, dancing propels human survival.

Movement repetitions are not always deliberately chosen, of course. It is unlikely that Siawoh considered other movement options before bringing a resonant cultural artefact into the room by throwing her body down into the dust when memorializing her friend's sister. Rather, she simply engaged in the known vocabulary of movement expression related to passage from this world to the next. Similarly, when our deceased security guard's sister opted to spike herself into the dirt—only to be ritually ignored by the entire village—her mode of bodily expression at the 40-day ceremony had been assigned her by the traditions of women survivors who had come before. The codification of these forms of expression and the codification of dance forms as techniques are designed to fulfill an almost identical purpose: to advance the power and duration of human memory in the face of inexorable forgetting. In the village, the woman aims to ensure her loved one a living embodiment there 40 days after his demise. Is it any wonder that this largely futile enterprise of sustaining the life's breath of one who is no longer breathing should be expressed in a transitory form that contradicts the entire immortality agenda? Dance and funeral rite would appear to be asking the same interwoven questions: In all of human history, where is the balance to be found between mobility and stasis? How feasible is it to realize our collective, universal aim to grasp being itself and fix it in place?

DANCING, THE ORPHAN BOYS OF KOINDU RECALL

The impulse to undo a history of ruthless devastation and loss, by symbolically immobilizing all potential judgment, guilt, and shame over participation in unthinkable violence, would become an ongoing theme in a DMT group that I launched for former boy soldiers in Koindu with three male Kissi-speaking paraprofessional supervisees. As I have documented elsewhere in significant detail (Harris, 2007a, 2007b, 2009, 2010), this group of a dozen teenage ex-combatants, all of whom had joined in one way or another in perpetrating egregious human rights abuses during their childhoods, underwent an incremental transformation in the course of 16 sessions over six months of dancing together. Masters of surviving adversity before coming to us, they were especially adept at suppressing disclosure of their innermost thoughts. Desensitized through direct involvement in both organized slaughter and more impulsive acts of mayhem, they would speak openly about such abuses from the start, but with great detachment and regardless of whether they had been targets or perpetrators of the crimes in question. They would not reveal the least capacity for empathy, in fact—for their victims or one another—until they had joined in several weeks of DMT. By gradually discovering in dance and movement the collective courage to mourn their own losses, they moved toward restoring their capacity for connection.

As was the case in Siawoh's DMT group for teenage females, each session of the former boy soldiers group—which took for itself the name PVK, *Poimboi Veeyah Koindu*, in Kissi, or Orphan Boys of Koindu—included improvised dancing to the beat of recorded Sierra Leonean hip-hop. In a calculated fusion of the African dance circle and what DMT innovator Marian Chace had developed with much older war veterans in the United States six decades earlier, the dancing would begin with a warm-up in a circular formation and devolve into all varieties of spatial organization, depending on the PVK youths' predilections in the moment. Typically, the youths' movement expression included powerful gesturing and numerous vigorous outbursts, but not without frequent ventures into quietude and intimacy.

From the very first session, in fact, the former fighters took advantage of what we called "The Circle Dance" to invest themselves in primary-process (Freud, 1958, as cited in Brenner, 1973) imaginings through which they engaged with pivotal aspects of their traumatic experience. Within minutes of starting to dance together, the former fighters began walking to the beat around the circle, counterclockwise, one behind another, then lunging, dipping, and eventually crawling, all the while maintaining the circle's protective enclosure. After a while I chose to play with qualities of time, deliberately slowing our pace. Soon everyone stopped, collapsing in place on the floor—with many of the ex-soldiers quietly cradling each other. I asked, "What are we doing now?" and a collective response came back, "We're hiding from our enemies." Despite the relative stillness, the former boy soldiers, in their very first hour of dancing together, had brought their wartime suffering into the room in the form of hypervigilance, a common post-conflict phenomenon. During their time with the rebels, staying constantly on guard had been an essential survival mechanism. Although this nervous system adaptation had served these survivors well, it was no longer beneficial—just one of the somatic markers (Damasio, 1991) of traumatic experience—that called for transformation through the DMT process. Opportunities for venting and modulating aggressive impulses, which to that point the former fighters little understood as their own patterned responses to systemic violence and devastating loss, would prove equally important.

At play as well in that first session's dance was an emerging, unstated sense of these dozen teenagers and four adult men as having banded together, not unlike the ragged platoons the youths had been part of when serving under rebel commandos. Survival tactics from that earlier time remained as habitual responses to danger and perhaps reinforced the youths' malleability in readily accommodating almost any verbal or nonverbal directive that we co-facilitators presented them.

Week after week, improvised dancing together—invariably with strong rhythmic synchrony, given a culturally ingrained capacity for collective attunement—enabled the PVK youths in-depth exploration of much that they could not then have verbalized about their lives or histories. Repeatedly, for example, in a number of early sessions they joined at some juncture in their improvising in stealthily trapping one or more of my limbs and, using their collective might, holding me down on the floor. The meaning of their joint effort to fix me in place was multilayered and may perhaps be considered emblematic of a tacit aspiration through dancing to defy human impermanence. The youths were certainly aware of the satisfaction I found in dancing freely, and by immobilizing me, they put a stop to it: I genuinely could not move. Their action also clearly amounted to a wartime reenactment, in this case, the symbolic capture of an enemy. Had the repetitions been performed as dull, unfeeling, robotic acts, rather than the energetic and sometimes rather spirited contests that I witnessed bodily, I would have worried that the youths were manifesting in such reenactment susceptibility to Freud's pathological "repetition compulsions" (Herman, 1992, p. 41). Even so, when the youths held me down, I wondered if they were unknowingly seeking a form of symbolic retribution for the abuses they had endured under the unscrupulous commandos they had served. At the very least, they could be seen as "killing off the leader" (Yalom, 1970) in order to wrest control over our gatherings. In fact, one of the PVK youths had by this stage in our process directed a role-play in session of having been forced by his commander to execute his own parents as a show of the boy's loyalty to the rebel cause. In the drama, which might have been based as much on imagination as history, the boy had afterward slain the commander himself in retaliation. At this stage in PVK's dances, inventive play deconstructed but rarely obscured memory's curse.

Indeed, a web of stark meanings emerged through primary-process embodiments during PVK's unstructured improvisations to music. It seemed more than likely to my co-facilitators and me, for example, that in holding me down, the ex-fighters evinced an unconscious desire to punish me for encouraging their individual and collective investigation of wartime experiences, an almost invariably taxing process. Further, my white skin made me an appropriate stand-in for the British soldiers who had defeated the rebel army and brought an end to the boy soldiers' pillaging of civilian communities. This desire for revenge was largely unspoken, as was an irrevocable association of whiteness with the rapacity and dehumanizing violence of centuries of colonial subjugation.

All of these meanings, and more, were likely operative in the PVK dance circle. Indeed, when I saw my own arms isolated under those of my captors, one arm sprawling atop another as if detached from our bodies, I could not help but envision what looked like a pile of hands spilled across the floor. This image, as my Kissi co-facilitators confirmed in one of our routine debriefings, appeared visually reminiscent of the heaps of severed limbs these child soldiers would have seen when their assaults on villagers had included forced amputations. In Sierra Leone's war, this had been such a common atrocity that few of the PVK youth could have managed *not* to witness it; probably some had joined, willingly or not, in committing such crimes. Recreating this haunting nightmare in play, certainly without forethought or intention, by no means represented a conscious coming to terms with the ex-combatants' horrific past. But just as surely, this rough, aggressive—albeit decidedly *not* violent—play helped these former soldiers transcend, or at least tolerate, the horrors that violence had engraved upon their memories.

Moreover, as everyone in the PVK group was aware but no one discussed openly, in our first weeks together one youth missed a group session in order to attend a funeral rite for his own mother. By magically fixing me in place, the Orphan Boys of Koindu were symbolically responding to the terrifying fear of abandonment by a caring adult, which all of them had experienced in quite horrific ways. By restraining me, the youths both neutralized my capacity to judge them for their crimes and likewise made it impossible for me, unlike their parents and grandparents, to die or disappear or desert them.

This freedom to embody among us such existential dread arose, paradoxically enough, given a restored sense of safety within the group's liminal space. When pinning me down, the youths were asserting power and playing with the threat of violent usurpation, and in doing so, engaging in a common adolescent behavior: testing unawares the limits of our acceptance, as if trying to coerce us into giving up on them and thereby endorsing their guilt-induced fear of their own worthlessness. The youths could not yet embrace me as a parental substitute; neither could they bear, then, for me to leave them before they would have a chance to bring appropriate closure to our prolonged dance together.

Throughout our process, the Circle Dance thus enabled the former child combatants to examine their collective history in ways that remained largely unspoken. Similarly, on occasion, individual PVK members, when joining in various group exercises, utilized gestural expressions that belied their growing, though still largely unformed, awareness of vulnerabilities shared between them and the people they had attacked. More than once, for example, a former fighter illustrated the liquidation of a military target by using one of his own hands as the cutlass blade with which he slit the person's throat. I was struck that the neck over which the blade was drawn was the PVK youth's own, such that when illustrating his killing of someone else he appeared to be demonstrating suicide. The disturbing duality in this gesture conveyed an implicit sense of oneness with the victim and unknowingly portrayed how gravely the child soldier himself had ended up mutilated by his own violent act. The youth may have meant to demonstrate his fearlessness as a fighter, but his body symbolism betrayed, instead, persistent subconscious regret.

The emergence of such burgeoning hints of self-knowledge undergirded the co-facilitators' commitment to advancing an agenda that paired unconditioned acceptance with enhanced personal accountability. The PVK youths had demonstrated mastery of unconscious symbolization in gesture and dance, embodying images of violent perpetrations, which implicated them in human rights crimes that went otherwise unnamed. Once the youths themselves began to talk frankly in sessions about how their rebel leaders had abused them, we co-facilitators opted to devise dance/movement exercises that might encourage the youths to find symbolic means of examining such leadership. Potentially, this would transition them from compulsively reliving a horrific and unnamable past toward eventual comfort in living in the here and now. Just as repetitive practices involved in learning traditional dance techniques allow for strengthening muscles and rerouting synaptic pathways so as to encode and later replicate complex movement sequences, so improvising together and exploring repeated wartime imagery in the process had enabled the building of ego strength and coping capacity.

Given such growth, during the group's ninth session, PVK as a collective endorsed the practice of a newly created exercise, which we facilitators had devised to enable mourning of their painful experience among the rebels. One by one, again in a circle, each of the former fighters would perform a gesture of his choosing, paired with a word, as representation of his own "suffering under someone"; his peers and we facilitators would immediately reflect that picture back to him. The ex-soldiers for the most part successfully performed precise and evocative gestures that allowed for overt expression of a decade's hidden sorrow. Upon thus fulfilling this first round's aims, the youths voiced consent to undertake a parallel exercise, which required depicting in gesture and word "how someone else felt when suffering under you." The PVK youths performed this distillation of empathy for a victim mindfully and with dignity. In turn, the attuned reflecting back of these same images rewarded each youth with a substantial sense of the group's acceptance, of communal support for tolerating long-buried guilt. A third exercise called on the dozen ex-combatants to both say and show how they had felt when victimizing others during the war, and how they had come in the course of PVK's few months to feel about that same victimization. In every case, the youths acknowledged remorse both verbally and nonverbally, something that to our knowledge they had never done before.

This tailored movement practice, performed with solemnity and purpose, had its desired outcome. Linking the unconscious, improvisatory exploration of primary process with the declarative understanding of secondary process, these dance-inspired exercises enabled the young men "to represent their ambivalence and confusion over the dynamic interplay of power and powerlessness in their lives" (Harris, 2010, p. 349). The practice afforded a creative means of *consciously* embodying insight into the duality that they had repeatedly portrayed unconsciously before: their simultaneous identities as both victim and perpetrator. Ultimately, performing these exercises proved to be crucial first steps toward the former boy combatants' surprisingly lasting reconciliation with the community that had shunned them for their part in the war's unspeakable atrocities (Harris, 2010).

SIMULATING RITES OF PASSAGE

The PVK group facilitators' conceptual framework for psychosocial healing was largely founded in conventions that have evolved in DMT, as developed and practiced over the last several decades in the United States. Among DMT's core premises is the notion that "the visible movement behavior of individuals is analogous to their intrapsychic dynamics" (Schmais, 1974, p. 10). When examining the meaning of the former boy combatant slicing his own neck when purporting to illustrate his childhood role in executing someone else, I drew on fundamental DMT assumptions that movement behavior reflects both personality and personal history or culture and sometimes discloses otherwise hidden attitudes about the self.

Over the last couple of decades, however, a critique of what is deemed an unnecessarily limited focus on intrapsychic matters, as defined in the global North, has emerged as a prevalent perspective among mental health practitioners serving survivors of war and organized violence from the global South (Harris, 2002). Beyond objecting to the "medicalization" of problems that might otherwise be understood in social, economic, or political terms, these psychotherapists, theorists, and researchers have chosen to "emphasise the social aspects of suffering and healing" (Bracken & Petty, 1998, p. 190). Accordingly, it has not been uncommon among international agencies providing services to demobilized child soldiers in Africa and elsewhere to avoid altogether mechanisms of "trauma healing," viewed as vestiges of colonialism, and to seek the support of traditional healers instead. Research suggests that sanctioned purification rites have, indeed, helped renew participating children's dignity and self-esteem while restoring their standing locally (Stark, 2006). Thus, without abandoning the intrapsychic altogether, I sought to deepen our work in Kailahun by grounding it in the district's foundational rites.

Accordingly, in many ways the PVK youths' understanding of the meaning of our shared process was informed by the ritual order into which they had been born. I recognized that within Sierra Leone and in many sub-Saharan African cultures "secret societies" had long been central to the transfer of local values, traditions, and expectations from one generation to the next (Peddle, Moneiro, Guluma, & Macaulay, 1999). Given my status as an outsider, I was far from privy to the operations of Kailahun's "societies"; even my co-facilitators had to respect the taboo against speaking to me about techniques and mysteries kept in utter secrecy.

It was clear, nonetheless, that for the former boy soldiers in our group the unthinkable had come to pass: 11 years of war had preempted participation in the local Poro Society's obligatory initiation rites such that the youths in PVK had been unable to undergo the rituals required to become adult men. While realizing that our circle dances lacked the ancestors' blessings, I posited that our gatherings resembled society initiations in certain significant ways, which my three local co-facilitators corroborated. In the absence of any sanctioned alternative to the Poro ceremonies, PVK offered an experience unique in the youths' lifetimes: our sessions brought together a dozen teenage males with adult men who offered guidance in ritualized dance and discussion within a time frame set apart from the ordinary activities and spaces of Koindu life, all for the expressed purpose of fostering lasting collective growth and transformation. By separating the youths from the routines of their daily lives and introducing them to a liminal ordeal rooted in bodily engagement, our DMT group primed its participants for the concluding reaggregation phase of their rite of passage. Altered for good by the PVK journey, the youths, when eventually returning to their community, demonstrated a readiness to reconcile, and their people accepted them back fully—as the transformed young men that they had truly become (Harris, 2010).

PROCESSING TOWARD THE FUTURE WITH THE PAST IN MIND

Van Gennep differentiated between two types of rites of passage: Beyond such life crisis rites as initiations, performed in hidden places and associated with status changes, he identified rites consecrated in public, as when a society as a whole confronts a major change as from plenty to famine, or peace to war (Turner, 1977a). Some such ritual performances linked to seasonal cycles or patterns observed in the heavens foster renewal and regeneration among numerous of the globe's traditional cultures by summoning celestial powers to frame what is otherwise time's overwhelming indifference. According to Turner (1977a), every type of society has its own "dominant mode of public liminality, the subjunctive space/time that is the counterstroke to its pragmatic indicative texture" (p. 34). Dance and DMT both offer incursions into the subjunctive realm that is the fertile soil of restoration and healing, as are seasonal rites and ceremonies in numerous cultural contexts.

Passing Crossroads

In 1989, I lived for a number of months in Antigua, Guatemala, a baroque relic of a city, where I witnessed the celebrated Holy Week processions. For generations, at the start of each *Semana Santa*, large crews of volunteer artisans have filled the colonial capital's cobblestone streets with vast *alfombras*: extraordinarily intricate "carpets" composed of seeds, flower petals, bark, and tinted sawdust and bedecked with astonishing abstract designs as well as true-to-life motifs of birds, flowers, and other natural marvels. Each Good Friday—the most solemn day in the Christian calendar, marking Jesus' surrender to torture and death at Golgotha—a parade passes over these dazzling, freshly completed displays of artistry. Scores of men dressed in robes styled after Renaissance images of biblical figures tread slowly together, while carrying on their collective shoulders massive wooden platforms topped with sculptured tableaux from the life of Christ up to and including the crucifixion. Invoking images of the Savior dragging his own cross, the costumed characters struggle under the tonnage of these ship-sized "floats." In order to avoid capsizing under the weight, the men rock side-to-side together, deliberately, and in striking unison as they move forward, step by step. While the disciples thus inch their way down the narrow streets, their sandaled feet trample the *alfombras'* gorgeous, ornate floral patterns into chance clumps of sawdust and seeds—degrading the exquisite into chaos. Watching from windows or adjacent sidewalks, community members cannot help but mourn in silence the brute passage of these processions for destroying the sublime creation of human hands. Paradoxically, the destruction performed in the streets is an emblem of rebirth. The liminal experience of Semana Santa cyclically reinforces the sacred mystery that the yearly celebration itself partakes of the eternal—the immortality promised all adherents of the faith.

Emblematic of the simultaneity of death and rebirth, of human and divine, these public rites roughly replicate the consecration of ephemerality that is inherent in dance as the most fleeting of all art forms. No one joining in Antigua's *procesiones* has to identify and verbalize the cosmological battle between death and everlasting vitality that is implicitly represented for it to yield a shared sense of hope and well-being: Communal healing is its reliable outcome for the faithful year after year.

Pluralism's Procession

In the Kailahun District, efforts spearheaded by our psychosocial counseling team in the town of Buedu culminated in a 2006 event that was at once a stirring, large-scale funeral rite and an anniversary commemoration in the form of a traditional procession. Emerging from a year-long community dialog—largely, a choreographic process—facilitated by the Buedu counselors under my supervision, this event bore profound implications for the community's post-conflict reconciliation and healing.

Around the globe, each June 26 since 1998, torture treatment programs have commemorated the date in 1987 when the Convention Against Torture entered into force (United Nations, 2019). Buedu's 2005 World Day Against Torture, as we called it, had brought together Muslims, Christians, and practitioners of traditional animism for a somber remembrance of the losses that torture and organized violence had imposed on the still divided community. In a town torn apart by religious intolerance, this meeting had been the first postwar occasion within memory when members of these three divided sectors had come together collaboratively to advance social cohesion.

As in many sites across Sierra Leone during the war, when the Revolutionary United Front held sway over Buedu, the corpses of countless civilian victims were unceremoniously dumped—without benefit of any of the obligatory rites for the dead. Such strategically deployed brutality amplified the impact of the slaughter itself by dispiriting the surviving populace to the point of paralysis. Accordingly, when planning the 2006 Day Against Torture observance as an occasion for honoring the dead and re-empowering the living, the three religious factions agreed that it take place at the site of one of three known mass graves within the Buedu town limits: an empty lot used for parking lorries in the years since demilitarization.

On the day itself, at the close of Muslim midday prayers, some 300 celebrants joined in processing to the abandoned gravesite. My team and I joined scores of participants moving through town as a way of marking—in the incongruously transient way that movement is invariably limited to—what could never be undone. Processing together, seeking as it were to still history's rampaging forgetfulness by honoring the fallen, we could not but feel the weight of the occasion's palpable grief.

Upon reaching the empty lorry park, the processional assumed a circular formation. No doubt, many of the survivors treading this circle did so in solemn remembrance of loved ones slaughtered and tossed into unmarked graves there years before. As a newcomer to this place, it was sobering for me to contemplate that somewhere deep in the rust-hued soil beneath our feet lay decomposing corpses of persons summarily executed during the war, and for no crime other than what the butchers had deemed wrongful allegiances: belonging to the wrong sect, the wrong family, or cultivating the wrong tract of land. In response, our collective, sharing a heightened state inclusive of both grief and defiance, pressed steadily onward, together sustaining the circle that had been the ageless soul of dances across the African continent and beyond for centuries. It was surely not incidental that our spectacle revived the unending form that since time immemorial has afforded entire peoples a chance to partake almost at once of catharsis and reflection.

At the procession's conclusion, religious observances completed the mass grave site's consecration, beginning with the acknowledgment that the very building in whose shade we stood had held a torture chamber. With this knowledge, the observant Muslims and Christians present paid close heed as the animist chief—a man known as Buedu's oldest living resident—poured libations to the ancestors for the innocent blood spilled on this spot. Before soaking the ruddy ground with the wine of purification and forgiveness, he shared his own eyewitness account of horror at seeing people who had been tortured and then killed thrown into a deep hole that had been dug here. Following his pivotal rite, Buedu's World Day Against Torture commemoration concluded with Muslim and Christian sermons. An imam condemned torture as wickedness perpetrated against innocent people and, praying for the victims, underscored the need to hold fast to the peace achieved in Sierra Leone. Christian parishioners lit candles around the gravesite in a large ring, and after a scripture reading, a Protestant pastor called for an end to stigma against persons who lacked benefit of proper burial following torture. Like the imam, the pastor emphasized nurturing the peace and urged all those wronged in war to continue to foreswear vengeance.

Had cultural anthropologist Victor Turner joined the choreographed Buedu spectacle that day, he would doubtless have deemed it exemplary of both a "metasocial" rite of passage for the dead and "a crisis rite," inhabiting the zone between the time of ruthless slaughter and the time of survival and reconciliation. "All performances require framed spaces set off from the routine world," he wrote. "But metasocial rites use quotidian spaces as their stage; they merely hallow them for a liminal time" (Turner, 1977a, p. 34). It is perhaps not unusual for a traditional rite to sacralize a space in the way that Buedu hallowed its lorry park. The ecumenism inherent in the Buedu procession, however, distinguished it from most traditional journeys into liminality. In the aftermath of terrible destruction and death, bringing together the community's three faith sectors through one pluralist commemoration of life's sacredness produced a unity perhaps feasible only within liminal space/time. Maybe only in the liminal realm are alliances formed that so effectively promote a people's safety and healing; only at ritual's threshold does the dance circle's communal harmony stay forever unbroken, an embodied vision of eternal oneness.

A CIRCLE WITHOUT BEGINNING, WITHOUT END

Dance/movement therapists seeking to collaborate with survivors from collectivist cultures of the global South in their effort to heal from the horrors of war and organized violence may draw meaningfully from an existential appraisal of DMT's foundational art form. As the foregoing observations on dance, understood inclusively, in the Kailahun District may attest, the art form's ephemerality may not so much impede as inspire the interplay and ultimate integration of memory in its implicit and explicit dimensions. The fact that dance's transitory character is not something that the participants in the DMT processes documented in this chapter would have identified explicitly does not make the form's implicit linkage to human impermanence any the less resonant on the unconscious level. To the contrary, as paradoxical as it may appear, coping in dance with unconscious reminders of human mortality seems to spur movement, animate achievement and interconnectedness, and generally build capacity for surviving. The growth evidenced among the former boy combatants and other DMT participants so deeply affected by their unimaginable losses during Sierra Leone's 11-year war may well have been informed in part by dance's distinctive evanescence: by the mystery that, in so many ways, people cannot help but find in dancing an embodiment of their lives as finite creatures with aspirations toward the infinite.

NOTES

1. Used with permission of University of California Press, from *Beyond Recognition: Representation, Power, and Culture*, Craig Owens (1992, p. 117); permission conveyed through Copyright Clearance Center, Inc. [Note: Gilles Deleuze published the original in 1968 as *Différence et répétition*.]
2. Pseudonyms are applied to protect confidentiality.

REFERENCES

Berger, M. (1972). Bodily experience and expression of emotion. *Writings on Body Movement and Communication, 2,* 191–230.

Berrol, C. F. (2006). Neuroscience meets dance/movement therapy: Mirror neurons, the therapeutic process and empathy. *The Arts in Psychotherapy, 33,* 302–315.

Bracken, P. J., & Petty, C. (Eds.). (1998). *Rethinking the trauma of war.* New York: Free Association Books.

Brenner, C. (1973). *An elementary textbook of psychoanalysis.* New York: Doubleday.

Cage, J. (1961). *Silence: Lectures and writings.* Middletown, CT: Wesleyan University Press.

Csiksentmihaliyi, M. (1975). *Beyond boredom and anxiety.* San Francisco: Jossey-Bass.

Damasio, A. (1991). Somatic markers and the guidance of behavior. New York: Oxford University Press.

Freud, S. (1958). Formulations on the two principles of mental functioning. In J. Strachey (Ed. & Trans.), *The standard edition of the complete psychological works of Sigmund Freud* (Vol. 12, pp. 215–226). London: The Hogarth Press. (Original work published 1911).

Harris, D. A. (2002). *Mobilizing to empower and restore: Dance/movement therapy with children affected by war and organized violence* (Unpublished master's thesis). Drexel University, Philadelphia, PA.

Harris, D. A. (2007a). Dance/movement therapy approaches to fostering resilience and recovery among African adolescent torture survivors. *Journal on Rehabilitation of Torture Victims and Prevention of Torture, 17*(2), 134–155.

Harris, D. A. (2007b). Pathways to embodied empathy and reconciliation: Former boy soldiers in a dance/movement therapy group in Sierra Leone. *Intervention: International Journal of Mental Health, Psychosocial Work and Counselling in Areas of Armed Conflict, 5*(3), 203–231.

Harris, D. A. (2009). The paradox of expressing *speechless terror.* Ritual liminality in the creative arts therapies' treatment of posttraumatic distress. *The Arts in Psychotherapy, 36*(2), 94–104.

Harris, D. A. (2010). When child soldiers reconcile: Accountability, restorative justice, and the renewal of empathy. *Journal of Human Rights Practice, 2*(3), 334–354.

Herman, J. L. (1992). *Trauma and recovery: The aftermath of violence—from domestic abuse to political terror.* New York: Basic Books.

Ogden, P., Minton, K., & Pain, C. (2006). *Trauma and the body: A sensorimotor approach to psychotherapy.* New York: W.W. Norton & Company Ltd.

Owens, C. (1992). *Beyond recognition: Representation, power, and culture.* Berkeley, CA: University of California Press, p. 117.

Peddle, N., Moneiro, C., Guluma, V., & Macaulay, T. E. A. (1999). Trauma, loss, and resilience in Africa: A psychosocial community based approach to culturally sensitive healing. In K. Nader & N. Dubrow (Eds.), *Honoring differences: Cultural issues in the treatment of trauma and loss* (pp. 121–149). Philadelphia: Brunner/Mazel, Inc.

Schmais, C. (1974). Dance therapy in perspective. In *Focus on Dance, 7* (pp. 7–12). Washington, DC: AAHPER.

Stark, L. (2006). Cleansing the wounds of war: An examination of traditional healing, psychosocial health and reintegration in Sierra Leone. *Intervention: The International Journal of Mental Health, Psychosocial Work and Counselling in Areas of Armed Conflict, 4*(3), 206–218.

Turner, V. (1977a). Frame, flow, and reflection: Ritual and drama as public liminality. In M. Benamou & C. Caramello (Eds.), *Performance in postmodern culture* (pp. 33–55). Madison, WI: Coda Press, Inc.

Turner, V. (1977b). *The ritual process: Structure and anti-structure.* Ithaca, NY: Cornell University Press.

UNICEF. (2000). Retrieved from www.unicef.org/

United Nations. (2019). *International day in support of victims of torture.* Retrieved from www.un.org/en/events/torturevictimsday/

van der Kolk, B. A. (1996). The complexity of adaptation to trauma: Self-regulation, stimulus discrimination, and characterological development. In B. A. Van der Kolk & A. C. McFarlane, & L. Weisaeth (Eds.), *Traumatic stress: The effects of overwhelming experience on mind, body, and society* (pp. 182–213). New York: The Guilford Press.

van der Kolk, B. A. (2014). *The body keeps the score: Brain, mind and body in the healing of trauma.* New York: Viking.

Winnicott, D. W. (1971). *Playing and reality.* New York: Routledge.

Yalom, I. D. (1970). *The theory and practice of group psychotherapy.* New York: Basic Books.

CHAPTER 19

AS THE DANCE WINDS DOWN
Coping with Aging as a Dance Therapist

Jane Wilson Cathcart

In dance/movement therapy, the role of dance is both central and unique. Central to our psychotherapeutic form is the dance, with all inherent expressive possibilities. The uniqueness of our work is how we use our whole selves always with dance as the starting place. It is our creative and physical home base. Most theoretical models offer the sequential phase of development, on one or two axes, similar to a series of still snapshots. However our way of knowing happens both sequentially and simultaneously. It is more similar to a hologram where you walk around and peruse with greater depth, larger surface and wider context. We see in space, time, weight and flow; in the personal kinesphere, the interactional space and the physical holding environment. Additionally, because of the dance our model is neither static nor flat.

There is no dance without the body: not the mind, not the spirit, not the words, and not even the pure body: the dancing body. This embodiment is our vehicle and instrument of sensing, observing, responding, interacting and healing. In our field we often refer to Freud's well-known statement in that the ego is first and foremost a bodily ego (1961). This is true for all humans. And dance/movement therapists value this particular definition of self in our schema of identity. Winnicott furthers this tenet when discussing the ongoing "basis for self in body" (1972). We realize, as van der Kolk (1996) states, the body keeps score. We know this within our profession and within our personal embodied selves. And if the body keeps the score of trauma and hurt, might it not also keep the score of masterful and pleasurable experience? This positive transitional phenomena can provide strength in times of injury and lessening of capacities due to aging.

While we develop and gain life experience intellectually, emotionally and physically our bodies remember . . . how it felt to skip, climb a tree, ride a bicycle, and dance on pointe. When we work with others we are invited to sense the other, to meet that separate self in a mutual space. We use our well-honed skills of mirroring and reflection to attune with others. This demonstrates our connection, empathy and understanding while offering a creative framework for perceiving a direct access to another's mental and emotional states (Damasio, 1999).

This is all well and good when we work at full physical and expressive capacities. But what of injury and aging? Perowsky (1991) helpfully reminds us that "Unlike professional dancers, dance/ movement therapists are not required to gracefully retire when the aging process takes its toll and increases vulnerability to injury. Therefore, they must consider how to function despite impairments due to age or injury" (p. 50). Both sides of the therapeutic relationship are affected. It used to be that I would extend or refine a patient's movement repertoire by offering my own. What happens now that my repertoire is diminished? How does the "call and response" shift? While I would "pick up" on the other's movement, now I have to modulate and regulate my response and offer dance that extends or refines without being able to necessarily physically offer my former full range of ways to cope with the internal and external environments (Bartenieff & Lewis, 1980). As a consequence the patient may not feel as strong a bond, as safe a holding environment, as rich a facilitating climate as before. The therapist may feel at the very least limited, possibly incompetent, maybe fraudulent, perhaps even as an invalid. There are many feelings and many challenges.

We as healers meet each person where they are and the excitement for this existential moment has not changed for me (Moustakas, 1966). But now what happens after that has changed dramatically. While moving together still elicits the dance elements, I can no longer offer the same expanded or focused ways to move the individual's "dance" along solely by my own physical expression. What happens subsequently has shifted and is more charged with probable limitations. I realized too much was changing much too fast when I worked with preschoolers into my early sixties.

Throughout my career, in sessions with individual children and groups I always utilized highly energetic, rhythmic and richly interactional dance. We would change levels: stand, squat, spiral, sink to the floor, rise again and so on. One day I was quite puzzled by the way the preschoolers were descending and ascending hesitantly and cautiously, as if elderly. I asked the staff for their thoughts. They pointed at me and gently said the children were mirroring me. The children could express fully all elements of the dance, while more often I could only suggest the intended movement.

At the same time in my private practice I was also unable to dance as fully as I once had been able. I began to utilize more of what I refer to as "mumbling". This is a way of reflecting in a more muted way the elements of movement. The name is derived from mumbling verbally, where there is a sense of what is being stated but also a lack of clarity in the expressed thought. I had begun using it decades earlier to purposefully reflect a diminished sense of what patients were presenting, but in a way where their greater abilities could be expressed as they showed me more fully what they were "saying" when I got it not quite right. Correcting me succeeded in eliciting from them what had been in them all along. Fischer and Chaiklin (1993) note this was a lesson learned from Marian Chace who "chose interventions which might elicit healing responses from each person" (p. 137). Our use of this Socratic model of health is one of our strengths, we are midwives to the strengths within those with whom we work (Cathcart, 2014).

Earlier in my private practice I devised the following technique with a particular patient while I was still able to dance fully. She was a young adult who was motivated to pursue dance therapy previously experienced in an inpatient facility. However, she would only talk and not dance in any way, shape or form. She finally agreed to walk around the dance therapy room. During one of these walks she said an image of a ladder would be helpful in our sessions. Ready to latch on to anything that might make me feel more effective as a dance therapist, I found one in a neighboring office. She directed me as to how to move with the ladder as a prop laid on the floor, and she remained unwilling to do anything but give directions and correct me verbally. I moved so badly (on purpose at the time) so that she was forced to embody her own experience while correcting me—this is always empowering for a patient. We continued this back and forth with her finally joining fully as a participant in her own healing dance.

I employ a mechanism I refer to as "mini-choreography". This usually involves my demonstrating in a reduced way the salient contrast under consideration in our clinical work. Sometimes it will be polar opposites: moving from the stuck feeling or emotion versus the desired expression, action, release as a healthier way of coping. One example of a common theme is the giving all and dispersal of self until there is nothing left to maintain uprightness. No "legs" if you will, to "under stand", or stand under and support. This uses a pun of "understanding" when the ability to support the self is depleted. It is contrasted with giving, reaching only so far as you are able to return to the stability of the self. At the very least, this dance expands ways of thinking and experiencing the patient's conflict; more often it widens their repertoire. The frequent result is a broadened expression to illuminate the "how" of that individual's experience in danced form. Here I am the mover, many times in a "call and response" with the patient in a subsequently embodied refinement or expansion. This structure supports their needs, and I am capable within my gesture and muted movement to offer and model these options. And they are able to try them on, make adjustments, and own what really has been their own dance all along. They may be experienced internally and invisibly, but felt nonetheless.

A useful pathway for these later years was also created well before injury, aging and the loss of mobility arrived and moved in. I decided that in order for mutual clarity about goals in private practice I would need to set the therapeutic goals with the client and to arrive at a structure that translated movement into words at the outset. This is in contrast to my agency work where treatment plans were the guide to goals, at the very least a starting point dictated by the institution rather than patient input. This simple innovative structure enabled me to suggest form for the individual's content and goal setting both verbally and nonverbally.

Most patients were desiring to dance and move within sessions. After all, they came into treatment with me precisely because I am a dance therapist. However, they also wanted to talk. The goal of dance therapy is not to make patients elegant beautifully moving expressive mutes. It is instead to enable their full expression, including and not incidentally verbal communication.

The structure of this exercise was simple enough. Once we introduced ourselves, I invited the patient to experiment. Would they go outside the room, close the door and when ready come back into the therapy room? There were two re-entries required using no words. I asked that I be shown first of all, how they felt coming into the room, into therapy and so on at this very moment. The second entrance would present how they thought they might feel entering the room for the last time when we were in agreement our work was satisfactorily finished. These demonstrations of before and after were then put into their own words. Bodily expression preceding the intellectual offered a glimpse of the parameters that would guide us in our therapeutic contract. This became a reference throughout our work as well as concrete transitional phenomena for the patient to take away between sessions. An additional, and major goal, was to facilitate understanding about how the body speaks, remembers and is present in all our living moments. Everyone who agreed to experiment with this structure completed both parts—except one woman.

She took a bit longer than most to prepare. As usual I was standing fairly close to the door. When the door opened I looked and saw nothing. No one was down the hall. But there she was, on her belly on the floor, crawling into the room. She stopped as soon as she was clear enough for the door to shut again. I joined her, face down on the floor on my belly. And so we spent our first session. Now, I would be unable to join her so quickly, move so readily and maintain that position due to old injuries, joint replacements and my aging body. I certainly could respond therapeutically, but at this point in my life it would be vastly different in energy, shape and level. For example, I now use gesture to shape what I once would have expressed in my whole body. Hands can replicate so many elements with dimension and dynamics. In sessions we are able to increase or decrease our expressive movement in shape, speed, height, force and flow. The hand is a universal communication tool that I now combine with my torso, limbs and whatever else is needed and able to engage in the dance. However, no matter how transformed, the intent for healing remains.

There is nothing permanent except change.

—**Heraclitus (2018)**

When we change, the dance changes. And the opposite is true. As my dance has changed, I have had to reset expectations about my abilities. I have reworked the definition of myself and my identity while looking for other constants. There are many stages in life. Stages of learning, developing a relationship and of development of our physical, emotional and thinking selves. In our work we are trained to apply our craft to the different life stages of our patients. But what of the different stages we clinicians traverse as we continue dancing through our own life cycles? Looking at the stages of the life cycle has been an extremely useful schema both clinically and personally.

Erikson (1959) provides a context of challenges for each phase. While his system describes a progression, it can also remind us how we revisit the issues over and over each time we face a similar situation There are eight psychosocial stages offered, of which I have found the first and the last two most enlightening for the purposes of this topic.

The earliest stage of development is trust versus mistrust, the latter of which I now experience predominantly on a body level. Is my "new normal" dance movement safe enough for me on a physical level, and adequate for my patients in a reflective, healing context? When referring to Terese Benedek's correlating trust with confidence, Erikson understandably negates confidence as a useful descriptor of an infant (p. 63). However, I see it as a useful naming of what I am personally revisiting in this time of waning ability. Indeed, I feel a mistrust, and am therefore far less confident in my dance movement repertoire. Often my struggles parry between embracing and overcoming the attendant mistrust. Yet trusting my instincts, intuition and current body response all lead to a revised, albeit abridged, sense of confidence.

Generativity versus stagnation is the next to last stage. And while he meant generativity mainly in a genital reproductive sense, he allowed a far wider definition:

> Generativity is primarily the interest in establishing and guiding the next generation, although there are people who, from misfortune or because of special and genuine gifts in other directions, do not apply this drive to offspring but to other forms of altruistic concern and of creativity, which may absorb their kind of parental responsibility.
>
> (Erikson 1959, p. 103)

This defines how I classify myself. I plan to continue my work life for the rest of my days.

Concomitantly, I am squarely in the integrity versus despair stage. For me, despair is largely absent as an issue. Rarely in my life has it been present, even in moderation. Part of that is due to temperament. Another part must be clearly attributed to the transformative nature of dancing itself. We dance among the possibilities of response to life not only with our patients but within our own psyches, minds and creative bodies. Now is the time to renew our acquaintance with that source within us as we address our own needs. We have solved some of the very same crises we might personally face at times when treating others. This is a reverse treatment of the projected self: we remember how the challenge was resolved for another with our help, and we reach into that repository and now try it on as a possible solution to a current personal situation. Always we employ the elements of the dance to reintegrate this newfound sense of self.

Can you, can't you, can you, can't you, can you join the dance?
—**L. Carroll (1865)**, *The Lobster-Quadrille (paraphrased)*

Decades ago I sustained a knee injury from singly breaking up a fight among four adolescent boys yielding large pieces of wood as weapons. This marked the end of my ability to dance on pointe. I had always felt so fully engaged in my body and in space when dancing on pointe for my own pleasure. It was also as recuperation and self-care from my clinical work life. However, this loss was certainly not the end of being in the world as a dancer—not by a long shot! Edited? Perhaps. Nevertheless, I had no idea that this particular lesson in reduction would be in the service of my ego for this current stage of life.

Here we continue to talk about ability. Not desire. Not even will. The reality, however, is that the full-out physical response as a dance therapist is diminished. Sandel and Hollander (1995) might include aging dance movement therapists when they state: "Implicit in a dance/movement therapy session with the physically challenged is the expectation that people will attempt to move and that movement stimulates their feelings about their bodies and their physical limitations" (Levy, 2005, p. 115). Some aging dance therapists would dance and move less. Less is experienced as loss. Vigilance is needed to view the loss—to experience and move both with and through the attendant sadness. The emotional aspect of the work likely remains unchanged, with the patient remaining the central focus. The content of the goals and goodwill towards the patient has not shifted, but the emphasis in the "how" has. The physical reaction in the clinical setting might appear to be more offhanded rather than hands on. Perhaps one becomes more witnessing or directive than participatory in body. Perhaps the full-out dance has become the art of gesture and more muted expression. There are many possible responses for individual therapists facing their increasing years.

Does this new iteration of the aging clinician still have validity? If not, it would become invalid. Turn the adjective "invalid" into a noun, pronounce it with different emphasis and it defines one as "not strong" (from Latin, *invalidus*, from *in-* 'not' + *validus* 'strong'.) No one wants to be negated, and yet the ancient Greeks saw old age as a form of unconsciousness. They posited if you were infirm in your body the rest of you followed into a demise of the self. This is juxtaposed against the concomitant reverence of elders and their wisdom. If both of these notions, seemingly opposite, can be contained in the thinking of a great civilization, who are we to argue? We can be both diminished in physical capacity and wise and valued for our lived years. Our field assesses people from a strengths perspective. Turn this mirror on our aging selves to rediscover our capacity for being as vital and present as possible. Is there an inverse relationship to knowing in ways other than the physical abilities? Does the inability to move as freely as I once did force my antennae to tune in differently? Is my new type of full presence now also redistributed in a new way?

The privilege of a lifetime is being who you are.
—Joseph Campbell, *A Joseph Campbell Companion: Reflections on the Art of Living*

Many currently aging dance therapists were most fortunate to learn from the founders of Dance Therapy as a modern profession. Those women were also in their older years when they taught us what they had gleaned over their lifetimes. As I write these words, I realize that Marian Chace was only a couple of years older than I am now when I was in her last class at Bellevue. Similarly, Irmgard Bartenieff was around my current age when she taught my two-year certification program at the Dance Notation Bureau. I reflect on some of the differences of these particular dance therapists at the end. What now do I incorporate of them at that stage in their lives?

The work of Chace and Whitehouse was not mutually exclusive; rather it overlapped, forming a continuum of style and technique with healing expression at the core.

When I studied with Chace in the final months of her life, I was struck by how little dancing occurred as opposed to a concentration on meaningful gestural dance movement. Much of what I learned about adaptation was demonstrated by her clinical work just weeks before her life ended. She healed mainly from her seated position.

While I did not study with Mary Whitehouse, she was highly regarded and well known in the field. Her techniques were so different than those of Chace. I wondered how leading from a seated position due to her MS compared with Chace. Hendricks (2010) provides a window into the presence of Whitehouse, sensing "her trying on the movements in her body." She notes about Whitehouse teaching from her wheelchair "that consciousness communicates even when the physical realm has diminished" (P. 65).

As I reflect on my trajectory, I cannot help but think of these innovators as unwitting role models for this very moment in my life just by having been in their individual situations and stages of their lives. They have passed on. As I have incorporated what they offered to me I wonder what of our shared past experiences will have meaning for those with whom I have worked. I occasionally hear, but for the most part it remains a mystery. And I truly have no way to ascertain any part of it once my life ends. Earlier in my private work I had an unusual portend of what it might be like.

A woman in her early thirties was referred to me by a clinical psychologist specializing in eating disorders. While this therapist felt it was time to terminate work with this patient, she also recognized the need for the body to heal. I knew from the referral that there was a history of sexual abuse by her father. However, I was struck upon seeing her that her mother had also abused her. Nothing in the referral or our preliminary chat to set up an appointment had revealed this. I do not know how to explain this knowing. Perhaps it is because we dance therapists gather information on many levels simultaneously. Often we form impressions from visual, emotional expression and kinesthetic data more immediately than when we focus on one aspect of the interaction at a time.

One of the main challenges a patient may face is the intimacy of moving one to one with a therapist. Because there often can be a sense of intimacy with bodies moving, rather than sitting, feelings of discomfort can arise. Since there is only one other person in the room, and therefore no one else to rely on, a patient may fear for her safety. This can be intensely triggering when the perpetrator of the one to one traumatic event was the same gender as the therapist. The fear of doing something wrong, of not being perfect, of not meeting expectations, much less being violated, can contribute further to the anxiety already present just in seeking help from a therapist and bringing in the body, psyche and sense of self that has been so wounded.

We worked together with more space between our moving bodies than usual. Comfort and safety were paramount. This became even more explicitly understood when she eventually told me of the additional abuse by her mother. After more than a year of weekly sessions we mutually agreed that our work was coming to a satisfying conclusion. Our last session was unlike any other in my entire career. She declared she had a final dance of healing. I was delighted to hear this. What she said next was a huge surprise. She asked that I sit in the waiting area outside the dance therapy room while she did the dance.

I quickly assessed her mental state to assure myself she would not hurl herself out of the third floor window. She said she would lock the door. Oh dear, can I handle being shut out? Trust works both ways. So does feeling safe. And so it came to be. I sat in my waiting area, which was shared with other offices. Minutes ticked by. I waited. After what seemed like an interminable amount of time she unlocked the door and invited me into the space she had just blessed with her healing dance. We ended our work together on this note of empowerment and ownership of the health she needed only to witness herself. This now gives me a sense of what it is to be held present internally, while absent in the physical environment (Winnicott, 1958). This was an experience of mutual object constancy. And a preparation for my final absence.

> **Older women are like aging strudels—the crust may not be so lovely, but the filling has come at last into its own**.
>
> —Robert Farrar Capon (n.d.), *Brainy Quotes*

As an older therapist, you revisit the spiral of the stages of life many times over as they occur for you and in other people's lives. So you have kept gaining internal, emotional and intellectual experience even as your body responses are lessening. The balance shifts: you have less of one thing and more of another. But they still add up to the same percentage of you being a whole clinician. Now when people ask me how I'm doing, I usually quip: "I'm doing my best with what I have left." However, on reflection, I am doing just fine. Truly.

REFERENCES

Bartenieff, I., & Lewis, D. (1980). *Body movement: Coping with the environment*. New York: Gordon and Breach Science.

Capon, R. F. Robert Farrar Capon Quotes. (n.d.). *BrainyQuote.com*. Retrieved December 1, 2018, from Brainy-Quote.com Web site: www.brainyquote.com/quotes/robert_farrar_capon_111087

Carroll, L. (1865). *Alice's adventures in Wonderland*. New York: MacMillan.

Cathcart, J. W. (2014). 2013 Marian Chace lecture: Introduction of Fran J. Levy, lecturer. *American Journal of Dance Therapy*, *36*(1), 3–5.

Damasio, A. R. (1999). *The feeling of what happens: Body and emotion in the making of consciousness*. New York: Harcourt Brace and Company.

Erikson, E. (1959). *Identity and the life cycle*. New York: W.W. Norton & Company Ltd.

Fischer, J., & Chaiklin, S. (1993). Meeting in movement: The work of the therapist and client. In S. Sandel, S. Chaiklin, & A. Lohn (Eds.), *Foundations of dance/movement therapy: The life and work of Marian Chace* (pp. 136–153). Columbia, MD: Marian Chace Memorial Fund of the American Dance Therapy Association.

Freud, S. (1961). The ego and the id. In *The standard edition of the complete psychological works of Sigmund Freud, Volume XIX (1923–1925): The Ego and the Id and other Works* (pp. 1–66). London: Hogarth.

Hendricks, K. (2010). What I learned from Mary: Reflections on the work of Mary Starks Whitehouse. *American Journal of Dance Therapy*, *32*(1), 64–68.

Heraclitus. Heraclitus Quotes. *Quotes.net*. STANDS4 LLC, 2018.

Levy, F. J. (2005). *Dance/movement therapy: A healing art*. (2nd re. ed.). Reston. VA: National Dance Association, an Association of the American Alliance for Health, Physical Education, Recreation and Dance.

Moustakas, C. (1966). Introduction. In C. Moustakas (Ed.), *Existential child therapy: The child's discovery of himself* (pp. 1–7). New York: Basic Books.

Perowsky, G. (1991). Working with pain: A self-study. *American Journal of Dance Therapy*, *13*(1), 49–58.

Sandel, S. L., & Hollander, A. S. (1995). Dance/movement therapy with aging populations. In F. J. Levy (Ed.), *Dance and other expressive art therapies: When words are not enough* (pp. 133–143). New York: Routledge.

van der Kolk, B. A. (1996). The body keeps score: Approaches to the psychobiology of posttraumatic stress disorder. In B. A. van der Kolk, A. C. McFarlane, & L. Weisaeth (Eds.), *Traumatic stress: The effects of overwhelming experience on mind, body and society* (pp. 214–241). New York: The Guilford Press.

Winnicott, D. W. (1958). The capacity to be alone. *The International Journal of Psychoanalysis*, *39*, 416–420.

Winnicott, D. W. (1972). Basis for self in body. *International Journal of Child Psychotherapy*, *1*, 7–16.

INDEX

Note: Page numbers in **bold** indicate tables. Page numbers in *italic* indicate figures and boxed text.

mineness and 38–39; ontology of the body and 40–41; overview 2, 44; *Verfallen* and 36–37, *37*
Heimann, K. 90
Hendricks, K. 286
Heraclitus 284
Hervey, L. 124, 134, 179
High Intensity of Tension Flow Attributes 242, 247n9
Hijikata Tatsumi (Butoh dancer) xix, 233, 242
Hirai, T. 235–237
Hogushi 4
Hollander, A. S. 285
Holmes, J. R. 225
Holy Week processions 277–278
Ho, Rainbow T. H. 2, 115–116, 220
Huber, M. 121
human trafficking 4, 30, 208
Hwa-Byung disorder (Korea) 219–220, 222
hypertonia as Parkinson's disease symptom 194

"I can be" modality 44–45n3
id 43
image 9–10, 184–185, *185*
imagery 89–90, 92, 238–241, *239, 240, 241*
immediacy in experiencing body 55, 57n9
implicit memory 266
implicit relational knowing 15
impression 103–104, 106n3
improvisation 13, 14, 61, 62, 63, 128, *142, 143*, 143, 144, 145, 163–164, *163*, 273; exploratory/introspective 13, 14
improvisation/play mechanisms of DMT 128
impulses, symbolization of 193
Imus, Susan Dee 3, 118, 124
inauthenticity 37–39, *39, 40*, 41
Indian dance culture 3–4, 27; *see also* Kolkata Sanved; *Sampoornata* ("fullness") program
indirect space 228
individual vs. community 220–221
informed decision making mechanism of DMT 129–130
initiation rite 194, 276–277
"inner life" and dance 13
insight/action phase of creative process 147–148
insight and being moved 103
integration 129, *129*, 148
intention, setting 182–184, *183*
interaction versus solitude 144
interbeing, intersubjective 12
International Association for Analytic Psychology 235
International Labour Organisation (ILO) 208

International Online Survey with DMT Novices: art form of dance 62; background information 61; comparisons of novices and experts 66–70, **66**, *67, 68, 69, 70*; conclusion of 72; data collection with novices 63–64, 73n2; demographics 64, **65**, 66; discussion 70–72; experts and 64; future research and 72; healing activity of dance 62; integration of dance interventions and 68, *68*; limitations of 72; non-dance based techniques and 69–70, *70*; novices and 64; overview 2; participants 62–64, 73n2; personal background to DMT, importance of 66–67, *67*, 69, *69*; procedure 62–64, 63–64; professional background to DMT, importance of 67, *67*; results 64; survey 63–64, 75–81; therapeutic activity of dance 62–63; WEXTOR and 64
intersubjective interbeing 12
interventions, dance: description of clinical practice and 111–112, 117–121; goal of 98; health improvement and 62–63; integration of 68, *68*; of Kolkata Sanved 216; of *Sampoornata* program 215; structural components of clinical practice and 132–134; transformation and 138; *see also specific type*
intra-acting 158–159, 165, 176
intrinsic motivation 189
intuition 42, 46–47, 52, 88, 130, 182, 185–186, 284
invalid 282, 285
invisible condition of dancing body 50–53
irreal dimension 50
"*it* speaks" (*Ça parle*) 43
I've Lost You Only to Discover That I Have Gone Missing (dance) 164, *164*
Iwashita-Konan Method 242, **243**
Iwashita, T. (San Kai Juku dancer) 242, *243*

Jacobs, T. J. 245
jaleos 255
James, W. 99
Jamison, J. 180–181
Japan Dance Therapy Association (JADTA) 234
Japanese dance culture and DMT: background information 233; bathing culture and 234–235, *235*; belongingness and, cultural sense of 244–246; body traditions and 234–238; *Bon* 233, 238, *239*; *Bon Odoiri* 27; Butoh 233–234, 242–244; characteristics of 234; folk dance 27; historical perspective 233–234;